The Most Important Thing You Need to Know About *Making* Love

[Louis] Nizer* has written that the greatest single cause for family-unit destruction and divorce in [the United States] is a fundamental sexual inadequacy within the marital unit.

— Masters and Johnson, in the Preface to *Human Sexual Response*

But No One Could Tell You Until Now

---

* U.S. lawyer (1902-1994), a legal wizard who was an expert on divorce law.
— *Encyclopedia Britannica*

Sex As Nature Intended It

The Most Important Thing You Need to Know About Making Love But No One Could Tell You Until Now

Kristen O'Hara
with Jeffrey O'Hara

Afterword by George C. Denniston, M.D.

Turning Point Publications
Hudson, Massachusetts

Copyright © 2002 by Kristen O'Hara
All rights reserved. No part of this publication
may be used or reproduced in any manner whatsoever
without written permission from the publisher,
except in the case of brief quotations embodied in
critical articles and reviews.

Printed in the United States of America.

Turning Point Publications
P.O. Box 486
Hudson, MA 01749

06 05 04 03 02   6 5 4 3 2
Second Edition

Dialogue from Woody Allen's movie *Bananas* used with permission
©1971 United Artists Corporation
All Rights Reserved.

Figures 1-1, 1-2, 4-2, 4-4 used with permission
Hourglass Book Publishing.

Figures 2-3 and 6-1 adapted from Bud Berkeley.

Figures 4-3 and 14-1 courtesy of
Circumcision: An American Health Fallacy by Edward Wallerstein.

Figure 8-1 used with permission Urban & Fischer Verlag from *Atlas of Human Anatomy*, Vol. 2, 10th Eng. ed., 1983, by Johannes Sobotta.

ISBN   0-9700442-1-6

Library of Congress Card Number   2001-096326

Bookstore Category Suggestions:
   Relationships
   Sexuality
   Health

Dedicated to

John Strand

The man whose problem
(And whose tenacious persistence to get it corrected)
Inspired a solution
That sparked a revolution
Which will echo around the world

Contents

1. The Secret Enters the Spotlight — 1
2. Something is Missing — 19
3. Making Love Last: The Tie That Binds — 41
4. A Sexual Comparison of the Natural and Circumcised Penis — 52
5. The Gliding Mechanism of the Natural Penis vs. the Friction Action of the Circumcised Penis — 69
6. A Further Sexual Comparison of the Natural and Circumcised Penis — 81
7. Women Tell Their Personal Stories — 101
8A. Normal Thrusting Rhythm of the Natural Penis vs. the Abnormal Thrusting Rhythm of the Circumcised Penis — 117
8B. The Male Clitoris: Its Discovery, Pleasurement, and How It Affects the Thrusting Rhythm — 133
9. Why Does the Circumcised Man Thrust Hard or Bang and Pound Away? — 157
10. It's Over in a Flash! But What If It Lasts? And Desire Deficiency: Hers, His — 173
11. My Personal Story — 189
12. Joining the Foreskin Restoration Revolution and the Personal Stories of Two Men Who Restored — 203
13. A Survey of Women Sexually Experienced with Both Circumcised and Uncircumcised Men — 239
14. How Americans Came to be Routinely Circumcised — 281

15. 35 Reasons Why You Should Not Circumcise Your Son	291
16. Are There Valid Reasons for Circumcising Your Son?	302
17. Common Myths That Popularized Circumcision	305
18. Medical Myths Perpetuate Circumcision in America	323
19. Will the Jewish People Disavow Circumcision?	339
20. A Call to Reason	348
Afterword by George C. Denniston, M.D.	353
Appendix A How to Have a Vaginal Orgasm 99.99% of the Time	357
Appendix B How to Prevent Premature Ejaculation and a Simple Secret for Prolonging Intercourse	363
Appendix C A Solution for Those Circumcised Men Who Take Longer Than They Want to Reach Orgasm	365
Appendix D Sevely's Male Clitoris Theory Explained: Excerpts from *Eve's Secrets*	367
Appendix E Reprint from *BJU* (British Journal of Urology) *International:* The Effect of Male Circumcision on the Sexual Enjoyment of the Female Partner	371
Appendix F Survey Questionnaire	385
Glossary	393
Resources	398
Reference Notes	403
Index	419

Important Notice

The authors do not directly or indirectly dispense medical advice. All matters regarding your health require medical supervision. The ideas, procedures, and suggestions contained in this book are intended only to offer information to help you cooperate with your doctor in your mutual quest for health. Neither the publisher nor the authors shall be liable or responsible for any loss or damage allegedly arising from any information or suggestion in this book.

OFFICIAL WEBSITE

www.SexAsNatureIntendedIt.com

1

The Secret Enters the Spotlight

There is something missing in millions of bedrooms across America—something that has been a necessary part of humanity's sexuality from the very beginning, *yet, incredibly, its importance has been completely overlooked*—until now.

Its "discovery" will make such a superlative difference in the lovemaking experience of sexual intercourse, it is destined to capture our national consciousness and change the sex life and sexual attitude of America's men and women forever—for it will set us free to explore and experience our true sexuality for the first time.

If you are a man, it promises to bring you a new level of sexual pleasure beyond your highest expectations, allowing you to see your female partner with new eyes of appreciation. At the same time, it offers a newfound explanation for the sexual dysfunctions you may be experiencing.

If you are a woman, you, too, have much to look forward to, for it brings the promise of greater overall happiness between the sheets, and pages, of your life. Gentler sex, more sensuous sex, more satisfying sex, increased attainment of orgasm from intercourse, can be yours—giving you new insight into the joy that lovemaking can bring when nature is on your side. At the same time, it will give you a new perspective on the role sexual fulfillment—*true* sexual fulfillment—plays in the overall well-being of your relationship.

Not that long ago, women were thought to be lacking in capacity for sexual enjoyment. But in the early '60s, sexual researchers Masters and Johnson proved that women are anatomically and physiologically capable of experiencing sexual pleasure and achieving orgasm just like men. Yet, there must be something amiss, because the popular press reports that millions of American women resort to faking orgasm during intercourse, for they are often unable to achieve them. This is, in general, an indication that women are not experiencing the level of pleasure and arousal necessary to bring on orgasm. For too many women, the lure of would-be delicious sex often turns out to be a disappointing experience that leaves them hungering for something more.

Men, too, apparently have been left wanting for something seemingly out of reach. In his book, *Male Sexuality*, Bernie Zilbergeld, Ph.D., reports on a survey of over 52,000 people conducted by *Psychology Today* in which 55 percent of the men said they were dissatisfied with their sex lives and 39 percent admitted to various problems such as disinterest in sex (1). Other men said they have relatively good sex but complain that "it's not all it's cracked up to be" and wonder "if they're missing something." "Is it possible," they ask, "that there is some new position, partner, practice, or gimmick which would bring sex up to expectation?" (2)

This book will disclose the cause and solution to the "missing something" by revealing a sexual *truth of nature*—a truth of nature so elemental and yet so enabling, it will not only bring you and your partner a more satisfying sex life, but, in the process, will reach into the very heart of your marriage or relationship and bring a deeper meaning to the word "love."

To delve into the secret, we must now keep an open mind, at this crossroads where the future touches the past, and look closely at the fundamental structure of the male sex organ as nature designed it. In so doing, we will come to find that America's obsession with circumcision—*the surgical alteration of the penis's structure* by removing its foreskin—has untold adverse effects on the sexuality of both the man and his female partner and profound detrimental consequences on the way they experience intercourse, diminishing their pleasure to an astounding degree.

This concept, at first, may seem hard to believe, and in the end its implications may be even harder to accept. Nevertheless, it will soon be the whisper on everyone's lips that the foreskin of the penis is the key that unlocks the mystery door, behind which we'll find the real sexual pleasure America's been searching for. Real sexual pleasure, as nature intended—tender, softly-smooth, and sensuous—so much more delicious and rewarding than the sex experienced in the circumcised bedroom. As we shall soon see, the foreskin—*ultra-erogenous tissue, and the penis's only moving part*—not only makes a dramatic difference in a man's sexual pleasure, but its presence during intercourse makes a doubly dramatic difference in a woman's pleasure and substantially enhances her ability to achieve coital orgasm (an orgasm from the movements of intercourse).

Bringing the importance of the foreskin into the spotlight would seem to present an insolvable problem since most American men don't have a foreskin because they are circumcised. There is, however, a solution to this problem: foreskin restoration. Luckily, virtually any circumcised man in America can now "grow" (restore) a new foreskin for his penis through various non-surgical techniques. But why will a man want to restore his foreskin? And why will his wife or lover desire—or even insist—that he do so? That is the primary focus of this book.

The idea of foreskin restoration may immediately strike you as strange and bizarre. But as this issue inevitably rises to national prominence, and you come to realize the paramount importance of the foreskin to the sexual pleasure of both partners (and the love bond that is borne from sexual union), it will begin to seem a very reasonable solution for today's circumcised men. Case in point, *The Wall Street Journal* featured a front-page article on foreskin restoration on December 28, 2000.

Nature designed the penis, with a foreskin, over millions of years of evolution, and every infant boy is born with one. Although the foreskin serves to protect the penis head during infancy, boyhood, and manhood, its real function is in adult sexuality, where it plays a definite, delicate, vital role during the lovemaking movements of intercourse, adding immeasurably to the comfort and pleasure of both partners.

Yes, the heretofore disregarded, discarded foreskin has a purpose—a sexual purpose—and a reason to live, to lust, and to love.

During intercourse, the foreskin performs several specialized functions. These functions allow a man and woman to experience intercourse in accordance with nature's sexual plan—tenderly, gently, and lovingly—as they mutually surrender to an enrapturing ecstasy that binds them so close it's as if the two were one. But when the foreskin is missing, the sex act becomes something entirely different. When circumcision removes the foreskin, the sex act becomes less—much less—than nature intended.

We are standing on the threshold of America's bedroom door. Looking in, we see that a revolutionary change must soon take place because circumcision significantly alters the penis by removing highly erogenous tissue, thereby preventing a man from achieving his true potential for sexual ecstasy. Moreover, the surgically altered circumcised penis has substantial negative effects on the female partner and reduces a woman's pleasure and arousal *throughout* the intercourse experience, thereby diminishing her orgasmic capabilities. As we will see, male circumcision is injurious to the sexuality of both partners.

Why haven't you heard about the sexual aspects of circumcision before? In effect, this is the first time this subject has been brought to the attention of the general public in such detail. There is a time and place for everything as humanity progresses along the path of enlightenment. The absurdity and tragedy of circumcision is simply an issue whose time has come. As a result, the controversy that clouds the decision-making dilemma of millions of American parents—to circumcise or not to circumcise—will soon be over, and, in the not-too-distant future, America will join the vast majority of nations that do not routinely circumcise. It is a little known fact, but **most of the world's men, approximately 80%, are *not* circumcised** —only about 20% are circumcised. The primary circumcising countries are America, Israel, some African countries, and the Arab and/or Moslem (Muslim) nations. Virtually all remaining countries of the world do not routinely circumcise. (Figures 1-1, 1-2 show important differences between the two types of penises.)

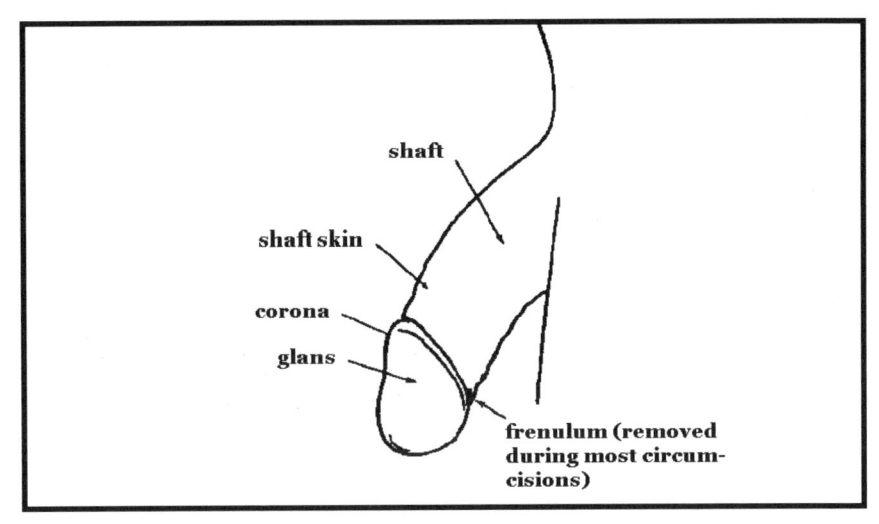

Figure1-1. Flaccid circumcised penis. The foreskin has been surgically removed, leaving the penis head exposed as an *external* organ. The frenulum (the highly erogenous tissue that connects the foreskin to the glans) is also partially or totally removed during most circumcisions.

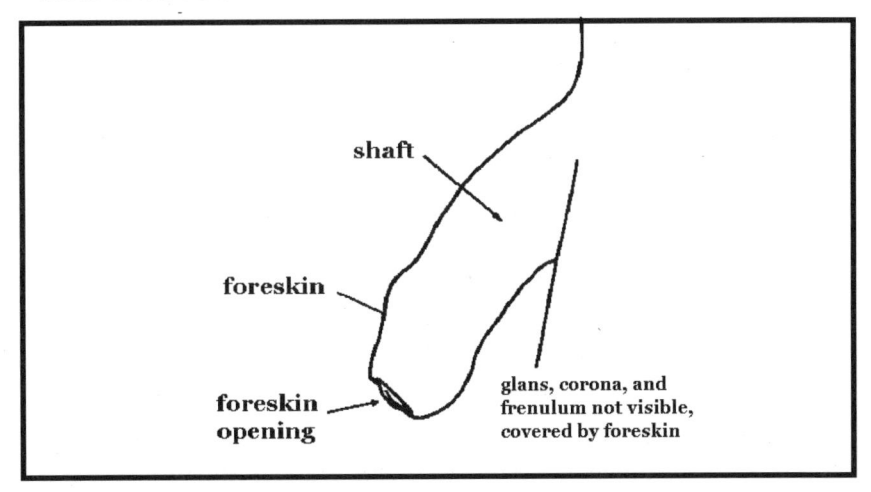

Figure1-2. Flaccid natural (uncircumcised) penis.* A foreskin covers the glans of the natural penis, making the penis head an *internal* organ. The foreskin retracts upon arousal.

* For greater simplicity and clarity, and to avoid the possibility of confusing the terms "circumcised" and "uncircumcised," this book will hereafter refer to the uncircumcised penis as natural (as provided by nature).

THE NEXT SEXUAL REVOLUTION HAS BEGUN

There is a quiet revolution now going on in this country: The Foreskin Restoration Revolution. More and more, as men begin to read and hear that it is now possible to restore their foreskin, they are choosing to "undo" their circumcision and become "uncircumcised" again. You don't hear about these men in the course of your everyday life because foreskin restoration is not exactly a top-ten topic of discussion. Nevertheless, these men, and the organizations that support them, are out there, and their numbers are rapidly increasing.

If you are a circumcised man, reading this book will give you a totally new perspective on circumcision and its relationship to your sex (and love) life. As a result, I believe you will come away eager to "grow" a foreskin of your very own to cover the head of your most prized possession.

Right now, however, you may understandably be having your doubts. You may be thinking that your sex life seems to be going along just fine. You don't want to think about the possibility that your sex life might not be the "real" thing. And you don't want your wife or lover to start thinking that you're not giving her the real thing. You don't want to rock your sexual boat and become part of some silly revolution—"Grow a new foreskin!? Not this guy!"

But the decision for a man to restore, or not to restore, isn't just a man's sexual issue. It's also a woman's issue, because a woman is on the receiving end of the penis during intercourse, and when the penis has been stripped of its foreskin, the sex act is *astoundingly abnormalized*, not only for the man, but especially for the woman.

Indeed, when the insights of this entire topic have permeated our national consciousness and all debate has been reconciled, the circumcision issue will have been reduced to a natural law—a sexual truth of nature: The foreskin is an inherent part of the penis, and during intercourse, a man and woman can only hope to experience their true potential for sexual ecstasy when the foreskin is present, allowing the penis to function and feel as it should, according to nature's design.

The foreskin is alive with sensory-pleasure nerves that give the natural (uncircumcised) penis more "feelings." As a result, the natural penis is more "tuned in" to the total intercourse experience; consequently, it thrusts the vaginal walls more delicately, more gently. To put it another way, the natural penis is more sensitive to the intercourse experience, which in turn affects the tenderness with which it thrusts—all to the delight of the participating woman.

Even the length of a man's stroke is affected by the foreskin's presence. The pleasure zones of the natural penis are focused in the upper penis, especially in the foreskin and its attached frenulum, both of which have a multitude of erogenous nerve receptors that love to be titillated with short, rapid stroking. *These short strokes, deep within the vagina, cause the male pubic mound to make gentle, rhythmically rapid, almost-constant contact with the woman's clitoral mound**—her primary pleasure zone— exciting her to higher and higher levels of passion.

In effect, the thrusting rhythm, and gentleness of the natural penis's thrusts, have a positive, sensuous effect on a woman's pleasure *throughout* the intercourse experience, resulting in a high degree of orgasmic success. Indeed, **the foreskin of the penis is the key to a woman's sexual ecstasy.** For it allows the penis to function and feel as it should.

In contrast, circumcision results in the desensitization of the penis because it is missing the erogenous tissue of the foreskin (and usually the frenulum as well). To compensate for this reduction in sensitivity, circumcised men tend to thrust with rougher, tougher strokes to elicit more feeling from the penis. In addition, by diminishing the amount of skin on the penis, circumcision causes the erect penis head and shaft to become *compacted*—abnormally hard and overly stiff—which not only detracts from the woman's feelings of pleasure, but may actually cause her various degrees of discomfort during active coital thrusting.

* I use this term to refer to the entire area surrounding the clitoris (the outer vulval lips, the female pubic mound) and the clitoris itself.

A woman who has experienced only circumcised intercourse does not realize that her pleasure is adversely affected, nor does she realize the extent to which she is discomforted because she has never experienced the comparative comfort and *pure* pleasure of "natural intercourse." She comes to accept the various negativities of circumcised intercourse as a normal part of having sex and simply tries to make the best of the situation, never realizing that her pleasure, responsiveness, and orgasmic capabilities are significantly compromised. (The same applies to circumcised men. Because they have known only the one type of experience, they do not realize that their pleasure, and the pleasure of their partners, is unduly inhibited.)

Moreover, compared to the natural penis, the circumcised penis often thrusts with longer strokes. Because it is missing the pleasure receptors of the foreskin (and usually the frenulum), its sexual focus is *not concentrated in the upper penis*, but is instead diffused along the entire penile shaft. As a result, the circumcised man tries to bring pleasure to his entire shaft by thrusting with elongated strokes. *These elongated strokes cause the male pubic mound to become detached from the woman's genital area.* Consequently, the circumcised man makes considerably less contact with the woman's clitoral mound, decreasing her pleasure and potential for orgasmic success. (A detailed explanation of the differences between natural and circumcised intercourse appears in Chapters 4-11.)

If you are a woman, reading this book will give you an entirely new perspective on what circumcision does to a man's sex organ and its harmful effects on your sex (and love) life. Once you realize how important the natural penis is to *your* sexual pleasure, you will undoubtedly want your circumcised husband or lover to begin restoring his foreskin without delay.

Yet, right now, most American women have no idea how important the natural penis is because they have never known the true sexual experience of natural intercourse—most American women have only experienced intercourse with circumcised men. Still, I hope to explain the differences between the two types of intercourse in such a way that women will be able to comprehend the foreskin's vital importance even though they have never experienced sex with a natural penis.

Like many women, I too, at one time, didn't realize that the circumcised penis was the cause of much of my dissatisfaction with intercourse, but because I had the good fortune to become sexually intimate with a man who had a natural penis, my eyes were opened to the simple truths affirmed herein. My story detailing my personal involvement with this issue appears in Chapter 11. After I came to realize that natural intercourse was an infinitely more gratifying experience, I was curious to find out how other women felt about this subject.

In this regard, I conducted a survey of women who have had the comparative experience of intercourse with both types of penises. The vast majority of these women agreed that there is indeed a definite, discernible difference between circumcised and natural intercourse. Natural intercourse is decidedly superior—gloriously better.

Please allow me to speak now from the woman's point of view those words which women will later come to speak themselves.

As a woman, you deserve to discover your true sexuality with a man who has a natural, whole, fully functioning penis. You deserve to experience the *tenderness* of "real" intercourse—to experience the ecstatic, gentle-grinding rhythm of natural thrusting, which places an almost constant, *gentle* pressuring on your clitoral mound. You deserve to have real orgasms instead of faking them. You deserve to experience the full range of sensations nature intended. You deserve to know the tender, gliding thrusting that *only* a penis with a foreskin can give you, instead of what you are now getting from circumcised intercourse—an abnormally hardened penis head and shaft, along with rougher, tougher, *even bang-away thrusting*, as a result of the penis's missing foreskin and its various vital functions.

Once women come to realize how important the natural penis is to their sexual happiness and love relationships, and that the restored penis will allow them to experience new joys of intercourse that will make them feel "born again," sexually, they will want their men to have foreskins.

Although this issue concerns men and their bodies, paradoxically, women's voices may have to lead the way. For my experience has taught me that when the sexuality issues of circumcision are broached with men, most say, "I'm circumcised and I'm fine." Due to the psychologically disturbing nature of this topic, circumcised men are reluctant to look this issue straight in the eye, and understandably so. This is why women's voices will be so important. Women will be more likely to view this matter with an open mind and quicker to acknowledge the merits of the natural (and restored) penis. *As the insights of this issue unfold, male circumcision and foreskin restoration will become one of the most important women's issues of our time.*

But certainly, circumcision is, first and foremost, a men's issue, for men are its primary victims; they are the ones who bear its physical and emotional scars. Some circumcised men have consciously realized all along that they don't like being circumcised, ever since they became aware that part of their penis is missing. Others intuitively feel that something isn't quite right about the intercourse experience, but they've never made the conscious connection that the sexual disappointments and problems they are experiencing could be related to their circumcision. For example, many circumcised men complain about discomforting erections or soreness during or after intercourse. Many have difficulty maintaining an erection, and some have to work too hard at achieving orgasm. Magazine articles have recently reported that some men are now admitting to faking orgasm. These and other problems, such as premature ejaculation, may very well be related to circumcision. Ultimately, as a circumcised man, you will come to realize that you, too, deserve more. You deserve to resurrect the sexuality that was stolen from you by circumcision and to experience the "born again" pleasures of sex as nature intended it.

You deserve to discover the exquisite sensitivity of a penis head, the nerves of which are kept keenly fresh and alive in the *warm, moist,* sheltered environment of the foreskin. You deserve to experience what the erect penis shaft feels like when the foreskin slips back over the head, giving you the "extra" shaft skin you need for a more comfortable erection. You deserve to experience the sensuous massage the foreskin gives as it glides back and forth over the penis head and shaft during intercourse. You deserve to know the relaxed tenderness of a vagina that is truly pleasured into ecstasy—a vagina that is *truly* loving every moment of your gentle, grinding rhythm; that thrills to the ecstatic, *gliding*-thrusting motions that only a penis with a foreskin can give... There are so many wonderful things a circumcised man can look forward to after his foreskin is restored.

Once the public becomes enlightened about the foreskin's functions and importance, circumcised men, in growing numbers, will decide that they'd really like to get back their protective little "jacket" and experience, as well as give their lovers, "real" sexual fulfillment. They'll want to join The Foreskin Restoration Movement and will ultimately be happy they did. The rest will become history—the controversy, the psychological pain, the denial, and the anger over circumcision will all gradually fade away, as time distances us from the realities of the present.

For circumcised men, natural sex with a (restored) foreskin is an idea whose time has come. And for their female partners, it is also an idea whose time has come—"vaginally."

Yet, "vaginal" orgasm is not the be-all and end-all of the total sexual experience. What really matters is the big picture, the overall picture. Of course, the climactic ending of orgasm is important, but, by analogy, we don't go to a movie just to experience the ending. We go for the fantasy, the plot, the special effects, the characters, and the passion—pleasures served to us during the *time focus* of the movie.

Sure, the story of sex would fall flat without an orgasmic ending. But the "middle time" of intercourse (between insertion and orgasm) is really where it's at. Therein lies the best pleasures of the show. For the beginning is only a tantalizing prelude. And the ending is over in an all-consuming flash. But the middle time is where the love story develops. That's where we are swept away in passionate eroticism. The middle time is where the lovemaking couple is transported to higher and higher states of ecstasy, passion, and love. *And this is where the natural penis excels*, with its ability to bring a man and woman to heights of pure pleasure and passion that are truly indescribable.

But when the foreskin is missing, everything changes. The intercourse experience is profoundly abnormalized for both partners. There is no easy way to say this: When the foreskin is missing, the penis is not a complete sexual organ. Consequently, it cannot function like the real thing. Nor does it feel like the real thing to a woman. It's like taking a ride in a car with the tires taken off. Though it's possible to drive a car on its metal wheel rims, it won't give a quality ride. Without the tires to cushion the ride, the experience will be completely different from what the car manufacturer intended. Similarly, without the foreskin's abundance of extra skin to cushion the intercourse ride, the experience will be completely different from what nature intended. (The foreskin constitutes 33-50% of the penile skin system (3)(4). This means that the circumcised penis has only 50-67% percent of the penile skin nature intended. The result: an overly tight, non-cushioned erection.)

We have a grave sexual problem in this country—men without foreskins—and this issue must be brought to the forefront of America's sexual consciousness.

The vast majority of the world's men live in countries where a penis with a foreskin is virtually the only kind of penis. The famous French lovers have them, the legendary Latin lovers have them, the Swedes, Danes, and the men of all other European countries have them, as do most of the men throughout the rest of the world.

In contrast, relatively few countries practice mass routine circumcision, primarily for its presumed health benefits or as part of an ancient cultural tradition. For others, like Israel and the Muslim nations (primarily in the Middle East, North Africa, and Pakistan), religious beliefs play a prominent role.

The Jewish and Muslim people have been practicing circumcision for thousands and many hundred of years respectively—passed along virtually unquestioned from generation to generation. Until now. In light of the information contained in upcoming chapters, I believe the present generation of Jews and Muslims will reconsider this ancient custom and decide to discontinue it. Non-circumcision is an idea whose time has come, for all races and creeds.

But why is the U.S. one of the major circumcising countries? America does not practice circumcision for religious reasons or as part of an ancient cultural ritual. In fact, before 1900, circumcision was virtually nonexistent in this country. And yet, by 1980, doctors were routinely circumcising almost all American boys. How did circumcision first take hold of the American medical community? And why did its practice become so routine? (The above topics will be briefly discussed below and expanded upon in Chapter 18.)

Nature must have put a foreskin on every human male for a reason. No matter how many are cut away, every infant boy continues to be born with one. What is Mother Nature trying to tell us? Can we presume to be wiser than nature by cutting away a vital part of a man's sexual anatomy for reasons of so-called medical "benefit"? Benefits which will be exposed in later chapters as virtually nonexistent.

Over the years there has been considerable controversy regarding circumcision within the medical community. In 1971 and again in 1975, the American Academy of Pediatrics officially announced that routine circumcision lacks medical justification, saying in their Task Force report that: "There is no absolute medical indication for routine circumcision of the newborn." *

---

* This position was changed slightly in 1989 when a new position paper from the AAP equivocated: "Newborn circumcision has potential medical benefits, as well as disadvantages and risks." But in 1999, after studying the issue for two years and analyzing 40 years of medical research, they issued a new policy statement: "Existing scientific evidence demonstrates potential medical benefits of newborn male circumcision; however, these data are not sufficient to recommend routine neonatal [i.e., infant] circumcision."

Despite the above reports, the overall medical community continued to recommend circumcision, and the circumcision rate in the United States continued largely unabated. It is currently (1998) about 60 percent, with the highest percentages in the East and Midwest and lower percentages in the West (5).

How did circumcision get started in America? As incredible as it may now seem, medical circumcision became popularized at the turn of the century as a "cure" for masturbation (6). Later, when this reason was refuted and dropped, another came in to replace it—purported cause of cervical cancer in women. But this, too, has been rejected by those who have seriously studied the facts (7). As the cervical-cancer myth lost credibility, other non-valid reasons popped up to replace it. Circumcision seems to be a surgical operation in search of a reason, which in reality does not exist.

The origination and perpetuation of circumcision by the American medical community is a historical fact that cannot be denied. With all the miracles of modern medicine, we sometimes forget that the medical profession is capable of making mistakes and that the science of medicine is still in the process of developing.

Only 200 years ago, it was common for doctors to practice "bloodletting" (draining various amounts of a patient's blood) in an attempt to cure various illnesses. It is a historical fact that a team of doctors was responsible for bloodletting our first president, George Washington, an act which no doubt hastened his death. By today's standards, the above practice seems incredibly primitive.

Only 100 years ago, medical circumcision gained acceptance because doctors thought it discouraged masturbation, which was at that time believed to be linked to a wide variety of physical and mental illnesses, including insanity (8). In retrospect, this belief seems incredibly silly (for today, as every teenager learns, masturbation can only lead to blindness—and for this reason, most of us only do it until we need glasses).

The medical thoughts and techniques of yesteryear were completely different from those of today. But that doesn't mean that today's thoughts and techniques are infallible—or even that we're headed in the right direction. A hundred years from now the practice of medicine will look completely different from the way it looks today because, as stated, medicine is still in the process of developing.

Throughout the 20th century, the American medical community's emphasis seemed to be focused on looking for reasons to remove the foreskin, when it should have been looking for reasons for the foreskin's existence. For most of the 20th century, the American pro-circumcision element had its way. But now things are beginning to come around full circle, as evidenced by the fact that the circumcision rate has dropped almost 30% since 1980. America's experiment with circumcision is approaching its end.

With all the medical advancements of the 20th century, society has come to look upon doctors as demigods. But, of course, they are not; they are human beings and are capable of making mistakes. Circumcision was, and is, one of their biggest mistakes. But we must resist the temptation to point all the fingers of blame at the medical community, for until somewhat recently, sexual topics and the study of sexuality have been taboo. In a country where both the general population and the medical profession are unduly inhibited about discussing the sex organs, and where the vast majority of the adult male population is circumcised, no one was looking for the sexual purposes of the foreskin. There is no one to blame for circumcisions of the "past"; it was just something that happened during the course of humanity's development.

With each generation, mankind gains more knowledge. We then use this knowledge to kindle the fires that light our way into the future. And the future, regarding the fate of the foreskin, is something that is being decided on now, as you read. You are part of the decision. And what will you decide?

I believe that once you become more knowledgeable about this issue, you will agree that the time has come to consign circumcision to the grave, alongside other historical oddities we've buried along the way, as we travel onward to a better world.

And yet, circumcision will not die an easy death because there is so much emotionalism, denial, and psychological distress surrounding it. Doctors may want to defend the circumcisions they've done and deny its negative effects. Men may want to deny that circumcision affects their, and their female partners', sexuality. And parents may want to deny that they made the wrong choice when they decided to have their son circumcised.

There is a great deal of emotionalism involved in the circumcision issue because of its medical and cultural entrenchment, and because to think of it as a mistake is a difficult thing to accept. In the end, however, mankind will decide to abandon the practice of circumcision. It is destined to become a dead issue because we're talking about living tissue, which wants to live and love on the penis of man.

As the importance of the foreskin gains public acceptance, members of the medical community will no longer recommend circumcision. Still, many readers may express anger and outrage toward them for circumcisions performed in the past. But we must remember that there is nothing to be gained from lashing out at mistakes of the past. We must move forward and put this dreadful era of medical history behind us. Similarly, sons should not place blame on their parents, nor should parents blame themselves for their sons' circumcisions, for up until now we did not realize that the foreskin mattered one way or the other. The mistakes of circumcisions' past cannot be erased, but through foreskin restoration every circumcised man can become "whole" again.

Will millions of American men really choose to restore their foreskins? How could they not? Once the sexual value of the foreskin becomes common knowledge, "Everyman" will want to have his very own foreskin NOW. Though it will take a little time to restore your new treasure, it will be time well-rewarded with the increased sexual pleasure you will ultimately experience.

Will your female partner understand and give support to you when you express your desire to restore? With the knowledge of its importance, yes, without a doubt, she will be cheering you on from the sidelines.

After all, what if the situation were reversed? How would she feel about it then? What if she had been the one who was circumcised? Female circumcision (an umbrella term used to denote the removal of various parts of the female sexual anatomy) is still performed today in some parts of the world, primarily in some Muslim nations and throughout parts of Africa. The most common form of female circumcision is clitoridectomy (removal of the clitoris). It is a little known fact, but there are an estimated 100 million circumcised women in the world. These female genital mutilations (FGMs) are usually done in childhood or early adolescence (not infancy), without anesthesia. Why is this incredibly cruel, ancient practice still in existence? Cultural ritual and superstition.

It may be hard for you to believe that there are so many circumcised women in the world. Since it is not practiced in this country, many of us are not aware of its current-day existence. You may be thinking that female circumcision is grossly barbaric and should be stopped without delay. You're right. And the United States Congress agrees. A federal law was recently passed (1996) outlawing FGM. (Immigrants to this country were requesting it of U.S. doctors.)

Women, how do you think you would feel if you had been the one who was circumcised? Try to imagine someone cutting away the foreskin that covers your clitoris. (Yes, women too have a protective foreskin.) Or cutting away your clitoris entirely. It makes you squirm just to think about it, doesn't it? Now that you have imagined the devastation of female circumcision, it will be easier for you to understand what it must be like for a man to have had a very important part of his penis removed, and you will undoubtedly be more compassionate about his desire to restore.

The very idea of female circumcision must surely strike a sensitive nerve; yet the practice of male circumcision is just as sexually insulting. When a man has been circumcised, he is deprived of an important and sensitive part of his manhood; an entire spectrum of erotic sensation and sexual function has been stolen from him. It must be said: Circumcision is sexual-reduction surgery.

Every year in this country approximately 1,200,000 screaming newborn baby boys are forcibly strapped to a Circumstraint Board, and without anesthesia, are routinely sliced, circumcised, and stripped of a very special part of their anatomy. Yet this excruciatingly painful 15-minute operation is only the beginning, for as will be explained, the denuded glans of the circumcised penis has harmful repercussions on a man's and his female partner's sexuality throughout their lives.

This book presents irrefutable evidence that male circumcision is, by definition, genital mutilation (MGM). Therefore, since genital mutilation of female minors is now prohibited by federal law, it follows that male children should be afforded the same protection. The 14th Amendment of the U.S. Constitution guarantees equal rights to both genders; thus it is mandatory that the present federal law prohibiting FGM be amended to prohibit male circumcision.

It is a self-evident, fundamental human right that one should be allowed to retain all the healthy body parts he or she is born with. When parents' have their child circumcised, it is a violation of the child's human right to retain the genitals he was endowed with by nature. It is the child's penis, not the parents'. Therefore, the child's human rights must be protected by law.

Surely the time has come for the cessation of both male and female circumcision. Surely there is truth in the statement that the practice of circumcision/genital mutilation—call it what you will—no longer belongs on the planet. Time and truth have a way of joining hands when the time for truth has arrived.

2

Something is Missing

>Woody: What do you mean, missing? Something is missing *from me?*
>
>Louise: Yes.
>
>Woody: Like what? Can you say what's missing from me?
>
>Louise: Well, no, but maybe if you could guess a few things, I could try.
>
>— Woody Allen and Louise Lasser
>from the movie, *Bananas*

How vital is the male foreskin to the sexuality of a man and his female partner? When the foreskin is missing, is the intercourse experience incomplete and unfulfilling, haunting the subconscious mind of both partners? Could the foreskin really make that much of a difference during intercourse? Yes, yes, oohhh yes, the natural penis makes a superlative difference in the lovemaking experience. Sex with a circumcised penis and sex with a natural penis are as different as night and day. They are as different as viewing the harsh, blinding light of the sun at noon vs. the softer, reflected light of the romantic midnight moon.

You may be thinking, "It can't really be *that* different. How could a 'little' extra skin make that much of a difference?" Later in this chapter, one of the foreskin's most evidential functions during intercourse will be overviewed. And, as you will later see in the survey chapter, the vast majority of surveyed women overwhelmingly preferred intercourse with a man with a natural penis. As one survey respondent commented:

> I experienced a huge difference between circumcised and uncircumcised men. Until I met my natural* husband, I thought that the rough, dry circumcised penis was the way it was supposed to be. WOW! I had been missing genuine, naturally satisfying sex and now have the utmost appreciation for the 'real thing.' There is such a remarkable difference, in all aspects of sex—from foreplay and fellatio to intercourse. In retrospect, I now consider the circumcised penis as a sort of unreal 'device' that made intercourse a not very pleasing experience that often left me sore. I now have orgasms that were very rare with circumcised men.

Once your man restores his foreskin and the two of you experience the ecstatic joy and thrill of a more fully functioning penis, I am confident that you will both agree that there is no comparison. Until you've had sex with a penis with a foreskin—ultra-erogenous tissue and the penis's only moving part—you haven't really had sex. You only think you have. In actuality, you've only had *circumcised* sex. Whatever pleasure you may or may not be experiencing from intercourse, only one thing is certain: When the foreskin is added, things will only get better—unbelievably better, exquisitely better. Sex without a foreskin is merely a three-letter word—sex. But when you add the foreskin, it becomes a four-letter word—sexy.

Perhaps the following "joke" will help to bring the point home more clearly: What does the French woman say after making love? "Oo La La!" What does the Italian woman say? "Mama

---

*The survey introduced women to the term "natural." Most respondents picked up on it and used it instead of the cumbersome term "uncircumcised."

Mia!" What does the American woman say? "Jim, the ceiling needs painting."

An article in *Cosmopolitan* that talked about couples who sought therapy for their relationship problems quoted Shirley Zussman, a marital counselor and sex therapist in New York City: "Sad to say, a lot of spouses have come to regard sex as just another chore. One statement I hear all the time is 'It's a hassle.' I don't often hear someone declare that sex is fun" (1).

Another article in *Cosmopolitan* opened with a depiction of a troubled relationship: "Three years into their marriage, Penny and Jason began bickering over such minor matters as who would take out the garbage, wash the dishes, walk the dog. 'Nothing my husband did made me happy,' says Penny, '...our relationship just didn't feel good anymore.' Jason agreed, 'We weren't considering divorce, but we did think *something fundamental was missing from our marriage*' " (2). (Emphasis added)

Could unsatisfactory sex have something to do with a couple's general dissatisfaction with one another, causing various degrees of nagging, whining, and bickering? Many people will see that this could be possible. But how many would suspect that circumcision could have something to do with it?

The information detailed in this book will show that circumcised sex doesn't measure up to natural sex. And it isn't simply a matter of one being good and the other being better. Circumcision cuts deeper; it is actually detrimental to the sex act. And its negative effects don't necessarily end at the sex organs.

I propose (and the survey results infer) that the incompleteness and dissatisfaction of circumcised intercourse can negatively impact the psychological attitude of one or both partners, which may lead to various levels of relationship unhappiness, and marital bickering and discord. This can gradually erode the relationship and may eventually set the stage for divorce.

The above may seem to be a drastic jump—from circumcision, to dissatisfaction in the bedroom, to non-sexually related quarreling in the living room, to divorce court—but as you read the remainder of this chapter, and chapters that follow, I think you will begin to see how circumcision could conceivably result in such a tragic progression of events. As this issue gains prominence, and is discussed and examined more closely, we will undoubtedly come to find that circumcision is a multifaceted problem with sexual, psychological, and sociological repercussions. The following comments from the survey give us a glimpse at the tip of the iceberg that lies hidden beneath the sheets of America's bedrooms.

> **"During my circumcised intercourses, I felt violated or used—like I was just a piece of meat—even with my husband.**
>
> **With my current natural partner, I feel warm, tender, soft, and beautiful. But during circumcised intercourse, I would often get aggravated emotionally. I have cried after many of my circumcised sexual experiences—feeling so empty and not knowing why. I have never cried or felt this way with a natural partner. I even once hit a circumcised man, and I couldn't help to ask if they 'got what they wanted' (to some of them) because I certainly didn't. I never made the connection between this feeling of hostility and circumcised sex until now [completing the survey]."**

> **"I felt hostile toward my circumcised partners because most of the time it felt like a selfish one-way experience with him not caring about me. I have never dug them with my fingernails during intercourse, but there are other things I thought of doing to 'unfeeling' circumcised men."**

Although various non-surgical methods of restoration are available, my husband had his foreskin reconstructed surgically, about 14 years ago. (His before and after story appears in Chapter 12.) Many a morning, while dressing, he says, "You know, getting a foreskin is the best thing that ever happened to me." And I agree. Getting his foreskin is the best thing that's ever happened to *me*. *And to our relationship*. But the thesis of this book is not based solely on our subjective experiences. There are many sound physiological reasons why circumcision disrupts the intercourse experience, which will be explained in detail in upcoming chapters. But for now, please let the following serve as an introduction.

HOW THE FORESKIN'S PRESENCE MAKES A DIFFERENCE TO A WOMAN DURING INTERCOURSE—A BRIEF

The glans (head) of the penis is designed by nature to be an *internal* organ, nestled inside the *moist*, protective covering of the foreskin. (Upon erection, however, the penis head emerges from the foreskin—like a turtle's head—and the foreskin is transferred to the shaft, allowing the glans to make contact with the vaginal walls.) As a result of the constant moisturizing afforded by the foreskin, the natural glans is pleasantly softened, and somewhat spongy to the touch, even when erect. Consequently, *the head of the natural penis feels softly-stiff to a woman during intercourse*. Nature herself designed it that way. This is the kind of penis head the vagina loves to have stroking its vaginal walls. Everything changes, however, when the penis is circumcised.

When circumcision removes the foreskin, the penis head is exposed to the open air and becomes a dried-out, *external* organ. Because of its dried-out condition and its constant exposure to the friction action of clothing, *the circumcised penis head becomes toughened, abnormally hardened, and "callused."*

During coital thrusting, the toughened, abnormally hardened glans creates a discomforting experience for the delicate lining of the vaginal walls. As a result, the intercourse experience is abnormalized for the participating woman. She may notice that she feels various degrees of vaginal discomfort and displeasure, which usually become more apparent as intercourse progresses (or as an aftereffect of intercourse). These detractions are, however, intermixed with pleasurable sensations, so the woman may or may not be fully cognizant that she is experiencing displeasure, because pleasure can override displeasure.

Perhaps you can better appreciate the significance of the moisturized natural glans vs. the abnormally toughened circumcised glans, and the discomfort it creates for the woman, through the following analogy. Suppose one man has a job of applying and testing moisturizing lotions to his hands all day, while another works outside digging ditches, causing his hands to be dried out, rough, and callused. Suppose these two men were to rub the sensitive skin of a woman's face with their hands, for however long she usually experiences intercourse. Which man's hands would create a discomforting and displeasurable experience for the woman's face? Which man's hands would provide a more sensual sensation?

Since most American women have known only the circumcised intercourse experience, they look upon various discomforts as just a normal part of having sex, since they occur virtually every time they have intercourse. They don't realize that these discomforts should not occur. Consequently, they try to ignore them and *concentrate* instead on the pleasurable sensations. A woman may think she is experiencing pleasure during circumcised sex, but her pleasure is actually a combination of pleasure and displeasure entwined. It is not an experience of *pure* pleasure.

This aspect of circumcised sex becomes more obvious when one has experienced natural sex as a comparison. But since most American women have never experienced natural intercourse, let me try to explain it this way. Circumcised intercourse is something like having a mosquito bite. When you scratch a mosquito bite, it feels pleasurable, but at the same time, it's discomforting. While you're scratching it, it feels good—*or does it?*

The circumcised man also experiences "mosquito-bite sex," for his pleasure, too, is intermixed with varying degrees of displeasure or discomfort (like a too-tight erection), even though he may not consciously realize it. Since he has never experienced anything but circumcised sex, he accepts mosquito-bite sex as normal. Like the woman, the man, too, tries to ignore any discomforting sensations and *concentrates* on the pleasurable feelings.

But sex, real sex, shouldn't be a frenzied lesson in concentration. Instead, it should be passionate (though relaxed) and dreamy. Floating. Nirvana. Out-of-this-world. This is the natural sex experience. Circumcised sex, however, is not this way. Instead, it is wide-awake, on-alert, muscles-tensed sex, with a narrowly focused concentration toward achieving orgasm.

ONE OF THE MOST SIGNIFICANT DISTINCTIONS BETWEEN THE TWO TYPES OF PENISES, AND HOW IT MAKES A DIFFERENCE TO A WOMAN DURING INTERCOURSE

In order to better understand the negative effects the abnormally hardened circumcised glans has on the vaginal walls, we must first observe the structure of the erect penis head in greater detail. (See Figure 2-1.) Notice that the penis head flares out from the shaft. I'll refer to this flared-out area as the *coronal ridge*. Notice that the coronal ridge causes the penis head to have a spear-like, hook-like shape to it.

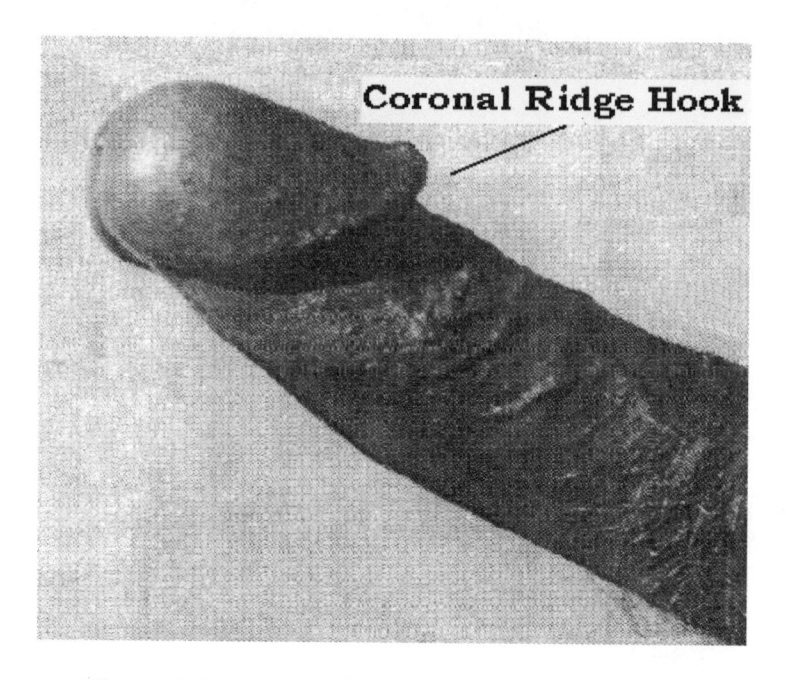

Figure 2-1. Erect penis showing the coronal ridge.

During coital thrusting, the tough, abnormally hardened coronal ridge of the circumcised penis acts as a hook-like scraper, which **scrapes the vaginal walls with every outward stroke**, *whether the woman consciously realizes it or not.*

This scraping action abnormalizes intercourse for the woman (we will discuss the male's side of this later), causing the vagina to fire off both pleasurable and displeasurable signals simultaneously—mosquito-bite sex—it feels good—or does it?

Some women, especially women in their 20s and early 30s who have not had as much exposure to circumcised intercourse and whose youthful hormones cause them to approach sex with frenzied excitement, may not consciously discern that they are experiencing discomfort. They simply accept the experience without dwelling on its qualities. *Yet, they may notice that there is something strangely bothersome or frustrating about the pleasure they're experiencing, even though they would categorize it, overall, as pleasure.* For other women, it manifests as a vague discomfort, either during or after intercourse. Some, however, notice definitively that they experience considerable discomfort. Below are the comments of two women from the survey:

> "I always experience vaginal discomfort with my circumcised partners—chafing—even enough to turn me off. I have also heard this from other women."

> "I feel very strongly that I experienced a lot of pain with my circumcised partner. The circumcised penis hurts. But with my natural partner, I have no pain, only pleasure."

I contend that the abnormally hardened, hook-like circumcised penis head lessens a woman's excitement capabilities and plays a prominent role in why so many women often cannot achieve orgasm from intercourse and, consequently, may resort to faking them.

But you might ask: "Doesn't the natural penis head also have a hook-like projection to it? Why doesn't it act as a scraper on the vaginal walls?"

That's a good question. Yes, it does have a hook-like projection, but the natural penis head does not act as a scraper because of the foreskin's various functions.

First, because of the foreskin's lubricating functions, the natural penis head is spongier; it has a yielding quality to it, similar to the sponginess of the tongue. This softer, giveable glans is kind and gentle to a woman's delicate vaginal walls during active coital thrusting.

Additionally, the foreskin plays another important role in the comfort of penile thrusting. The "extra" shaft skin it provides serves to cushion the effects of the coronal ridge hook. (See Figure 2-2.)

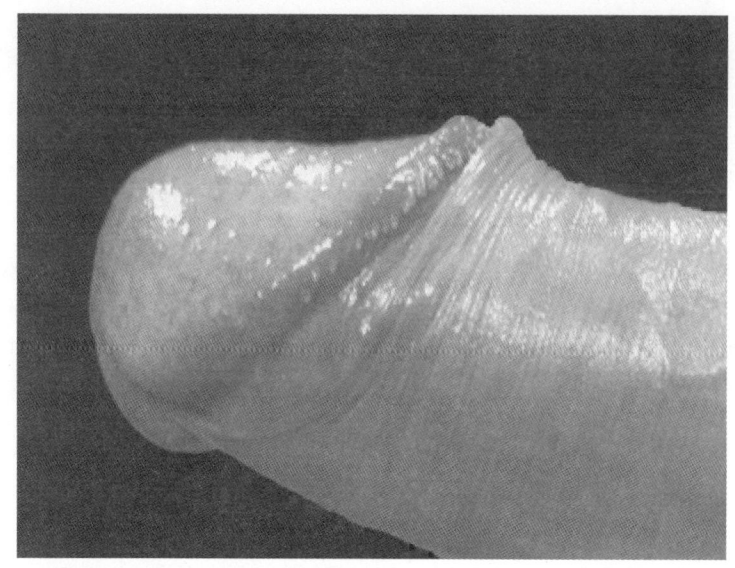

Figures 2-2: Foreskin cushions the coronal-ridge hook from scraping the vaginal walls.

During the outward stroke, this extra penile skin bunches up behind the coronal ridge, thereby providing a cushion of soft, pliable skin against the vaginal walls. (See Figure 2-3.)

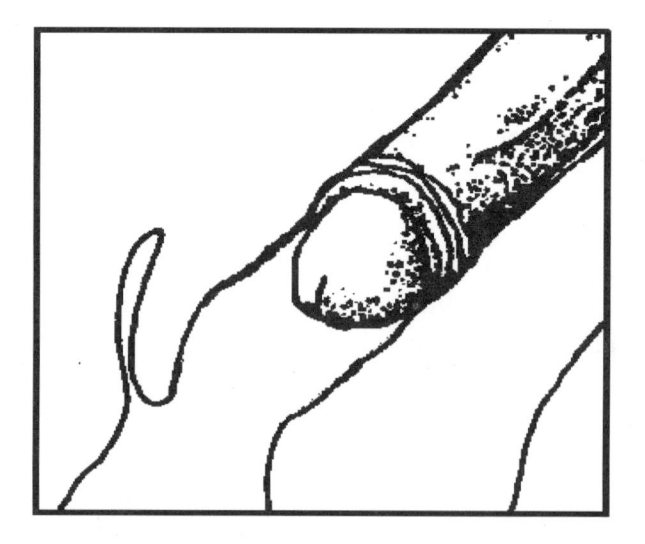

Figure 2-3: Foreskin bunches up behind the coronal ridge as the penis withdraws from vagina. (Adapted from Berkeley) (3).

(The preceding comparisons are only intended as a brief overview and are oversimplified. A more detailed analysis for both sexual partners, as well as several other differences between natural and circumcised sex, will follow in later chapters.)

Natural intercourse is an experience of sexual ecstasy and a relaxed surrendering to the simultaneous, mutual experience of sensually indescribable, blissful lust. The physical structure and thrusting motions of the natural penis give the vagina soft, smooth, sensuous pleasuring, and more often than not the woman experiences coital orgasm (according to the results of the survey).

Real sex, natural sex, is an incomparable joy ride without any lumps and bumps, like riding luxuriously in a Cadillac limousine with the man or woman of your dreams. In contrast, circumcised sex, especially for the woman, creates stress, discomfort, and frustration to the sex organs, and is, comparatively speaking, more like riding over a rough road in a Chevy Chevette.

During circumcised sex, the subconscious mind (and perhaps even the conscious mind) senses that something is wrong. Although each partner has his or her innate craving for sexual stimulation and its orgasmic release, which drives them to seek it out again and again, still, the body and brain seem to somehow know that "real sex ain't this way." Below is a comment from the survey.

> **My present husband is circumcised. He is very concerned about pleasing me, but during intercourse, the penis feels hard. I experience discomfort, and I often feel like I'm being pounded on.**
>
> **With my natural partner, whom I went with before I was married, intercourse felt gentler and more sensuous. I could sense that he got much more pleasure during intercourse than did any of my circumcised partners. He was more passionate, and sex with him was very stimulating and fulfilling. With him, I always experienced much more pleasure,**

and intercourse seemed more loving. I strongly feel that this is the way it was meant to be.

Perhaps you are beginning to feel angered, saddened, or dismayed that you were circumcised or that you are a woman married to a circumcised man. But relief from your distress or dismay is coming into view at the speed of insight.

The first part of any solution is to realize that there is a problem. This is not always easy to face. But remember, there is a solution for the millions of American men who are circumcised—foreskin restoration. Through the promise of restoration, every circumcised man—the guy next door, and men just like you—can now become "whole" again.

There is nothing we can do to change the past. But we can change the eyes with which we look at the future. The future—a foreskin for Everyman—is opening its door. And that door leads to greater happiness and satisfaction in the bedroom, which will in turn lead to greater overall relationship happiness.

You are standing at the very threshold of The Foreskin Restoration Revolution. It may now seem to be a strange place for you to be standing, but once you cross that threshold and join the millions of men who will be crossing over it with you, then—and only then—will you and your partner find the sexual "wholeness" that has been missing from your life. Then—and only then—will you be able to look deep within your wife's or lover's eyes and see "we."

SEX IS A CEREBRAL EXPERIENCE TOO

On the surface, the partners of a circumcised relationship may not be consciously aware that they are experiencing sexual dissatisfaction and frustration. They may think their sex life is "OK," or they may even think it's great, depending on youthful naiveté and individual libidos.

Some, especially younger people, may think that if sex has a lot of wild thrusting—a lot of action to it—then that's an indication their sex life is great. But I think that the frenzy of circumcised wildly active thrusting and whamming is actually a symptom that the sex organs are frantically seeking the sensuality they cannot achieve. Like if the partners thrust harder and faster, they'll get somewhere. I must stress that natural sex is entirely different. It's a much gentler intermingling. It's more of a tender blending—an enrapturement oozing with sensuousness—with both partners swooning in ecstatic surrender to the passionate, graceful dance of the sex organs. Circumcised sex simply cannot bring these feelings.

Sometimes a person may think his or her sex life is okay, even though they have it infrequently. But infrequent sex in a normal, healthy adult is a sign that one's sex life is actually not okay. I remember a conversation with a friend whose wife was talking divorce. I asked him point blank, "How's your sex life?" He replied, "Our sex life is okay—I mean, sex is great when we have it, but we hardly ever have it." How, then, can you say your sex life is okay? Sure, you're going to get into it when you have it, if you're only having it once or twice a month—because you're starved for it. It's like going all day without eating, you eventually become frantic to eat.

When the facts of this issue come to light, we may find that the real reason one partner, or even both, puts sexual activity on the back burner, having time for everything else, is because they actually find sex displeasing on a conscious or subconscious level.

Still, many people probably have sex with some regularity. As stated, the couple is drawn back to it again and again—good, bad, or indifferent—because their innate need for sexual stimulation drives them to do so, and they mistake quantity for quality—equate orgasm with satisfaction.

Nevertheless, on a hidden subconscious level, the mind of both partners longs for the true sexual experience nature intended. This is essentially what the men of the *Psychology Today* survey (quoted in Chapter One) meant when they said, "Is it possible that there is some new position, partner, practice, or gimmick which would bring sex up to expectation?" If men are thinking these kinds of thoughts, are the innermost thoughts of women that much different?

Sexual intercourse, although experienced primarily in the sex organs, is as much a cerebral (brain-related) experience as it is a genital experience. And the foreskin is absolutely essential if the man and his partner are to enjoy the true genital *and cerebral* pleasure that nature intended as part of the total sexual/lovemaking experience. A woman who participated in the survey describes beautifully the cerebral experience of natural intercourse:

> **Intercourse with my natural partner is a totally wonderful, emotionally supporting/healing connection. I feel the natural penis sets up a whole current between us. We cross the threshold of being male/female opposites into experiencing the union, the similarities, and the complete dropping away of mind, of fears, and of thoughts that reinforce our separateness.**

In contrast, we shall see that circumcision's modifications to the penis interfere with a man's and woman's ability to both give and receive pleasure during intercourse. And, as mentioned, I contend that the negative effects of circumcised sex don't end at the sex organs. There are psychological and sociological repercussions as well.

When the sex organs do not experience the true feelings they were designed by nature to experience but are instead subjected to intermixed feelings of discomfort, displeasurement, and disappointment, either or both partners may become annoyed, frustrated, or angered—not necessarily during sex, but as an *aftereffect* of sex—not necessarily immediately after sex, but hours later, or the day after.

An example, though admittedly extreme, is the recent, highly publicized John and Lorena Bobbitt case, in which, you may recall, the couple had sex over 900 times within a three-year period. Shouldn't this much sex—*lovemaking*—draw a couple closer and closer together? Yet, what did the Bobbitts experience? John (whose circumcised penis was shown in a subsequent adult video) increasingly mistreated his wife as the relationship progressed, and Lorena became so angered she cut off his penis. Why did she focus her anger on his penis?

Of course, Lorena's act was outrageous and bizarre. I mention the case primarily because it is familiar to so many people. I'm not saying that the Bobbitts are typical of what is going on in circumcised relationships around America. But the case does clearly indicate that sex for the Bobbitts was not creating the kind of "emotionally supporting/healing connection" that the survey respondent above was experiencing with her natural lover.

Scientists are beginning to find evidence that romantic love has a biochemical basis, and that sex creates biochemical changes that not only bring on feelings of physical pleasure and orgasmic satisfaction, but also emotions—feelings of peace, love, closeness, contentment, and emotional security (4).

From this, I theorize that during natural intercourse the pleasure centers of the brain receive positive biochemical messages, which bring about these feelings of love and closeness. But during circumcised intercourse, the pleasure centers of the brain receive a deficiency of these biochemical messages, or an aberration.

How could this be so? First, biologically, the foreskin is profusely endowed with erogenous nerve endings (5). The circumcised male is missing these pleasure sensors; he has no foreskin, so he has no foreskin pleasure sensors. This causes him to miss out on much of the pleasure he should be getting both during foreplay and during intercourse. Second, as will be later discussed, the pleasure sensors of the penis head itself become atrophied and desensitized due to its exposure as an external organ (6). *In effect, the circumcised penis cannot send the "right" messages to the brain because many of its sexual nerves are either missing entirely or have become deadened or dulled.*

As a result, during intercourse, the man's brain receives an incomplete message from the penis, a message of partial frustration. It's as if the brain were saying, "Where are all the pleasure sensations from my missing foreskin and desensitized penis head? I'm not receiving the right biochemical messages. Something is missing."

Yet, you might say, "But the circumcised man does orgasm, and certainly, his orgasms are pleasurable." But this experience, too, may not be everything it could be, for men circumcised in adulthood often report that their circumcised orgasms are not as intense, nor nearly as satisfying, as the ones they experienced when their penis was whole (7).

I submit that circumcision's alterations to the penis cause the pleasure centers of the brain to "miss out" on the "right" biochemical messages throughout all phases of the sex act. Consequently, the mind becomes discontented and frustrated by the incompleteness of the experience, whether the man consciously realizes it or not.

I further theorize that this frustration has a negative psychological impact that can manifest itself in aftereffects of discontentment, irritability, or anger, which are carried far beyond the bedroom door.

The above may seem farfetched at this point in your reading, so, for the moment, let me simply say that the positive biochemical messages that the brain *should* receive during intercourse are very important to the brain's mental "attitude." And when these biochemical messages are denied to the brain, it may develop an "attitude problem." Perhaps the following will help to explain what I mean.

A few years ago, comical "word-saying" T-shirts were all the rage—humorous reflections of our "philosophies" on life. Perhaps you remember sayings like "I can't be overdrawn, I still have checks," "Visualize Whirled Peas," "Born to Shop," "I owe, I owe, it's off to work I go." Among the more popular sayings was the T-shirt that exemplifies the point I'm trying to make: "Sex is a misdemeanor. The more I miss, de meaner I get." There just might be some truth in these twisted lines. But it could just as easily say, "Circumcised sex is a misdemeanor. The more real sex it causes me to miss, de meaner I get."

Though the above discussion focused on the male side of this issue, there is also the female side. The abnormalities of circumcised sex also result in an incomplete and frustrating experience for the woman, especially when she doesn't achieve orgasm.

As will be elaborated upon in later chapters, circumcised sex causes discomforts and detractions to a woman's pleasure. This negatively impacts the pleasure centers of her brain, whether she consciously realizes it or not (but I think many women realize that something isn't right). Even if a woman does achieve orgasm, her copulatory pleasure (the "middle time" of intercourse—from insertion to orgasm) is adversely affected throughout the experience by the negativities of the thrusting circumcised penis.

If she repeatedly has sexual sessions with her partner where her pleasure is compromised or she does not achieve orgasm, she may begin taking out her dissatisfaction and frustration by belittling him, or nagging him about his faults, or by being argumentative and bitchy toward him—"Dammit, Joe! You left the cap off the toothpaste again. How many times do I have to tell you"! Another of those popular T-shirt sayings comes to mind: "Life's a bitch, and then you marry one."

(Of course, not all circumcised marriages are outwardly antagonistic. Many couples may learn to control their tempers. Still, the partners may lack a genuine affection for one another and may work at staying out of each other's way to avoid confrontations and intermingling. Though they have sex from time to time, one would hardly call it a love-filled marriage.)

The influence of the penis on the relationship can be so subtle it can often go unrecognized. Drs. Phyllis & Eberhard Kronhausen addressed this ***transference effect*** in their book, *The Sexually Responsive Woman*:

> We can well understand why women who do not experience orgasm gradually lose interest in sexual relations and come to find intercourse unpleasant.... One should not therefore be surprised to hear that failure to achieve sexual happiness is likely to have an adverse effect on the woman's total relationship with her partner and may lead to the breakdown of their relationship.
>
> *This does not mean that such a couple would themselves be aware of the sexual roots of their problem.... In many cases, the couple do not quarrel at all about their sex life, but may violently disagree on a variety of irrelevant matters* (2). (Emphasis added)

In America, about half of all marriages end in divorce. We can safely assume that in many cases, a great deal of discord and disharmony takes place before the couple finally decide to leave one another.

Could the sexual dissatisfactions associated with circumcised intercourse be an unrecognized contributing factor in relationship discordance? I propose that it is, even though sex itself may never be mentioned in these domestic spats.

This idea should not seem implausible. After all, the desire for sexual satisfaction is a primal drive, and sexual relations are an important part of an intimate relationship. When sex is consistently disappointing or unsatisfactory (including infrequent sex and sex that's over too quickly), it's going to wear on the relationship. At some point, one or both partners begins to associate their partner with the lack of fulfillment and negative feelings that accompany circumcised sex. Once this association is made, the person (subconsciously or otherwise) may develop a certain kind of resentment toward their mate, including a disrespect for their partner's sexuality, and may begin to take on a general negative attitude toward the partner overall. This is reflected in the couple's everyday interrelationship beyond the bedroom door, manifesting itself in various degrees of nagging, needling, bickering, and discord. I propose that the physiological and biochemical effects of circumcised sex, and the negative emotions it generates, engenders discontentment and disharmony, which serve to drive a wedge through the heart of a relationship.

I formulated this hypothesis when I realized the positive effect the foreskin and natural sex had on my marital relationship (after my husband's restoration), as well as from my premarital relationships with both circumcised and uncircumcised men, and from the eye-opening results and comments of the survey. Additionally, my observation of circumcised and natural relationships around me further reinforced my opinion that circumcised sex does not bring about the kind of communion in a relationship that natural sex brings. Please jump ahead momentarily to page 165 and read one woman's thought-provoking comments on this subject.

As the book develops, it should be easy for you to see how circumcision causes serious damage to the male organ and drastic alterations to the sex act. But could circumcised sex actually be a negative experience for the brain's pleasure centers? Could it really result in resentment and hostility toward one's partner, leading to everyday arguments and quarreling over "little" things? Could this cause a general loss of respect, which in turn causes the relationship to gradually (or quickly) fall apart at the seams? Listen closely to women's quotes throughout the book, like the ones below, and decide for yourself.

> "When I didn't achieve an orgasm, I felt cheated. Oftentimes I would just fake it or lie there until he was done. I would also feel guilty because I didn't feel anything for the man after he was done with me."

> "With my natural man, I always glow after intercourse, but with circumcised men, I couldn't wait to get dressed and get away from them. I never glowed."

The negative physiological and psychological effects of circumcised sex are clearly not the only cause of relationship discord, disharmony, and divorce. Other factors undoubtedly play a role. There is no denying that financial hardship, alcohol abuse, drug abuse, unfaithfulness, etc. can be contributing factors to putting a marriage on the rocks. Nevertheless, America's divorce rate is more than double that of Western Europe, where men are not usually circumcised (8). When the final truths of this issue emerge, I am certain that we will find that circumcised sex plays a significant role in America's high divorce rate.

The following humorous (though tragic) dialogue between the characters played by Woody Allen and Louise Lasser (who in real life were married at the time and divorced soon thereafter) in the comedy movie, *Bananas,* points out how the missing foreskin can affect a couple's relationship without them being consciously aware of it.

Louise: I have to tell you something, and I don't know how to break it.

Woody: Why, is there something the matter? Have you seen x-rays of me?

Louise: (Laughing) I saw x-rays of you.

Woody: I fail to see the humor in this.

Louise: You didn't see the x-rays.

Woody: ...What? Tell me what's the matter? (Nervously) I'm white. You know how your heart beats. My heart is beating.

Louise: I know.... I just don't think that we should see each other anymore.

Woody: Oh, really?! Why, what's the matter?

Louise: ...There's just something missing...and....

Woody: What do you mean, "missing"? Something is missing *from me?*

Louise: Yes.

Woody: What do you mean? Like what? (Emotionally distraught) Can you say what's missing from me?

Louise: ...Well, no, but maybe if you could guess a few things, I could try.

Woody: What do you mean? Can you say? .... Can you tell me?

Louise: Something is missing and I don't know what it is.

Something is Missing

Woody: Is it personality, or looks, or something like that? Or I'm not smart enough? Is that what you're saying?

Louise: Well, no.

Woody: It's not something to do with height, or something like that?

Louise: No, it has nothing to do with the fact that you're short.

Woody: Cavities?

Louise: No, it has nothing to do with the fact that you're not bright enough. And it has nothing to do with the fact that your teeth are in bad shape....

Woody: So what, then? What could it possibly be? I don't understand. Has it got to do...? It's not my personality.... Do you have fun with me?

Louise: No, but it's not that. I mean it's not that I don't have fun with you when I'm with you.

Woody: We laugh. Don't tell me that we haven't laughed. 'Cause we laughed a lot.

Louise: Yeah. No, it's not that. It's not that we've laughed or haven't laughed. We've laughed a lot.... I can't put my finger on quite what it is. Something's missing, that's all.

Woody: ...Whatd'ya mean, missing? (Impatiently) Well, what's missing?

Louise: Well, the relationship isn't going anywhere.

Woody: Well, where do you want it to go?

Louise: Well, where could we get it to go?

Woody: Well, that's not.... I don't know.... I LOVE YOU. I mean, what matters is that I love you and you love me.

Louise: And it's not because I don't love you.

Woody: (In excited anticipation) Then you love me?

Louise: No, I don't, but that's not the reason why. Just something is missing....

Woody: (Lost for words and looking perplexed.)

Louise: It's no use.... It's just not going to work out. I'm sorry. Bye. I'm sorry if I hurt you.*

This chapter began with the question: When the foreskin is missing, is the intercourse experience incomplete and unfulfilling, haunting the subconscious mind of both partners?

Woody wrote the above dialogue himself and it says precisely, "Something is missing *from me?*" I believe he sensed that she longed for something fundamental that he just wasn't able to give her. And it was the hidden, unspoken factor leading to her breakup with him. Could the "missing something" be the sexual fulfillment and connectedness that natural intercourse provides? Could they both know this intuitively, yet be unable to verbalize it, leading her to say "something is missing," and him to say "*from* me?" Interestingly, years later, Woody composed a scene in *Shadows and Fog*, wherein a group of mohels (Jewish ritual circumcisers) are deported. Then, in a subsequent movie, *Deconstructing Harry*, he wrote a scene in which his character explains to his son why the boy doesn't have a circumcised penis like his father. Evidently, this issue plays in the inner recesses of Woody's mind, though he is undoubtedly not aware, on a conscious level, of circumcision's devastating effects to the sex act.

* To better appreciate the relevancy of the above dialogue, I recommend renting the movie and replaying the scene over a few times.

3

Making Love Last: The Tie That Binds

> [A]lthough the particular dimension, shape, or peculiarity of the penile end never figures prominently in the complaints of women who apply for divorce—the charges being everything else under the sun—it can safely be assumed that this organ and its condition is the silent unseen, as well as unconscious, power behind...the whole business in a great many cases.
>
> — P. C. Remondino, as quoted in *Sex in Civilization* (1929)

"It's just not going to work out. I'm sorry. Bye. I'm sorry if I hurt you."

The words uttered to end a relationship are among the saddest words you'll ever hear. The hardest to take. They're so unyielding. So final. You listen to them in disbelief. Your heart sinks into your stomach. You suddenly feel weak. Your mind aches.

You awaken the next day—after a fitful sleep—and the words seem to stab your mind again and again... You don't feel like eating. You don't feel like going to work. You can't concentrate. You feel sick. You are. Love sick.

Your life will never be the same. You're sure of it. You really wanted the relationship to work out... Thoughts of the singles scene start drifting through your mind. You don't want to think about it. Instead, you start thinking about the girl who has just broken up with you. You wonder what went wrong. You can't believe she's doing this. You really wanted her to care for you. You've had a couple of spats in the past, but you've always gotten back together within a day or two. Perhaps if you call her, maybe you can still work things out. You reach for the phone. Your heart is pounding. She answers. You try to act like nothing has happened, but she's cold, distant. Suddenly, you blurt out, "Listen, why don't we meet for coffee and talk things over?" She's hesitant... You're squirming... She says it's over. She's sorry. There's nothing to talk about.

It hits you like a ton of bricks. It's over. It's really over.

What happened? What went wrong?

You really liked being with her. You had so much in common. You seemed to have fun together, but somewhere along the way...

You stare out the window, wondering...thinking. The sky is gray. You feel so blue. It feels like rain, but grown men don't cry. You think about something she said a week or two ago. The words linger in your mind. You should have seen it coming. Yeah, you sort of knew it was coming. You're angry, sad, confused, and empty, all at the same time. It hits you over the head again. It's over. She no longer wants you.

So you start to think—maybe it's best that things turned out this way. You'll just forget her. She's just a girl. It's not the end of the world. You'll get over her. You'll get on with your life. You'll meet someone else. Maybe next time it'll be different. Maybe next time things will work out. Maybe next time it'll be the real thing.

Miles away, *she's* thinking... Why didn't things work out? He was such a nice guy. He seemed to really care for her. He was thoughtful and kind. He sent her a dozen roses last Valentine's Day. He was easy to talk to. They shared some good times together.

And yet, something about the relationship just didn't add up. She asks herself: What is it that she wants that he wasn't giving her? Is she being too fussy? Has she been reading too many romantic novels? Are her ideals of the perfect mate unrealistic? Why wasn't the chemistry there? What is this thing called love?

Where is the guy who will fit her like a glove? Her mind is crowded with questions. Questions with no clear answers.

The sky is blue. It should be gray. After all, she's just ended a relationship that could have developed into something. Or could it? She just doesn't know. He seemed to really care for her, but something about their sexual relationship just didn't feel right. It didn't seem to be what lovemaking should be all about—it seemed to be more like *sexmaking*—like they were just satisfying their young, urgent, individual needs instead of being a union of sensuous ecstasy and mutual pleasuring. She can't quite put her finger on it, but something... Even still, maybe she should give him a call—give it another try. Maybe if she really worked at the relationship, perhaps it could work out after all. She heads toward the phone. She ponders. She's confused. Her mind is racing with questions and memories. She sets herself down on the sofa and stares out the window thinking, wondering.

No. She decides it's no use trying to put the torn pieces of their lives back together. She'll just get on with her life. It's not the end of the world. She'll find someone else. Maybe next time—maybe next time it'll be the real thing. She's going to hold out for Mr. Right, and that's all there is to it.

After all, even though more and more of her friends have been settling down, many of them are already having problems. Some of them are already talking divorce, and they haven't even been married that long. She's determined not to let that happen to her. She won't settle for second best. She's going to hold out for Mr. Right—that's it, and that's that. She wants to hear those bells and whistles ring. And she wants them to be in tune.

She sets her mind on the future. Miles away, he too sets his mind on the future, both of them hoping that tomorrow's sunrise will bring a better day.

It's a sad tale. Both end up going their separate ways, though both wanted the relationship to work out. It happens every day across America, thousands of times.

But what if they had gotten back together? What would have happened if the girl had called him back and they had patched things up? Deep down, somewhere in the back of their minds, they would both feel a longing for that missing "something." He would be plagued by feelings of a vague inadequacy because of their previous breakups, and she would have a recurring sense of being unfulfilled.

Sure, they could get back together and work at the relationship. They could commit—get married. They could buy a house in the suburbs with a white-picket fence and get a couple of cats and a tail-wagging dog. They could have sex 2.3 times a week, have a couple of kids, watch TV together in the evening, enroll the kids in karate or dance class, and join the PTA. And yet, peeking out from the back of their minds, from time to time, the haunting thought would return—maybe your mate doesn't truly love you, and maybe you don't *truly* love him.

Why? What's wrong? You've got all the comforts and securities of life. You've got the kids and the house in the suburbs with the white-picket fence. You've got the cats and the tail-wagging dog. Why, then, are the bells and whistles out of tune? What's missing?

The foreskin! That's what's missing.

The foreskin is the magic, secret, sexual ingredient that helps build a deep, lasting love bond between a loving couple—"the tie that binds." Lovemaking with a natural penis sends special biochemical messages to the brain that put a sparkle in a woman's eye, a bounce in a man's step, and gives them both a feeling of mutual loving closeness. Each subsequent lovemaking experience renews this biochemical language of love and restrengthens the love bond. The seasons come...the seasons go...through all your life, your love still grows...

Does this mean that the foreskin is a panacea that can save every relationship from troubles or the tragedy of breaking up? No, I'm not trying to say that the relationship of a couple experiencing natural sex is guaranteed to last a lifetime and that they can't have troubles in their relationship. Nor am I saying that a couple experiencing circumcised sex can't love one another and that their relationship is doomed to failure.

However, great sex can go a long way toward making a relationship more loving, helping it to run more smoothly. If the vast majority of survey respondents are correct in their concurrence that sex with a man with a natural penis is decidedly superior, then a couple experiencing natural intercourse is more likely to have a mutually rewarding sexual relationship, and this increases its chances of lasting a lifetime.

Of course, there is more to a man than just his foreskin, and just because a man has a natural penis doesn't mean that every woman is going to fall, and stay, madly in love with him. We all know that men and women are attracted to each other on several levels—personality, intellect, looks, interests, etc. And yet, beyond those attractions, sexual attraction surely exists. It is the sexual chemistry between two people that puts the frosting on the cake of love.

While it's true that many non-sexual factors are part of a couple's attraction to one another, the importance of sexual compatibility and fulfillment should not be minimized, for this is where our hearts are truly filled with a special kind of joy. And without sexual fulfillment, there is a certain void in the pages of our lives.

When a man and woman become fond of one another, they will naturally want to become sexually intimate. When this happens, intercourse brings the relationship to a higher level of meaningfulness. The ecstasy of delicious natural sex is the foundation upon which an intimate couple builds a mutual sexual admiration for each other. The wonderful sex they experience promotes the development of deep biochemical "love roots," from which blossoms a mutual love bond that may, in many instances, last a lifetime.

Of course, sex isn't everything. There is more to a relationship than the time spent between the sheets. But if it isn't right up there in the top three, maybe it's because the penis is missing its foreskin, causing it to feel and function completely abnormally, which in turn causes the sex act to lose its magical appeal, especially for the woman.

The recent Laumann study in the *Journal of the American Medical Association* found that approximately 1/3 of the 1,500 women studied lacked interest is sex (1). On a similar note, a study conducted by sociologists Cameron and Fleming (2) asked a representative sampling of people of both sexes ranging in age from 18 to 55 to rank in order 22 pleasurable activities on a five-point scale. Among males age 18 to 25, sex shared the number one spot with music. Among females of the same age group, sex ranked fifth, after music, nature, family, and traveling. Among males in the 26 to 29 age category, sex was at the top of their list. Females of the same age group listed sex and their jobs tied for fifth. Jumping to the 40 to 55 age group, sex gets somewhat of a bashing. Males listed it behind family, in joint second place with nature. Females in this group *listed sex 15th*, behind such mundane pleasures as sleeping, attending church, watching TV, and even housework! If this is typical, it means that a middle-aged housewife would rather fire up the vacuum cleaner than have sex. Could their lack of interest in sex be a consequence of the kind of sex these women were getting over the years?

In recent years, the problem of women being unable to orgasm from intercourse has come out of the closet. The famous Hite Report of the mid-70s surveyed over 3,000 women: 70% could not orgasm regularly from intercourse (3) *(70% is also the estimated number of circumcised men in the population at that time)*. Subsequent surveys by women's magazines reveal similar findings. Though percentages can vary, one thing is certain: There is a problem. And because of it, women are "faking it."

In one survey, actress/author Naura Hayden interviewed 486 women. The results were astonishing: 310 (64%) said they faked orgasm *every* time they had intercourse, 124 (25%) said they faked orgasm *most* of the time, and 52 (11%) said they faked orgasm some of the time. Naura says, "On call-in shows I received hundreds of calls from women, women married eight years, 20 years, 35 years, all telling me how they'd been faking it for all the years of their marriage" (4).

Why are all these women unable to achieve orgasm from intercourse and consequently faking it? Could the surgically altered circumcised penis have something to do with this problem?

In this regard, as mentioned, I conducted a survey of women who have had intercourse with both circumcised and uncircumcised men. Many of these women reported that they had considerable *difficulty* achieving vaginal orgasm with *circumcised* men. And yet, these same women had remarkable *success* achieving vaginal orgasm with unaltered men. **Considered as a group, women were nearly 5 times likelier to achieve vaginal orgasm when the man had a natural penis.** (See Appendix E.)

(This book defines *vaginal orgasm* as an orgasm that occurs while the penis is in the vagina, brought about by the partners' genital and pelvic movements and body pressure, with no simultaneous stimulation of the clitoris by hand.)

Why should there be such a difference between the orgasmic response of women having intercourse with unaltered men versus circumcised men? Because the circumcised penis is missing its foreskin—the VIP—Vitally Important Part—causing it to feel and function completely differently from the natural penis.

It is an incontrovertible, yet painful, fact that without a foreskin, a man doesn't have the sexual equipment nature intended. Consequently, he can't do the job "right," according to nature's design. As the facts regarding circumcision come to light, we will surely find that the inability of women to have vaginal orgasms is, to a great extent, directly related to circumcision and its negative impact on the intercourse experience. Indeed, in my mind, faking orgasms and circumcised sex walk hand-in-hand along the stormy, shoreline sands.

As more research into human sexuality is conducted, scientists are discovering that men and women are anatomically and functionally very similar in their sexual makeup and desires. When a man has intercourse, he expects the vagina to bring him to orgasm. Why shouldn't a woman expect the penis, and its accompanying body movements, to bring her to orgasm?

Doesn't it seem logical that the sexual organs of both partners

Doesn't it seem logical that the sexual organs of both partners should *mutually* pleasure each other to orgasm during the entwinement of intercourse? The female orgasm must be part of nature's sexual plan; otherwise, women's sex organs wouldn't be outfitted with orgasmic capabilities. Yet, the inability to climax during intercourse is the second most common sexual complaint of women—behind lack of sexual desire (5).

Women feel the need for vaginal orgasm,* otherwise they wouldn't bother trying to achieve them or to fake them. Let's face it—women *want* vaginal orgasms, and according to the survey's results, women are *having* them—with *unaltered* men. But with circumcised men, women achieve orgasm much less frequently because their sexual excitement is progressively lessened by the scraping action of the penis's unbuffered coronal ridge "hook," as well as other negative factors, which will be discussed in detail, beginning with the next chapter.

When a woman doesn't achieve vaginal orgasm, she may instead fake it, because she doesn't want to upset her partner's ego or have him think that something is sexually wrong with her. Indeed, if she has had sex with several men who have been able to give her 5-15 minutes of thrusting and she finds herself unable to orgasm, she would tend to think that it's *her* fault and not the man's. **She doesn't suspect that his surgically modified penis may really be the cause of the problem.**

---

* Although there is considerable controversy concerning use of the term "vaginal orgasm," I decided to use it despite its controversiality because I wanted a familiar term women could use when discussing this issue among themselves. Coital orgasm was a possible alternative, but it didn't conjure up the intended mental image, and I was concerned that women would feel uncomfortable using this term because it is largely unfamiliar to them. At the same time, since the type of penis and its role in bringing a woman to orgasm were major points of the survey, I did not want to simply use the general term "orgasm" because it could include cunnilingus (orally-induced) orgasms, or orgasms induced by stimulating the clitoris by hand, or some other means of inducing orgasm. I am not contending that one form of orgasm is superior to another, only that a vaginal orgasm, as previously defined, was significantly more achievable by women when the man had a natural penis.

When a woman is unable to have a vaginal orgasm,* it can lower her self-esteem. And even though she feels reassured when she reads the many articles written about the high percentage of women who have the same difficulty, these same articles often indicate that women desire vaginal orgasms and persist in wishing they could have them.

Men, too, indicate that they would like women to be able to orgasm from intercourse, and many men feel they have failed if they can't last long enough to bring a woman to climax. However, when a man is able to give a woman 5-15 minutes of thrusting, he may feel that there is something wrong with *her* if she can't have an orgasm. He doesn't realize that her ability to have an orgasm is impeded because *his* penis has been surgically altered.

I know. It hurts—deeply. It isn't easy for circumcised men to let themselves think that there is something wrong with their penis. It is a devastatingly painful thing to discover and accept. This entire issue is devastatingly painful for everyone involved—for circumcised men and the women married to them.

The "Case of the Missing Foreskin" and the "Case of the Missing Vaginal Orgasm" are not easy topics to bring into the spotlight. But now that the problems caused by circumcision are being brought into the open,** isn't it better to be aware of the problem and to know that there is something you can do to correct your situation? Isn't it better to face up to this situation now, before the two of you possibly end up as a divorce statistic, and you have to start all over again with someone else, only to find out that your new marriage is just more of the same—looking hard into your new lover's eyes, you still see it—that empty surprise.

After overcoming your initial denial and conceding that there is a problem, you will be glad you have finally found the root of

---

* See Appendix A for my suggestions on the best position and technique for achieving vaginal orgasm virtually every time.

** *Men's Health,* July 1998; *Men's Fitness,* September 1999; *Esquire,* January 2000; *GQ,* February 2000; *Hustler,* March 2000, *Penthouse,* June 2001 the problem. You'll begin to feel happy about growing a little "jacket" for your most prized possession. You deserve it, and so does she.

Once you've gotten over your denial, and your subconscious "tells" your conscious mind that something really is missing, it will be a time for grieving. But after a time, you must let yourself get over it, because you *can* restore your foreskin. Everything isn't as bleak as it might now seem, for restoring your foreskin and giving real sexual satisfaction to your female partner, while you, yourself, experience new levels of pleasure beyond your highest expectations, is the best thing that's ever going to happen to you in this lifetime.

To borrow an adage from the '60s, "Today is the first day of the rest of your life." You've got the rest of your life ahead of you and the best part of your sex life is yet to come.

Your new foreskin is going to put a sparkle in your eye and a springtime bounce in your step. You're going to look deep within your wife or lover's eyes and see "we." It's going to give both of you a new sense of self-esteem, and a new sense of sexual fulfillment. Both of you are going to be relieved that you finally got to the bottom of that empty, gnawing feeling—that feeling that something was sexually wrong, that feeling that you don't desire your mate as often as you think you should, or that unexplainable feeling of dissatisfaction, subtle hostility, or even outright anger toward the one you love.

The negative aftereffects of circumcised sex have created an invisible barrier which has prevented America's men and women from perceiving and experiencing our true interrelationship with one another. It has kept us apart, at arm's length, despite our attempts to overcome our differences. It is always between the lines of what we are really trying to say—always in the way of what we really want to be to one another. Circumcision not only separates a man from his foreskin, it separates the sexes by abnormalizing the sex act, and hence the very *making* of love.

But all this is about to change for the better. Soon millions of circumcised men will begin the process of growing "it" back.

And when it's all said and done, the men and women of America will be enriched because of it. The whole white-picket-fence picture will be more in focus. It's a story with a happy ending, but not without some crying along the way.

Up until now, circumcision has been mostly a silent topic, talked about in whispers, or talked about with embarrassment or indifference. But now that sexuality has entered the spotlight, it is sure to become coffee-table conversation and a talk-show topic like no other. For it affects the lives of almost all adult men and women in America and the younger generation just behind.

This discovery by Americans en masse—that the foreskin is a necessary part of our sexuality—is destined to become one of the great burning issues of our time as it lights the twin revolutionary fires of greater sexual quality/equality and greater love between the sexes.

The next wave of the sexual revolution is about to sweep us all off our feet by surprise. Better sex, more satisfying sex, more gratifying sex, is just around the bend. With it will come a new respect for women's sexuality and for women as sexual partners. With it will come a new respect for men's sexuality and for men as sexual partners. With it will come a new respect for America's women in the eyes of men. And with it will come a new respect for America's men in the eyes of women.

4

A Sexual Comparison of the Natural and Circumcised Penis

Nature marches to the rhythm of a drumbeat that she alone hears loud and clear. She hears this rhythm in the fluttering of a moth's wings, flying hundreds of miles to meet its mate. She hears it in the opening of a flower's petals, wishing to bask in the warmth of the sun, and in the closing of those petals when the chilling rain comes. And she hears it in the insistence of the incoming tide, rushing in to kiss the shoreline sands, on a precise timetable with destiny.

She has counted many revolutions
Of the Earth around the sun
Seen millions of daffodil springs come
And watched billions upon billions of autumn leaves fall,
And through it all
She has gained a wisdom
We can only hope to comprehend

Though we may be inclined
To think of her as our foe
When the icy winds of winter
Blow shifting drifts of snow,
Even still,
In the end,

We shall think of her as our friend...
Somewhere down the road...
Just around the bend...
As we unravel her many mysteries
One by one
And gradually blend
Into the harmony of her heartbeat
And the melody that expectantly comes
With the early morning robin
And the rising morning sun
While she dances along in unison
To the rhythm of her drum...

Nature perfected the natural penis over millions of years of evolution. Mankind, on the other hand, "fashioned" the circumcised penis in relatively recent times by removing the foreskin with knives, scissors, and clamps, amidst simultaneous screams and spurts of blood. Who do you think you should trust?

At one time, it was common for doctors to remove the tonsils, adenoids, or both, as a remedy for childhood throat infections. They later came to realize that these organs have a vital bodily function and should only be removed in rare circumstances. This is the situation we now find ourselves in regarding the foreskin. We have been stripping our newly born infant boys of a vital part of their anatomy without understanding the foreskin's sexual functions.

Like the controversy over removing tonsils and adenoids that came before it, the pendulum of the circumcision controversy is about to swing—full swing—in the anti-circumcision direction. When the clouds of controversy have cleared, the new call of the day will be, "Let the foreskin live—and above all, let it make love."

The term "lovemaking" is used so casually these days we seldom stop to consider what it really means—the *making* of love.

As mentioned, scientists are beginning to discover that love has a biochemical basis and that sex induces biochemical and hormonal changes that not only bring on feelings of pleasure and orgasmic satisfaction, but also feelings of love, contentment, closeness, and emotional security.

We can be sure of one thing: When it comes to the sex organs, and the millions of years that these have evolved, nature did not make a mistake. For the sex organs are not only the means by which the species is procreated and perpetuated, but also the means by which the love bond is repeatedly re-cemented—the sex organs are, in effect, the generators of love. And love is an elemental part of the human condition, helping to ensure that a couple stay together and work cooperatively in caring for the offspring of sex—children—during their long period of dependency, thus helping to ensure the survival of the species. It seems a self-evident truth that the sex organs must have been designed perfectly.

It is only logical that natural genitals—the sex organs as designed by nature—are an essential ingredient if the love*making* experience is to take on its rightful dimension. But when the penis is stripped of its foreskin, everything changes—the intercourse experience is abnormalized. Consequently, the lovemaking process—*the making of love through sex*—is, in turn, abnormalized. And this can adversely affect the well-being and emotional health of the relationship.

THE SOFTLY-STIFF NATURAL PENIS HEAD VS. THE ABNORMALLY HARDENED CIRCUMCISED PENIS HEAD

THE SOFTLY-STIFF NATURAL PENIS HEAD

As overviewed in Chapter 2, the glans, or head of the penis, was designed by nature to be an *internal* organ (Figure 4-1). This chapter will expand on this concept and its significance.

Foreskin — **Penis Head (Glans)** — **Frenulum**

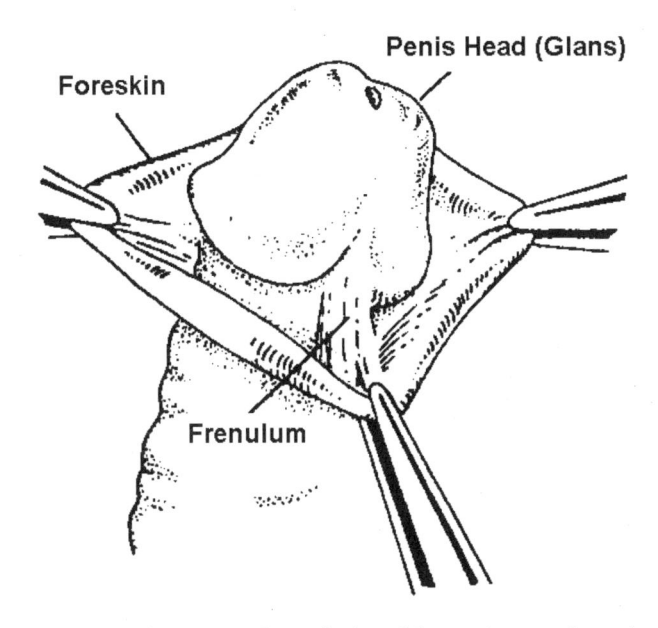

Figure 4-1. The natural penis head is an internal organ.

Just as the tongue is an internal organ of the warm, moist environment of the mouth, similarly, the penis head is designed to rest protected inside the warm (98.6⁰), moist environment of the foreskin.

In addition to the 98.6⁰ warmth provided by the foreskin, the foreskin's inner lining, which is mucous membrane, continually moisturizes the penis head with a lubricating lanolin-like substance that I suggest we call *lanofore.** This constant moisturizing results in a glans which is giveable and somewhat spongy to the touch, even when erect. The *softly-stiff, giveable glans is part of nature's sexual plan and is what nature intended for a woman to experience* during intercourse—it is kind and gentle to the vaginal walls.

The constant warmth and moisture afforded by the foreskin *provides the proper environment for the development and maintenance of the penis head's nerve-endings,* analogous to the way warm, moist soil allows the roots of a plant to thrive.

---

* Smegma is another substance entirely and will be discussed in a later chapter.

Although the foreskin enwraps the glans, the glans itself is covered by only a thin, delicate layer of moist, satin-like skin. (By running your tongue along the inside of your cheek, you will get an idea of the texture of the natural glans.) This thin-layered skin feature is important because during intercourse, it allows the nerve-endings of the penis head to fully feel the sensations of coital thrusting—which in turn play a role in the tenderness and gentleness of its thrusts. This is the kind of penis head the vagina was born to kiss and caress.

THE ABNORMALLY HARDENED CIRCUMCISED PENIS HEAD

In contrast, the head of the circumcised penis is a constantly exposed, *external* organ. As a result, the glans becomes dried out and abnormally hardened due to lack of moisture, analogous to the way a sponge hardens when water evaporates from it.

In order to better appreciate the significance of this to the man, imagine your tongue hanging outside your mouth, all dried out. You may have experienced this occasionally upon awakening. Now imagine your tongue never being able to return to the protective, moist environment of your mouth—constantly exposed, constantly dried out. Then imagine someone rubbing a coarse fabric across your tongue every waking hour. Doesn't sound like a lot of fun, does it? And yet, for a man denied his foreskin due to circumcision, this is what life for his penis head is like, as it is chafed by coarse underwear, bedding, and the man's own wiry pubic hair, day in and day out. The glans of the circumcised man never gets to experience what it is like to live as an internal organ, sheltered inside the moist foreskin. (Like the female vulva stays constantly moist.)

Moreover, the skin on the circumcised penis head becomes abnormally thickened and toughened because of its constant contact with clothing, etc. Continual stimulation caused by this constant contact is bothersome and annoying to the penis head's nerve-endings. Consequently, the body builds excess layers of keratinized (unfeeling, callused) skin (1) over the nerves in order to shield and desensitize them from this unwanted stimulation.

By the time a circumcised male reaches his late teens, the skin on his penis head will be up to 10 layers thick and its nerve-endings (the pleasure sensors) become buried, or smothered, under the excess layers of skin (2)(3). (This is evinced by observing that the glans of the *natural* penis is purplish-red in color because the blood runs closer to the surface, whereas the glans of the circumcised penis is an anemic pale pink, or whitish in the light-skinned person—or a muted, chalky-brown in the dark-skinned person.)

The skin on the circumcised glans is essentially "callused," and its sexual nerve-endings become deadened, dulled, and atrophied for three interrelated reasons—lack of moisture, lack of 98.6^0 warmth, and the frictional action of clothing. The end result is a desensitized glans—a penis head that has lost much (or nearly all) of its sensibility, especially for delicate stimuli.

Even though the circumcised male may have enough feeling in his overall penis to achieve orgasm during intercourse, he is denied the full, true sensual experience of the sex act because his penis head is desensitized.

This deficiency in glans sensitivity is one of the reasons why the man thrusts rougher and tougher in an attempt to elicit more feeling from his penis. Unfortunately, because the man's glans is desensitized, he doesn't realize that his thrusting actions are too rough, causing his partner varying degrees of discomfort, or at the very least, decreasing the woman's pleasure. The following is a comment from a woman who participated in the survey:

> **In general, except for the ones who orgasm quickly, circumcised men seem to work awfully hard to get an orgasm and seem to need a lot more violent thrusting to achieve it. I always thought sex was painful until I had sex with a natural man.**

Also, because the circumcised glans is *abnormally hardened* due to lack of moisturizing, and covered with callused skin, as discussed, its abnormal texture—dense and overly firm—adds to the woman's discomfort as the penis thrusts roughly against the vaginal walls.

Another reason why the circumcised penis feels too hard to a woman is because the penis's tissue, including its head, becomes *abnormally compressed* due to the fact that the circumcised penis is missing 1/3 to 1/2 of its skin, due to removal of the foreskin. (This will be explained in the next section.) The penis head can be so tightly compressed, I'd equate it to an overly hard foreign object repeatedly penetrating the vagina. Totally unlike the softly-stiff caresses of the natural penis head.

The woman who has known only the circumcised intercourse experience becomes accustomed to the abnormally hard penis head and the penis's hard, forceful, even bang-away thrusting style. On the surface, she may even seem to enjoy circumcised sex, because she is driven to it—good or bad—by her innate drive for sexual stimulation. But, in actuality, it is a combination of pleasure and displeasure inextricably entwined. Not knowing any better, she accepts it for what it is and makes the best of it, not consciously realizing that intercourse shouldn't really feel that way. However, on a subconscious level, she is dissatisfied and aggravated by it, and this may ultimately serve to drive a wedge through the heart of the relationship, as discussed.

If you are a circumcised man, reading the above may be emotionally disturbing for a variety of reasons. But keep in mind that foreskin restoration offers a viable solution. After you have "grown" your new foreskin, your penis head will gain more sensitivity as its previously deadened nerves reawaken, which will greatly enhance your pleasure. And because your thrusting will be done with a softly-stiff, giveable, velvety-smooth glans, your partner will experience an intensified pleasure you were incapable of giving her with your circumcised penis. Your sexual strokes will become more gentle; your sex organs will dreamily swoon and "melt" into one another; you won't know where your sex organ ends and your partner's begins because they will feel a sensual connectedness they've never experienced before; she will truly love it, and will love you more because of the sexual pleasure you will be giving her. Here is a survey comment:

> **I realized there was a difference the first time I had sex with a natural man, who is now my husband. I wouldn't have been able to put in words the difference at first, but over time I discovered that sex is smoother, gentler, and more sensual. I orgasm almost effortlessly.**

It may be difficult to believe that the vagina can be affected by the difference between the softly-stiff natural penis head and the harder circumcised penis head, but if you try this simple experiment, I think you will understand how this could be so. Using your index finger, lightly stroke the inside of your cheek about a dozen times. Next, apply finger pressure against the inside of the cheek and stroke it another dozen times. Notice that stroking it with a firm pressure against the cheek creates subtle feelings of discomfort. These feelings of discomfort are similar to the sensations the vagina emits when it is stroked by a penis head that is overly firm. Even though these negative sensations can be overshadowed by the pleasurable sensations the vagina is experiencing, still, they detract from the woman's enjoyment of intercourse, even though she may not consciously realize it.

THE CUSHIONED **SHAFT** OF THE NATURAL PENIS VS. THE ABNORMALLY HARD, NON-CUSHIONED **SHAFT** OF THE CIRCUMCISED PENIS

THE CUSHIONED **SHAFT** OF THE NATURAL PENIS

The previous material focused on the penis head; this section focuses on the penile shaft.

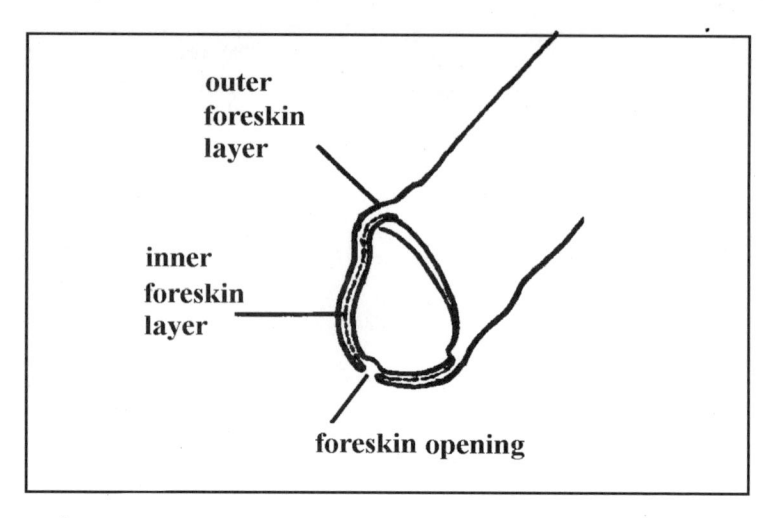

Figure 4-2. Hidden view of the inner and outer foreskin.

The foreskin of the flaccid (not erect) natural penis usually covers the entire penis head, often extending beyond it. The foreskin is actually a double-layered fold of skin having both an inner and outer layer, similar to the lined sleeve of a jacket. The inner layer is highly erogenous mucous membrane, rich in nerve-endings (4)(5). The outer layer is a continuation of the penile shaft skin. (Figure 4-2.)

During erection, the outer layer of the foreskin slips over the penis head, onto the shaft. As erection continues, the inner layer also unfolds onto the shaft, giving the shaft *a third to a half more shaft skin* (6). (See Figure 4-3.)

Notice that the erect natural penile shaft has *both* its original skin *and* the foreskin. This results in a shaft skin that is relatively loose and mobile. The penis *needs* this "extra" skin to stretch into as it advances to erection.

The extra shaft skin afforded by the foreskin is another part of nature's sexual plan, for during intercourse it acts as a thin, spongy cushion on the erect penis shaft (similar to the extra cushioning you would get if you put a thin innersole in your shoe). Moreover, because the shaft has ample skin to accommodate its

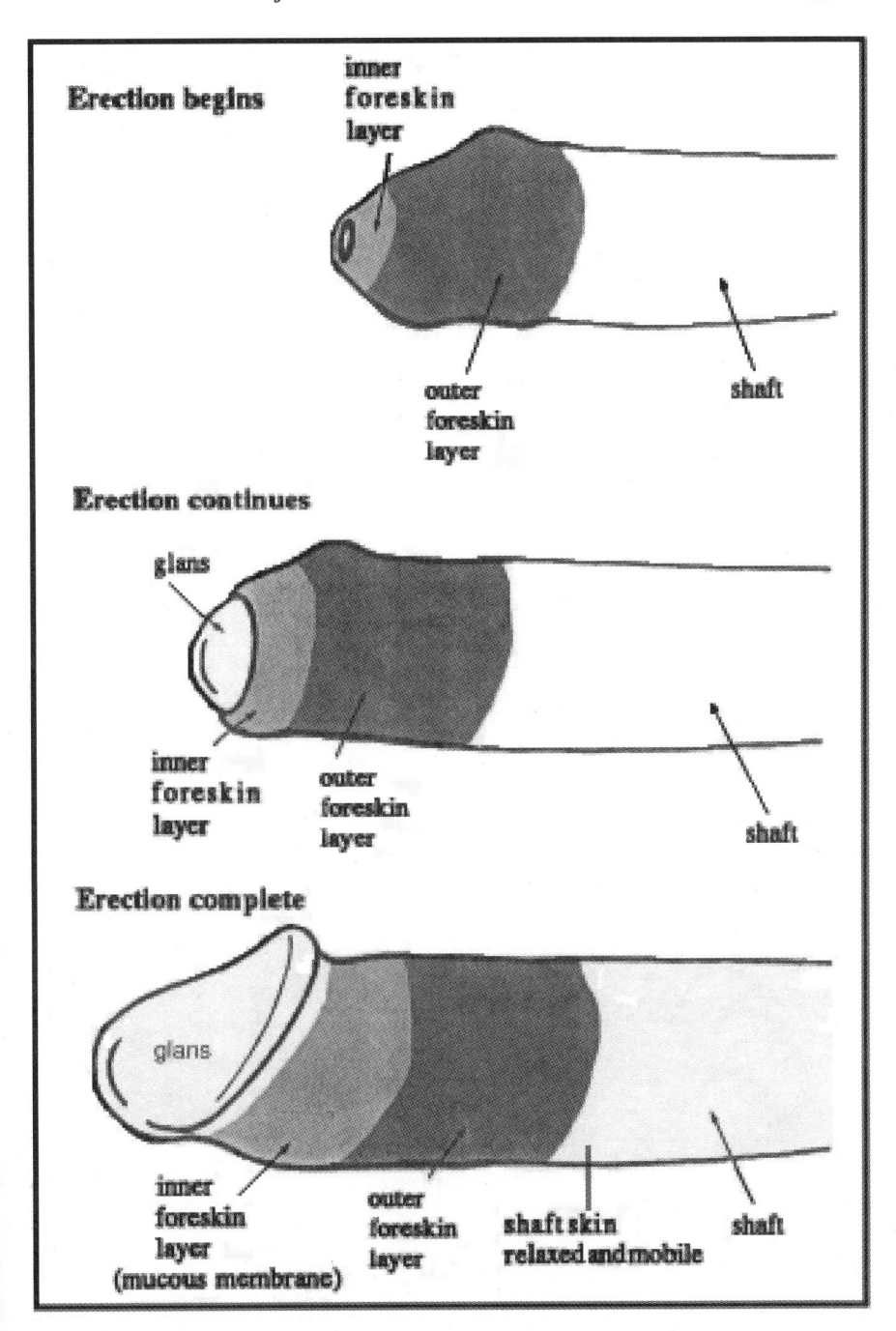

Figure 4-3. Erection process of the natural penis.

erection, *it does not compress the shaft's tissue*, thereby adding to the cushiony giveability of the natural penis.* This cushioned shaft feels delightfully comfortable to a woman's vaginal opening and walls during coital thrusting. This is the kind of penis shaft the vagina was born to love and adore. This is the kind of penis shaft the vagina was born to caress and possess. This is the kind of penis shaft... Excuse me, I have to go see my husband about something...

THE ABNORMALLY HARD, NON-CUSHIONED *SHAFT* OF THE CIRCUMCISED PENIS

The tight-skinned shaft of the circumcised penis is quite different from the cushiony shaft of the natural penis. The circumcised penis may have enough skin when it is flaccid, but upon erection, the shaft skin is forced to stretch itself too thin in order to accommodate the fullness of the erection. Like blowing up a balloon, as more air is forced in, the balloon gets stretched thinner and thinner, and becomes tighter and firmer.

The circumcised erection may feel discomforting, or even painful, to the *male* depending on the tightness of the original circumcision. Many circumcised penises are so tight-skinned that when erect, they are deformed, bowing upward or downward, left or right, whereas the natural penis seems to be more of a straight-out shape.**

During erection, the shaft skin of the circumcised penis is tight, taut, and stretched to the limit, causing it to *abnormally compress* the shaft's tissue, making it feel abnormally hard to a woman during coital thrusting. Women seem to be able to discern this extra hardness, because when women of the survey were asked if

---

* Please do not misinterpret the term "cushiony giveability" (or previously used "softly-stiff") to mean that the natural penis does not have a firm erection. The natural erection is solid and erotic, but not abnormally hard like the circumcised penis (discussed in next section). One woman commented: "...like it's covered with velvet, but firm and solid underneath."

** You can confirm this by looking at several male-oriented "beefcake" magazines at your local newsstand.

the circumcised penis shaft feels discomfortingly hard during intercourse thrusting, an astoundingly high percentage of them agreed that it did.

During intercourse, the abnormally hard, compressed shaft frictionizes the vaginal walls and opening, causing various amounts of discomfort to become intermixed with whatever pleasure the vagina and penis are receiving—"mosquito-bite sex."

As discussed, when you scratch a mosquito bite, it feels pleasurable, but it's discomforting at the same time—it isn't an experience of *pure* pleasure. Similarly, the various negative physiological aspects of circumcised intercourse cause a couple to experience a mixture of pleasure and displeasure simultaneously, instead of pure, unadulterated pleasure. The partners accept these discomforts as a "normal" part of the sexual experience.

CIRCUMCISION REMOVES MORE THAN JUST A LITTLE SNIP OF SKIN

The amputated* skin removed during circumcision may seem small on an infant, but as the baby grows, so does his penis. The tiny foreskin of the infant penis will eventually "grow up" and become the foreskin of the average 6-inch erect adult penis. That "little snip" of skin amputated at an infant's circumcision results in the loss of at least one-third (and according to recent research, more like one-half) of the adult penile shaft skin system (7). *A piece of skin about the size of a 3"x 5" index card* (8). (See Figure 4-4.)

The average adult foreskin is about **2.5 inches long**—from its base (at the coronal ridge), to its tip, and then back again (for the inner layer). The foreskin also surrounds and encloses the average 1.5-inch diameter of the flaccid glans, which computes to approximately **4.7 inches in circumference.**

---

* While some readers may consider the term "amputation" an exaggeration, it is neither inappropriate nor inexact. The American Academy of Pediatrics, itself, defines circumcision as "amputation of the foreskin."

Thus, the skin surface of the average adult foreskin is about 12 square inches (**4.7 x 2.5** = 11.75). *A piece of skin equivalent to the area enclosed in the Circumcision Skin Removal Chart below.*

Circumcision's Skin Removal

**Erect Adult Penis Surface
Skin Area (square inches)**

	Natural Penis	**Circumcised Penis**
Shaft Skin	21	21
Foreskin	<u>12</u>	<u>0</u>
Total Skin	33	21

**Approximate Percentage
Skin Loss in Circumcision**   =   12/33   =   36%

Figure 4-4. Adult penile skin loss due to circumcision. (Source: Thomas J. Ritter, M.D., *Say No To Circumcision*)

The average erect adult penis is 6 inches long, with a shaft of about 4.5 inches and a circumference of about 4.7 inches. The shaft skin of the erect circumcised penis, then, is about 21 square inches (4.5 X 4.7 = 21.15), compared to approximately 33 square inches (21.15 plus 11.75) for the natural penis (9).

It is the loss of this skin that makes the circumcised penis shaft abnormally hard when erect because too much swollen tissue is packed into too small a packaging of skin.

During intercourse, the circumcised penis does not have the cushiony, giveable ride that the natural penis has. Instead, it can feel overly hard and discomforting to both the man and the woman.

In my childhood, my mother and father often had heated arguments. She was clearly dissatisfied with him for several

A Sexual Comparison
of the Natural and Circumcised Penis

reasons and was always saying, "You just wait until these kids grow up, I'll divorce you so fast it'll make your head spin." She eventually did divorce him. However, I was very close to my mother and I know that she really wanted to love my father, but she didn't really like having sex with him (she talked about it quite openly to me). Now that I know what I know, I believe that with good, natural loving, she could have become putty in his hands. Instead, she took out her sexual frustration and resentment in periodic arguing and bickering. It's so sad to watch how love goes bad when it could have grown into a beautiful thing.

During one particular argument (it was long after my bedtime and I'm sure they thought I was asleep), my mother shouted, "I wish I'd never married you. I should have married John. I'd be happy now, instead of being miserable with you." My father growled back, "Oh, sure...John this...John that... You wouldn't have been happy with him." To which my mother yelled back, "Yeah, well at least when I had sex with him, it didn't feel like he was shoving a broomstick in and out of me, like it does with you."

I was about 9 years old at the time, and those words left quite an impression on my young mind. From time to time, in my adolescent years, I would relive that argument in my thoughts, asking myself, what did those words mean? Is that what sex is like? Why did she yell out those ugly words, in such an ugly tone?

In time, I came to understand what her words meant and why the words of a circumcised-marriage argument are surely the cruelest words of all. They come hurling out of the subconscious with one intention—to cut like a knife—it's payback time for all the sexual frustration, displeasurement, and resentment.

As discussed, I contend that the circumcised penis is the underlying cause of many marital arguments (not necessarily just sexually related arguments) because intercourse is frustrating and unfulfilling to both sexual partners, even though they may not be aware of it on a conscious level. With time, these dissatisfactions exert their subtle influence on the everyday relationship and may lead to "circumcised arguments," wherein a couple needle, bicker, or argue about a variety of irrelevant and trifling matters to vent their frustration.

During circumcised intercourse, the abnormal hardness of the penis head and shaft displeasures the woman's vaginal walls and opening. Hard, tough penis pounding away against the soft, delicate vagina, which is frustratingly hungering for something more, something out of reach—something entirely different from what it is experiencing. Something the woman may not be able to identify until she has experienced natural sex as a comparison. Here is what one survey respondent said about discovering the difference:

> **In general, I love sex, but most of my life I've picked 'the wrong kind' of man because a lot of my circumcised intercourse experiences were rough, with him banging and pounding with a penis that felt like hard plastic at times.**
>
> **The one natural man I had was unique. Oh, what a wonderful experience. Often we made love for over an hour, four times longer than my typical circumcised session. Yet all the while, his penis felt so comfortable in me—smooth, pliable, and untroublesome—it seemed to fit me more naturally, like it was better matched to a woman—probably because that's how it was designed.**

As noted, a woman who has experienced only circumcised sex may know that she is in some measure dissatisfied with the experience, but she may not be able to put her finger on exactly what is wrong. She may mistakenly think that the discomforts are just something women normally endure during sex. Or she may blame herself, thinking that she just doesn't like sex that much. But if she were to experience the comfort and sensually soft pleasures of natural intercourse, she would soon realize that the two experiences are distinctly different and would be better able to identify how circumcised intercourse causes her to be discomforted. Here is another woman's comment:

> **With my circumcised partners, just about all the time I had intercourse I experienced discomfort, even pain. I was glad when it was over. Back then, I didn't know it could be any better. But when I finally experienced intercourse with an uncircumcised man, I found out it was more gentle, more enjoyable, and less demanding. I could relax and get into it, once I realized that it wasn't supposed to hurt.**

Earlier in this chapter, we learned that the desensitized penis *head* causes the circumcised man to thrust rougher and tougher. He also thrusts rougher because his *shaft skin system* lacks a vast number of nerve-endings, due to its missing foreskin. If his penile shaft skin system had its full complement of erogenous nerves, and the sensitivity that goes with it, it would "tell" the penis to stroke more gently.

The following is a comment from a survey respondent:

> **A circumcised man's thrusting is harder. I think this is due to the fact that the circumcised penis is less sensitive, so circumcised men push harder to compensate for this lack of sensation.**

Unfortunately, because the circumcised penis lacks the keen-sensitivity awareness of the foreskin, the man does not realize the harshness of his strokes. (Any circumcised man who wants to get an idea of the erogenous sensitivity of the foreskin should run his finger *lightly* over his circumcision scar, which is, in effect, where the would-have-been foreskin joins the penile shaft skin.

Many men are probably not aware that they have a circumcision scar that runs circumferentially around the penis shaft, and is usually noticeably darker in color.)

Because the circumcised penis is missing twelve to fifteen square inches of highly erogenous tissue, during intercourse the man's brain receives only a partial message from the penis—an incomplete message—which, I contend (as explained in Chapter 2), can lead to a sense of frustration. If we were to draw an analogy to music, we would say that the "extra" sensory nerves of the foreskin allow a man to listen to a symphony of stimuli, able to hear all the musical notes and experience the full richness of a live orchestra. But for a man whose penis is circumcised, not having his foreskin causes him to miss many notes and sounds and much of the dynamics of the orchestra. His experience is more like listening to an orchestral symphony on a portable transistor radio that keeps fading in and out. Even though he hears the symphony, it is not the true, full experience the composer intended. Similarly, even though a circumcised man can derive pleasure from intercourse and have an orgasm, still, the sexual center of his brain is denied the true pleasure of intercourse.

Yes, "Requiem for the Departed Foreskin" is a very sad tune to hear, but it must now be listened to so that future generations will not have to hear its mournful sound.

5

The Gliding Mechanism of the Natural Penis

vs.

The Non-gliding Friction Action of the Circumcised Penis

GLIDING MECHANISM OF THE NATURAL PENIS

Upon erection, the foreskin is transferred to the penile shaft and becomes part of the total shaft skin system. This results in a loose, moveable shaft skin that provides the penis with a gentle gliding mechanism. During intercourse, *the natural penis shaft actually glides within its own shaft skin covering. This minimizes friction to the vaginal walls and opening, and to the shaft skin itself,* adding immeasurably to the comfort and pleasure of both partners. In the words of one survey respondent:

> **The foreskin is the best thing God ever invented for us women. It feels so good to have the feeling of the man's foreskin in my vagina...it glides easily. Once a natural penis is in your vagina, you wish it could stay forever. It makes you feel like you're on top of the world. You will only know if you've had sex with a natural man.**

Because of its special gliding function, the foreskin steals the show and plays the leading role during the performance of intercourse—it's the SUPERSTAR of the sexual connection between a man and woman.

The interaction of the foreskin, penis shaft, and vaginal walls is passionate, sexual poetry in motion. The natural penis's coital "glide-ride" gives both partners a thrilling lesson in sensual schooling they shall not soon forget. Ah, the unforgettable foreskin—that's what you are. How I do love thee and your unforgettable ways, daydreaming of you as I do on this delightfully warm Spring day...

...But daydreams must eventually give way to reality, so below is a comparative example, which will help you to understand the foreskin's gliding mechanism. (See Figure 5-1.)

1. Take the first finger of your left hand and hold it in front of you horizontally, as if you were pointing at something to your right, but with your *knuckle skin facing up*.

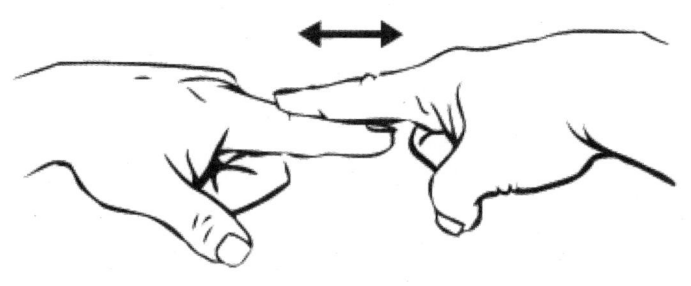

Figure 5-1. Finger simulation of natural intercourse.

2. Next, take the fingertip of your right-hand first finger and place it, flatly, on top of your left-finger's center knuckle. In this example, your left finger represents the penis; its loose knuckle skin represents the extra skin on the natural penis shaft. Your right finger is the vaginal wall, and its fingertip is the vaginal opening.

3. Now move your left finger (penis) forward and backward to the extent your knuckle skin allows. Notice that although the "penis" is moving in and out, it is, however, actually *gliding* on its own skin. Because it is gliding on its extra skin, there is no friction to the "vaginal opening" (right-hand fingertip).

(IMPORTANT: Note also that because the penis shaft is able to move forward and backward within its own skin, the skin itself, relative to its position against the vaginal opening, virtually doesn't move. *This allows the vaginal fluids to remain within the vagina because they are not dragged out with every stroke.*)

In actuality, of course, the adult penis is much bigger and has much more mobile skin. The important point you should gain from the example is that, because of its gliding action, the natural penis is infinitely more kind and gentle to the lower vaginal walls and opening, and the penis's shaft skin as well.

The 2½-inch average foreskin, once extended onto the erect shaft, provides mobility to the *entire* shaft skin system, from the coronal ridge to the penis base; thus the shaft skin can glide easily up and down the shaft. Or, inversely, if the shaft skin were held stationary, *the shaft can easily glide forward and backward inside its own skin.*

Once the penis is in the vagina, the purposeful vaginal-wall wavy-ribbing structure (Figure 5-2) "grasps" the loose skin of the shaft and *virtually holds it in place* while the thrusting penis

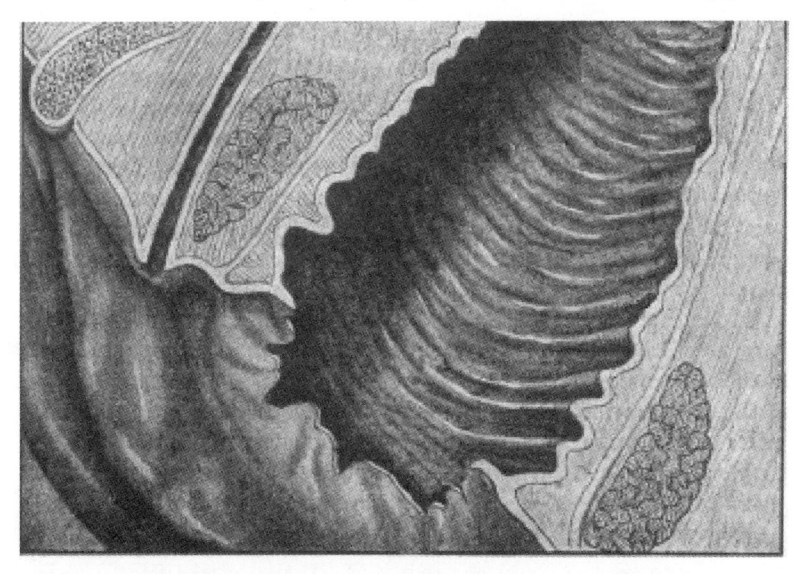

Figure 5-2. Cross-sectional view of the vagina showing the wavy-ribbing structure. (Adapted from *The Illustrated Encyclopedia of Sex* by Drs. Willy, Vander, and Fisher.)

shaft glides within its own shaft skin, thereby minimizing irritating friction. One survey respondent described it clearly and simply in this way:

> **A circumcised penis creates more friction, while with the natural penis, once inside me, the penis skin doesn't seem to move back and forth, only the penis inside the skin slips back and forth and the skin stays pretty much in the same place.**

Friction is not entirely eliminated during natural intercourse but is largely eliminated. Friction can take place in the lower vagina, but only if the man uses a stroke that exceeds the (forward and backward) gliding range of the shaft's extra skin. And in such a case, there will be friction only to the extent that the shaft exceeded its extra skin, which is uncommon, since the natural penis has a propensity for short strokes.

(Primarily, it is the penis head that makes frictional contact with the vaginal walls. But this takes place in the upper vagina where there is ample lubrication. *Importantly, during natural intercourse, lubricating fluids tend to remain inside the vagina, because when the loose shaftskin of the penis bunches up on the outward stroke, it creates a seal that holds fluids in.* This beneficial factor, combined with the giveable, softly-stiff characteristics of the natural penis head, allows it to sensuously caress the vagina rather than rubbing it irritatingly, as does the circumcised. We will learn later that the structure of the circumcised penis works to pump fluids out of the vagina.)

The gliding principle of natural intercourse is a two-way street—the vagina glides on the shaft skin while the shaft skin massages the penis shaft as it glides over it. Since the gliding mechanism is an intrinsic part of natural intercourse, we must assume that the sex organs were designed to experience intercourse in this way. Glide in. Glide out. Glide in. Glide out. Smooth as silk. Sweet, tender, gentle, loving stroking. Poetry in motion.

I would like to emphasize this essential point: When observing the natural penis's stroke during a sexually explicit video, it appears, on casual observation, that the penis shaft is frictionizing as it thrusts in and out, but this is largely an illusion. On closer observation, you will notice that the shaft is actually moving forward and backward within its own skin while the skin stretches on the outward stroke and collapses on the inward thrust.

Here is another comparative example that will demonstrate what happens as the natural penis thrusts (Figure 5-3).

1. Grasp your hand around your forearm about an inch above the wrist bone.

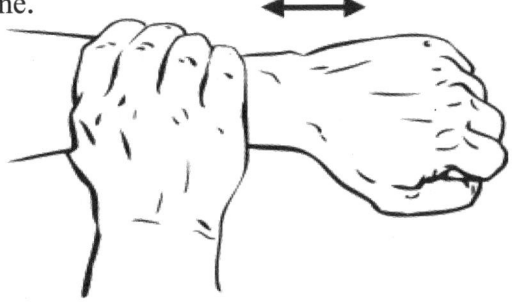

Figure 5-3. Forearm simulation of the foreskin's gliding mechanism

2. Now, move your hand forward and backward several times. As you do, notice that the area above your wrist gets longer and shorter even though there is no frictional movement underneath your hand. It simply happens because the skin is stretching and collapsing.

3. If you imagine that your grasping hand is the vagina and your forearm is the penis, you can easily see that the penis shaft can move in and out of the vagina with minimal friction.

The gliding mechanism is also an important factor during masturbation or foreplay because it allows the penis shaft to be stroked comfortably. During foreplay, when a woman grasps the penis with her hand to stroke the penile shaft, *her hand and the shaft skin move as a unit,* up and down the shaft. The hand does not frictionize the shaft skin because when the hand moves, the mobile shaft skin moves with it, to gently massage the shaft tissue within. When oral sex is performed, the gliding feature allows her to stroke and stimulate the shaft while simultaneously caressing the penis head with her mouth. This doubles the man's pleasure.

THE NON-GLIDING FRICTION ACTION OF THE CIRCUMCISED PENIS

The circumcised erect penis usually has little or no slack skin on its shaft. As a result, it has no gliding mechanism, and during intercourse the tight-skinned penis and the vagina experience an abnormal degree of friction.

Let's go back to our finger comparison for a moment to see how this lack of shaft skin changes the feeling of intercourse (Figure 5-4).

1. Connect your left knuckle skin and right fingertip as in the previous example.

2. Next, turn your bottom finger over so that the undersides of both fingers are touching.

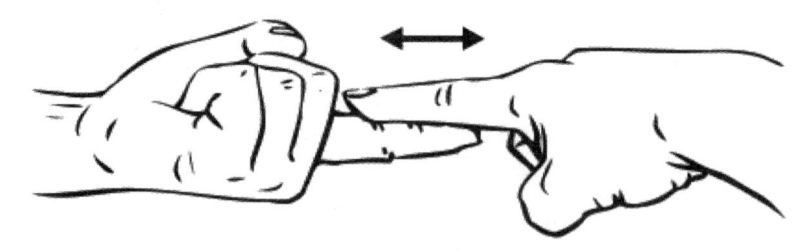

Figure 5-4. Finger simulation of circumcised intercourse.

3. Now *slide* your "penis" finger back and forth 15 or 20 times.

As you do, you will notice frictional discomfort because skin is rubbing against skin. This feeling of skin *sliding* against skin is entirely different from the comfortable *gliding* action you got on your knuckle skin in the previous example.

With circumcised intercourse, there is *constant* friction. The penile shaft continually frictionizes the lower vagina and vaginal opening because there is no foreskin to provide a gliding mechanism. Even the upper vagina is adversely affected because lubrication is reduced. In the upper vagina, where it is normal for friction to take place, *the projecting coronal ridge of the circumcised penis head works like a one-way valve to pump lubrication from the upper vagina into the lower vagina, where the penis shaft drags it out into the open air to evaporate.* Whereas, with natural, as you recall, the bunched-up foreskin creates a seal that works to keep fluids in the upper vagina.

Also, no slack skin is a problem during circumcised foreplay or oral sex because it is difficult to stroke the penis shaft without pulling on the skin too tightly. The hand cannot glide freely up and down the shaft; *instead, it frictionizes it.* Using an artificial lubricant can help, but stopping to apply a lubricant detracts from the spontaneity of sex, and once it has been applied, one usually wants to avoid mouth contact. The problems created by the lack of a gliding mechanism are very well expressed by the following survey comment:

> **I could never figure out the technique of touching a circumcised man. I recently found out the key was to keep a jar of massage oil by the bed. The man who I was with suggested this to me and asked me to keep his penis oiled. With the bottle of oil present, we could share more, but it seemed weird and unnatural. I felt it got in the way...because I had to keep this oil bottle in one hand while we explored together.... It doesn't make sense that a circumcised guy has to be kept oiled just to keep him turned on.**

The constant friction of circumcised sex causes the skin of the vaginal opening (and the penis shaft skin) to abnormally heat up. As the skin heats up, so does the vagina's lubrication, causing the already diminished vaginal fluid to thin out and lose its lubricating usefulness.

Perhaps the following analogy will help to bring the point home more clearly: Suppose you have a car whose crankcase holds four quarts of oil. Suppose the engine starts to burn oil. Soon the crankcase will be down one quart, then two. At this point, there is not only inadequate lubrication, but the engine oil will change in density and become "thinned out" because of added friction heat. The engine may still run with inadequate, thinned out, overheated lubrication, but it's not good for it to do so. If the engine could talk, it might cuss you out to alert you to its discomfort. But, instead, it's polite and just lights up the dashboard warning light.

During coital thrusting, the constant friction and diminished lubrication of circumcised sex interferes with the sexual pleasure of both partners, whether they are consciously aware of it or not, and may cause either or both partners to become increasingly discomforted as intercourse progresses. In contrast, the gliding feature of the natural penis minimizes friction and conserves vaginal fluids, thereby maximizing both partners' pleasure.

Many survey respondents made comments similar to this woman's:

> **Circumcised intercourse feels like a friction burn. With the natural penis, the extra skin makes it go smoother...my vagina doesn't get sore.**

When abnormal amounts of friction are combined with the circumcised penis's abnormally hard texture and its characteristic rougher, tougher thrusts, the intercourse experience is completely abnormalized for both partners. Though each partner tries to make the best of the situation and does experience some degree of pleasure, still, if they really think about it, there is something about the constant frictionizing and the roughness and toughness of circumcised thrusting that doesn't quite make sense. One woman had this comment:

> **With the circumcised penis, the vaginal tissues can get rubbed raw and sore from abrasion, painfully so. But with a natural penis, there is no abrasion—intercourse is much more comfortable and sexually stimulating.**

Lovemaking should feel tender and gentle. Yet the circumcised couple experiences hard sex, rough sex, tough sex, as the penis shaft frictionizes itself against the vaginal walls and opening. Friction in. Friction out. In. Out. In. Out. In. Out. The vagina begins to feel assaulted and becomes tenser and tenser. Friction in. Friction out. In. Out. In. Out. In. Out. "Finish already—this is beginning to hurt."

Here are some comments from surveyed women:

> "The circumcised penis often leaves me feeling chafed on the inside."

> "Sometimes, too often, I got sore after circumcised sex. It felt like my insides were all moving.... Yes, sometimes I would classify it as pain."

> "Rubbing, in an absence of moisture, that leaves you sore is a real problem with circumcised penises."

> "I had one lover who was into setting a Guinness record, and after 30 minutes I would start to feel as if he were sandpapering me down there" (1).

In my own personal experience, the vagina involuntarily reacts to this abnormalized sex by tensing and tightening up, thereby compounding the friction problem. As I look back, I always remember circumcised sex as discomforting, even though I derived pleasure from it and was able to achieve orgasm. In my 20s and 30s, the discomfort was minimal, yet still annoying. But by my 40s, it caused me to develop *vaginismus*—a condition where the vagina tightens up so much it makes intercourse painful or virtually impossible. Fortunately, my vaginismus was cured after my husband became restored. Sex is now completely enjoyable with no discomfort whatsoever. (I discuss vaginismus and its relationship to circumcised intercourse in Chapter 11.)

A woman who has experienced only circumcised sex may not realize that her vagina is abnormally tensed and tightened. Only after she has experienced the relaxed vagina of natural sex will she realize the true extent of vaginal tenseness during circumcised intercourse.*

I believe that the abnormalities of circumcised sex can ultimately cause a woman to produce less sexual fluid as she ages, which augments friction irritation. It is well known that many women produce less vaginal fluid as they age, but this may be due to more than just the biological changes that come with aging—the abnormalities of circumcised sex may be a contributing factor. With the passage of time and repeated sexual encounters, the woman's brain increasingly associates sex with the displeasures and dissatisfactions she experiences. This in turn reduces her anticipatory sexual excitement and passion for sexual activity; hence, she produces less vaginal fluids.

Young women may or may not understand the concept of vaginal-dryness discomfort. They may be able to produce copious amounts of lubrication despite the fact that it gets exposed to evaporation with every outward stroke. But as these women repeat the circumcised intercourse experience again and again,

---

* Importantly, it may take several sessions with the natural or restored penis before the vagina truly learns to relax. In effect, it takes time for the vagina to "unlearn" the tensing and tightening reflex actuated with the circumcised penis. Still, I think a woman should be able to notice some degree of vaginal relaxation right away.

I contend that over time its abnormalities will condition a response where they get only minimally aroused, producing minimal amounts of lubrication.

In order to overcome a lack of vaginal lubrication, many couples may resort to using synthetic substitutes such as K-Y Jelly. But the need for man-made lubricants should be largely thought of as a man-devised reparation to compensate for a man-made problem—the friction action of circumcised intercourse—which shouldn't exist in the first place. Admittedly, artificial lubrication may be needed in certain situations, but I suspect that its use will decline considerably once circumcision is a thing of the past.

The dried-out-vagina syndrome of circumcised sex is not a comfortable topic to talk about. However, it must now be discussed so that circumcision can be brought to a halt, and future generations will have the freedom to enjoy one of nature's greatest gifts to mankind—the pure, nominally-frictional, gliding action of natural intercourse.

Yet remember, *today's* generation is not totally lost and abandoned, because foreskin restoration offers a real solution. In the words of my restored husband, "Restoring your foreskin is the best thing that's going to happen to you in this lifetime."

With The Foreskin Restoration Revolution in mind, then, let us proceed to the next chapter where we will learn the solution to a puzzling anatomical riddle—why nature designed the penis head to flare out in a "hook-like" projection, and why its presence is proof that nature fully intended the foreskin to play a pivotal role in a couple's mutual pleasuring of one another during the act of lovemaking.

6

A Further Sexual Comparison of the Natural and Circumcised Penis

The following is an excerpt from a letter written to Dr. Lawrence E. Lamb, whose syndicated column on health and medical advice appeared in many newspapers around the United States in the 1970s.

> Dear Dr. Lamb: I am pregnant...if the baby is a boy, my husband and my doctor both want to circumcise him. My mother says...a man needs the foreskin for slack during sex. Furthermore, [she says] a man will lose most of his sensitivity and he needs the protection [of a foreskin].

Below is an excerpt from Dr. Lamb's reply:

> Whether a man is a good lover or not usually is unrelated to the presence or absence of the foreskin. Men who retain their foreskin have just as much sexual enjoyment as men who do not have one. The factors that influence sexual activity are far more complex than merely the presence or absence of a little piece of skin. During the sex act, even in a man who is not circumcised, the foreskin normally retracts in back of the head of the erected penis. There really isn't much to the thought that a man needs this extra skin for slack.... Considering the mechanisms of the female sexual response, it is *inconceivable* that it really makes any difference to a woman during the sex act whether or not her husband has been circumcised...(1). (Emphasis added)

Dr. Lamb's response is probably typical of the attitude and opinion of most American doctors, most of whom are circumcised themselves, and thus have no personal familiarity with the foreskin's possible importance. As the information detailed herein indicates, this opinion is both ill-conceived and naive.

THE CUSHIONED CORONAL RIDGE OF THE NATURAL PENIS VS. THE CORONAL RIDGE "HOOK" OF THE CIRCUMCISED PENIS

The most easy to understand sexual difference between the natural and circumcised penis is what I call "*the hook*," which was briefly overviewed in Chapter 2. This chapter will delve into this concept and its importance with considerable new information.

As you will notice from re-examining Figure 2-1 (see page 26), the penis head projects out from the shaft. This projection, where the penis shaft flares out to the rim of the corona, is referred to by some as the sulcus. Sexual researchers Masters and Johnson, and others, have used the term "coronal ridge." *Dorland's Medical Dictionary* defines a ridge as "a projection or projecting structure." I consider "ridge" more descriptive, so I will refer to this area as the *coronal ridge*. On close observation of aforementioned Figure 2-1, you will notice that the coronal ridge is hook-like (barb-like) in appearance. This "hook-head" feature is conspicuous on both the erect natural and erect circumcised penis.

Since both types of penile heads look the same upon erection, how then could they feel different to a woman during intercourse? The reasons are as follows.

THE SUPERIOR RESILIENCY OF THE NATURAL GLANS ALLOWS THE CORONAL RIDGE TO BEND AND FLEX DURING INTERCOURSE

Earlier we learned that the tissue of the natural penis head has a spongy giveability, even when erect, due to moisturizing, whereas the circumcised head is considerably harder. Using a simple analogy, I would characterize the erect natural glans as having the resiliency somewhat like Jell-O or bubble-pack, *firm yet giveable*, whereas the erect circumcised glans has virtually no resiliency, like an unripe tomato—overly firm and compacted.

The giveability feature of the natural glans allows it, and its coronal ridge, to bend and flex as the penis thrusts the vagina. I must emphasize how essential this is to a woman's comfort—and pleasure—during intercourse. We will find out later in the chapter why the circumcised glans lacks this flexibility feature.

THE BUNCHING-UP, CUSHIONING ACTION OF THE FORESKIN

The comfort the natural penis head provides is further enhanced by the shaft's abundant skin system, which interacts with the vagina to cushion the force of the coronal ridge during intercourse.

The vaginal walls are structured with wavy ribbings (2) (see Figure 5-2, page 71) that have a one-way action, which allows the penile shaft (and its mobile skin covering) to move into the vagina easily on the *forward* thrust. But, when the shaft of the penis moves backwards on the *outward* stroke, its flexible skin covering is "grasped" by the wavy ribbings and virtually held in place. As the penis head moves backwards, the projecting coronal ridge "plows" against the constrained shaft skin (foreskin) and collapses it into a bunch, buffering and cushioning "the hook's" impact on the vaginal walls. (See Figure 6-1.)

Figure 6-1 (below). The bunching-up action of the foreskin. (Adapted from Berkeley) (3).

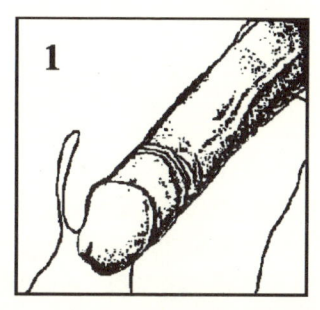

1. The penis is fully inserted in the vagina.

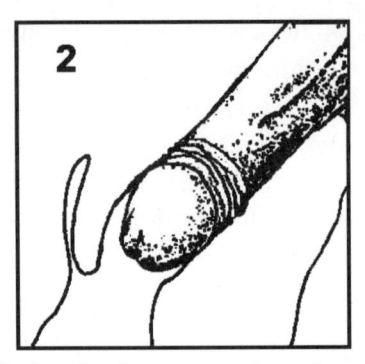

2. The penis begins its outward motion.

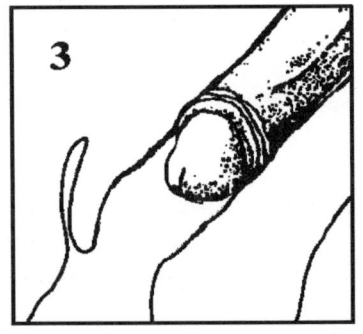

3. The penis continues its outward motion and as it does, the shaft skin is virtually held in place by the wavy ribbings of the vaginal walls, which are designed to grip only on the outstroke. Because the penis head is in motion, the foreskin bunches up behind the protruding coronal ridge.

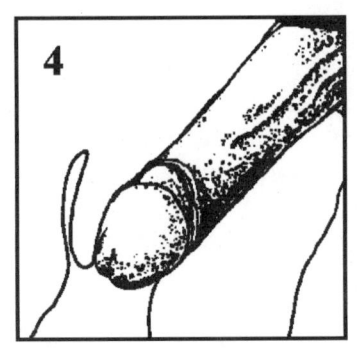

4. During the next inward thrust, the vaginal ribbings relax their one-way grip and the forward movement of the penis causes the foreskin to unbunch.

The action of the vaginal-wall ribbings works similarly to the fur on a cat. If you stroke a cat in the same direction as the fur lays, your hand will slide smoothly. But if you stroke the cat in the opposite direction, the fur grain will impede your hand. In much the same way, the vaginal-wall ribbings let the penis's mobile shaft skin move smoothly into the vagina on the inward thrust but impede its withdrawal on the outward stroke.

In the process of bunching up, the foreskin may sometimes slide over the coronal ridge, onto the head, but even when this happens, the vaginal walls are protected from the coronal ridge hook because the foreskin buffers it.

THE BUNCHING AND UNBUNCHING FEATURE HAS OTHER SEXUAL BENEFITS

As beneficial as the bunched-up foreskin is in cushioning the coronal ridge to make intercourse more comfortable, it seems that its real purpose is to pleasure and sexually excite both the penis and the vagina. Some survey respondents commented on this:

> **"I believe the shaft skin of the natural male has more mobility. I found that I could 'move' the skin on the natural penis shaft with my vagina and enhance our mutual pleasure. But with the circumcised penis, this was not possible."**

> **"During intercourse, the natural man has sensually softer sexual movements...which I attribute to the man getting more pleasure because of the stimulation from the foreskin's movement back and forth."**

Author's note: These women's comments might seem confusing, unless you understand an essential point mentioned earlier: The vaginal walls hold the shaft skin virtually in place, and from the vaginal walls' perspective, the foreskin virtually does not move. However, from the perspective of the penis shaft (which is constantly moving inside its own shaft skin), the foreskin does move up and down. Our perception of the foreskin's movement is influenced by our observations during foreplay where the shaft is stationary and the hand moves the shaft skin up and down over the shaft. But during intercourse, it is the shaft skin that stays virtually stationary, while the shaft moves like a piston, back and forth, inside its own skin.

THE BUNCHING AND UNBUNCHING FEATURE ENHANCES A MAN'S PLEASURE BY EXCITING THE NERVES OF THE FORESKIN'S INNER LINING

One of the ways the foreskin's bunching-up action increases pleasure for the penis is by alternately covering and uncovering the erogenous nerves of the foreskin's inner lining (and frenulum).

As you will recall, the foreskin is comprised of both an inner and outer layer, similar to the lined sleeve of a jacket. The foreskin's inner lining becomes exposed only upon erection, when it unfurls onto the upper shaft, allowing it to make direct contact with the vaginal walls. This inner-lining tissue (and frenulum) abounds with nerves that are highly responsive to touch and are easily excited sexually. These nerves are so exquisitely sensitive that continuous touch is too much stimulation for them. The foreskin's bunching-up action allows them to receive touch sensations *alternated with a period of rest*, rather than constant, continuous stimulation.

On the inward thrust, while the foreskin is in the process of unbunching, it gradually uncovers the supersensitive nerves of the inner lining (and frenulum), allowing them to be titillated by the vagina's loving caresses.

During the outward stroke, as the foreskin bunches up, it rolls over and covers most, or all, of the (frenulum and) inner-lining nerves, allowing them to rest from stimulation.

A brief rest period is important to a nerve because it allows it to recharge itself so that, on the next stimulation, it can again fire off a new sensation of pleasure. That's why wine tasters rest their taste buds in between sips, so they can better experience the next sensation of taste. Similarly, resting the nerves of the inner lining (and frenulum) allows them to recharge so that when they are uncovered on the next inward thrust and are re-exposed to the vagina's caresses, they can fire off new sparks of pleasure. Think of the bunching and unbunching of the foreskin as nature's way of enabling these nerves to sip on the vagina's sweet caresses. (This rest/recharge concept is explained more fully in Chapter 8A.)

THE FORESKIN'S BUNCHING AND UNBUNCHING ENHANCES A MAN'S PLEASURE BY EXCITING PRESSURE-SENSITIVE NERVES

Another way the foreskin's bunching-up action excites the penis is by *applying pressure* to nerves that are embedded within the coronal ridge area. These interior nerves are erotically turned on by the pressuring action of the bunched-up foreskin, as explained below.

In the nervous system, nerves have specialized sensory functions—some register taste sensations, others smell sensations, and others touch sensations. Touch-sensitive nerves are further specialized into distinct varieties programmed to respond only to certain kinds of tactile stimuli. For example, some nerves pick up only the feeling of light touch, as do those located on your ear lobe. Others register temperature sensations, as when you touch a hot stove or dip your toe into the cold ocean. Others respond only to pressure, like the sensations you feel when your lover massages your body. Similarly, the coronal ridge's inner-tissue nerves are sexually excited by pressure. When pressure is applied and then released, *alternately*, they not only become excited, they become ecstatic.

If you are a man, you can test this pressure sensitivity concept on yourself. Place your hand around the upper shaft of your erect penis. With your thumb on the coronal ridge, press down with moderate pressure. You will feel a sensation of pleasure. Now release the pressure for a couple of seconds and press down again briefly, then release again briefly (during the release period, the nerves recharge so they can fire off anew). Do this press/release experiment for about a minute and notice that it causes you to get sexually excited. It is through this principle of *alternately* applying and releasing pressure that the foreskin's bunching-up action works to heighten the male's sexual pleasure.

Here is what happens during intercourse: On the outward stroke, the bunched-up foreskin applies pressure to the pressure-responsive nerves embedded within the tissue of the coronal ridge area. On the inward thrust, the foreskin unbunches and pressure is released. This alternation of pressure/release in the coronal ridge area is one of the many reasons why intercourse is more pleasurable for the unaltered man than for the circumcised man. Here is a survey comment:

> **What I noticed was that my natural man got a lot of pleasure from deliberate slow insertion and backing out because his foreskin would fold back and forth, which would excite me also.**

THE BUNCHING AND UNBUNCHING FEATURE ENHANCES THE WOMAN'S PLEASURE, TOO

The alternating pressure/release feature of the bunched-up foreskin also works to increase a woman's sexual pleasure and is one of the many reasons why natural intercourse feels better to her.

Located behind the vaginal walls are essentially the same erogenous pressure-responsive nerves as the coronal ridge's inner tissue (4). Each time the foreskin bunches up, it increases the diameter of the penis significantly enough to apply pressure to the pressure-sensitive nerves located behind the vaginal walls (5). When the foreskin smoothes out on the next inward thrust, pressure is released. When it bunches up again on the outward stroke, pressure is reapplied. Each time the foreskin bunches up, the pressure-sensitive nerves behind the vaginal walls emit sensations of pleasure. Below are two comments. The first is from a survey respondent; the second is from a man who wrote in to a men's magazine:

> "**Natural penis is softer, more pliable.... The foreskin bunched up toward the vaginal opening is great.**"

> "**I finally got my foreskin restoration, and none too soon...my wife of twenty-five years is happier and we respond to each other like youngsters.... By the way, there is a little trick I learned in intercourse.... If I hold her tightly when I am inside her, I can feel my cap [glans] going in and out of the foreskin. She likes the feeling of the shaft sliding in its foreskin case against her vaginal walls.... I can tell you that my modified tool has brought a new dimension to her interest in me.**" [signed] **Old Dog with New Tricks (6)**

In summary, a woman receives special pleasuring with every erotic stroke of the natural penis. Its softly-stiff, spongy head gently caresses the vaginal walls, and the foreskin provides ample, supple shaft skin to cushion the thrusting coronal ridge hook. Meanwhile, the vagina's pressure-sensitive nerves are also pressure-pleasured by the changing diameter of the magical FUNskin as it rhythmically bunches and unbunches.

THE CIRCUMCISED PENIS LACKS THE FORESKIN'S CUSHIONING ACTIONS

In contrast, the circumcised penis lacks the cushioning action of the bunched-up foreskin, and, on every outward stroke, its coronal ridge acts to scrape the delicate lining of the vaginal walls.* One woman commented that her partner's circumcised penis made her feel like she was being "fucked by a doorknob." Moreover, the coronal ridge is additionally discomforting to a woman because the circumcised glans is abnormally hardened, as discussed. And there is yet another reason why the glans and its coronal ridge are too hard.

THE CIRCUMCISED PENIS HEAD IS ABNORMALLY HARD BECAUSE ITS TISSUE IS TOO COMPACTED

Circumcision may cut away so much penile skin that *upon erection, the skin of the shaft gets stretched so tightly it pulls down on the skin covering the glans. This causes the tissue of the glans to become compacted, thereby making the penis head, and its coronal ridge, overly firm, with little or no flexibility.* As a result, when the abnormally hardened coronal ridge makes contact with the vaginal walls and scrapes, scrapes, and scrapes again with every outward stroke, it can feel increasingly discomforting to the woman. Here are two survey comments:

> **"With the circumcised penis, I feel the...hard, tight shaft, and the glans,** *specifically the rim of the glans,* **is felt thrusting in/out." (Emphasis added)**

---

* There is some speculation that circumcision may cause the corona of the glans to become abnormally flared, thereby deepening the coronal ridge hook. Close observation of photos in various male-oriented "beefcake" magazines seems to bear this out. This, unfortunately, is not a situation where more is better, because the extra flare-out may cause additional discomfort to a woman during coital thrusting. Conversely, the *natural* penis may have less flare-out at the corona, which could be related to its constant covering by the foreskin, which somehow "tells" the corona (perhaps by the pressure of its elasticity) not to excessively flare out.

> "I have found sex with circumcised men to be rough, hard, and *abrasive*.... I found sex with natural men to be much more soft and gentle. I love the feeling of a foreskin sliding inside me." **(Emphasis added)**

However, every woman may not be able to actually discern definitively that her vagina is being scraped because the vaginal nerves are primarily pressure-sensitive (and only minimally touch-sensitive). In my own personal experience, I was simply aware that the thrusting penis was vaguely discomforting and that I experienced considerable discomfort after intercourse. It wasn't until I analyzed the structure of the penis that it dawned on me that the discomfort I was experiencing was due to the scraping action of the coronal ridge.

Sometimes, as mentioned, the pleasurable sensations of intercourse can be so overwhelming, a woman doesn't consciously realize she is being simultaneously displeasured. One time, a friend of mine came to work and said, "Joe and I sure had a good time last night, but boy, am I sore this morning." We must assume that since she experienced soreness the next morning, she must have been discomforted during the act; she just wasn't consciously aware of it because the pleasurable aspects overrode the discomfort (or she may have noticed some discomfort, but she ignored it and concentrated instead on the pleasure). Also, I theorize there might be another explanation, as follows.

IF CIRCUMCISED SEX IS SO DISCOMFORTING, HOW ARE WOMEN ABLE TO PUT UP WITH IT?

I theorize that the hook-scraping aspect of circumcised intercourse (along with excessive friction from the penis shaft) causes the vagina to send distress signals to the brain. In response, the woman's brain "orders" pain-relieving anesthetizing substances (endorphins) to be released to help desensitize the vagina from the discomfort it is receiving. These anesthetizers have a numbing effect, analogous to the Novocain you receive when you go to the dentist, but not, of course, so overpoweringly numbing as Novocain. The following information may help to explain how I arrived at the above conclusion:

> Eating hot chili peppers...can actually induce the brain to produce a rush of endorphins...according to researchers at the University of Pennsylvania. Scientists theorize that when you eat hot chilies, the capsaicin 'burns' the nerve endings of the tongue and mouth, causing them to send...pain signals to the brain. In response, the brain secretes endorphins, natural painkillers.... Another bite of pepper incites further release of endorphins, and so on (7).

In much the same way, the various discomforts of circumcised intercourse cause the brain to respond with pain-relieving endorphins. As a result, the vagina isn't completely aware of how much displeasure it is receiving during the nitty-gritty of circumcised sex because the endorphins' effects alleviate some of the vagina's discomfort. But at the same time, the positive pleasure sensors are also anesthetized, decreasing the woman's arousal capabilities.

I would like to emphasize that these anesthetizers are *pain-reducing, not painkilling*. A woman may still experience discomfort, but it is reduced, *not eliminated*. Still, it allows her vagina to accept greater amounts of abuse without her being completely aware of how much abuse she is actually receiving. Paradoxically, she may notice that she feels greater amounts of discomfort, even pain, *after* intercourse (or the next day) when the endorphin effect has worn off.

A woman may or may not perceive circumcised thrusting as discomforting in the first 2-3 minutes, but as intercourse progresses, the discomfort and displeasure of the coronal ridge hook, and the accompanying release of desensitizing endorphins, *lessen her sexual excitement* and hamper her ability to achieve vaginal orgasm.

Even if she is able to achieve vaginal orgasm, its buildup is accompanied by various degrees of frustration. It requires intense concentration to block out the discomfort and distress the vagina is experiencing, while simultaneously focusing on building up whatever pleasure she is deriving.

Or perhaps she may not be able to achieve an orgasm at all—and is it any wonder that she can't? For during the entire experience, the vagina is essentially traumatized by the frictional thrusts of the tight-skinned shaft, along with the scraping action of the coronal ridge. Indeed, she may end up faking orgasm just to get the session over with. When she doesn't climax, or doesn't fake it, the male usually ejaculates anyway, signaling the end of the session.

Hopefully, he gave her an oral or hand-induced orgasm before his orgasm, because he's not about to start giving her any form of sexual stimulation now. At this point, all he wants to do is roll over and go to sleep.

Meanwhile, the woman's brain stores up memories of the entire experience. Repeated exposures store additional negative memories. I believe these memories of displeasure and frustration ultimately lessen a woman's desire for her sexual partner. As one survey respondent put it, **"It's hard to 'get into something' if you know ahead of time that it's going to be rough and not that enjoyable—just like it's always been."**

CIRCUMCISED SEX MAY CAUSE THE VAGINA TO ABNORMALLY TENSE UP AND DECREASE ITS LUBRICATION

The negativities of circumcised sex, especially the scraping hook of the penis, cause the vagina to abnormally tense up—something like a boxer tenses his stomach in anticipation of a blow from his opponent. In this tensed-up condition, *the vagina does not have the loving softness it would have if it were receiving the cushioned, softly-stiff caresses of the natural penis.*

Several survey respondents noticed this. Here are two representative comments:

> "With circumcised men, my vaginal muscles tighten up. With natural men, my vaginal opening is much more relaxed and accepting of the penis."

> "I have noticed that the vagina is much more accepting of the natural penis. Once the head of the natural penis is at the opening of the vagina, it just kind of naturally slides in.... I notice that the vagina gets softer during intercourse."

In addition to the involuntarily tensed-up condition of the vagina, I theorize that in the process vaginal lubrication is decreased. It's as if the vagina were saying, "Look, I don't really like this all that much—well, I like it—I mean, I *want* to like it—but at the same time, it's somewhat annoying, irritating, and displeasurable. I think I'll stop the flow of lubrication to send a message that I want to bring this session to an end." As vaginal lubrication decreases, friction will increasingly build up. So what do we do? We grease up the circumcised penis with an artificial lubricant.

Here are two comments from the survey on this subject.

> "With circumcised intercourse, I dried out and suffered from post-intercourse irritation and soreness. I do NOT like lengthy intercourse with a circumcised man! During natural intercourse I don't get sore—there is no friction against me."

> "With my circumcised husband, initial insertion is dry and rough (unless we use artificial lubricants).... With prolonged intercourse, I get dry and painful.... Originally, I lost my virginity to a natural man ...dryness was never a problem."

THE CORONAL RIDGE HOOK MAY DISCOMFORT THE MALE

The projecting coronal ridge can also cause discomfort for the circumcised male, because with every inward and outward stroke, this non-resilient tissue is dragged and scraped against the wavy ribbings of the tensed-up vaginal walls. As a result, he may notice that this area is sore or irritated during, immediately after, or the day after sex. This is because the corona/coronal ridge area does not bend and flex as it should, and also because it is not buffered by the foreskin. In effect, the coronal area gets chafed during intercourse (assuming intercourse lasts long enough for irritation to develop).

The constant dragging of this hardened, projecting tissue applies too much continuous direct stimulation to this area. The application of *continuous* direct pressure to nerves isn't as sexually satisfying as alternately applied pressure, and it may even be discomforting or painful.

To prove this, males can try another experiment. With your hand on your erect penis as before, use your thumb again to press down on the coronal ridge area, but this time *hold the pressure; don't release it*. Notice, when you do, that initially you get a sensation of pleasure, but as you hold the pressure continuously, the feeling starts to turn into a discomforting sensation. Release and try it again. Hold the pressure. Feel the discomfort? Constant pressure and overstimulation is what the upper area of the circumcised penis is subjected to during intercourse. (In contrast, alternating pressure, which you experienced in the previous experiment, is what the natural penis experiences because of the foreskin's mediating actions. This concept will be explained more fully in an upcoming chapter.)

In addition, on every inward and outward stroke, the taut-skinned penile shaft is repeatedly frictionized, as discussed in Chapter 5. The degree of discomfort a circumcised man experiences during and after intercourse will depend on several factors, including the tightness of his shaft skin, the vigorousness of his thrusting, the duration of intercourse, and the amount of lubrication.

Like the woman, instead of sex being a sensation of pure pleasure, the circumcised male experiences pleasure intermixed with discomfort—mosquito-bite sex.

The circumcised male may say, "I don't know what you're talking about—I find sex exceedingly pleasurable." In reply, I can only say that the negativities of circumcised sex become clearly discernible after you've experienced intercourse with a restored penis. My husband says that before his restoration, he did consider sex to be pleasurable, but in retrospect, now that he has experienced the "real thing," he rates circumcised intercourse a 2 and natural intercourse a 10. That old car you rode around in as a teenager was great, but how many guys would give up a BMW or Lexus to go back to it?

On a conscious level, the circumcised man may not be aware of the degree to which he is being discomforted during sex because it is intermixed with so much pleasure. Nonetheless, the displeasurements and deficiencies that are the consequence of circumcision are still present and leave a negative imprint on his *subconscious* mind, influencing his sexuality and his attitude toward women.

CIRCUMCISION MAY CAUSE A MAN TO WORK HARDER TO ACHIEVE ORGASM

When the circumcised man has sex, he, like his female partner, must concentrate intensely on the pleasure he is receiving, while simultaneously blocking out displeasurements and detractions. Many women commented that their circumcised partners seemed to have to work too hard at building up to orgasm. The circumcised man's intense concentration on his own individual experience causes him to become physically and emotionally distanced from his partner. It's almost as if she isn't there. Indeed, she can sense his distance. Many survey respondents noticed this. Below are three typical comments:

> "My sexual experience with the circumcised partner seemed very one-sided. He was so intent on trying to achieve his own orgasm that he felt nothing towards me."

> "I have on occasion become aggravated with a circumcised man because there was so much necessary concern focused on his trying to reach orgasm that I have been forgotten. Not only is this frustrating sexually, but it is unsatisfactory, emotionally."

> "My first lover was a natural man. I didn't notice differences until later on, after I had been more sexually active with circumcised men. I remember being disappointed since they all seemed to focus entirely on their own penis sensations—very concentrated, while my natural man could enjoy several sensations including my responses."

Even though the circumcised man achieves orgasm, his *copulatory pleasure—the totality of pleasure experienced during intercourse, excluding orgasm*—is adversely affected by all the negativities we've discussed—his desensitized glans, his overall desensitized penis (which is missing a piece of highly erogenous tissue about the size of a 3" X 5" index card), too much direct stimulation and over-frictionization, along with factors yet to be discussed. Consequently, the pleasure centers of his brain are deprived of the positive biochemistry of "real" sex, even though he has an orgasm.

As we have seen, circumcised sex fails to give both partners the kind of stimulation their minds and sex organs desire and crave. They never get to experience the true pleasures of intercourse and the nirvana-type physical/emotional experience natural sex brings. And this ultimately affects a person's sexuality—how they identify themselves with sex and their sexual self-image.

In her book, *Eve's Secrets*, sexual researcher Josephine Lowndes Sevely states, "The genital/brain connection is... a two-way flow, back and forth, each influencing the other (8).... [B]y repeating experiences...[we] 'create' a neural pathway. Each person's sexuality is linked to the awareness of his or her genitals" (9).

The idea that circumcised intercourse imprints the brain's memory centers with negative biochemical messages—memories of discomfort, frustration, and dissatisfaction—was brought up earlier, but I bring this concept up again because now that you are more cognizant of circumcision's negative impact on the intercourse experience, you can better see how the following could arise.

Circumcised intercourse frustrates and even angers the primordial subconscious, which somehow knows innately that "real sex ain't this way." Each new circumcised experience builds upon the negative-memory imprints of the past, and over a period of time, the subconscious and the conscious mind become more and more annoyed. After repeated sexual encounters with the same partner, the brain begins to develop negative feelings toward the partner that are ultimately carried far beyond the bedroom door, into the everyday relationship. The partners may belittle each other, purposely aggravate one another, and start quarrels over everyday little things. The relationship may even become outwardly hostile. And eventually, the couple may decide that divorce is the only solution.

The partners of a circumcised relationship enter marriage with the enthusiastic optimism of youth, thinking everything will be a bed of roses, but sadly, the bed of roses has a thorn—the coronal ridge *hook*.

Could circumcised sex erode the love bond between a man and woman and be an important factor in America's alarmingly high divorce rate? This question, of course, cannot be answered that readily because other socioeconomic factors undoubtedly contribute to a couple's decision to go their separate ways. But in response, I pose another question: Other things being equal, which couple is more likely to stay together—one enjoying delicious, satisfying sex, or one whose sexual pleasure is being compromised in many ways?

CIRCUMCISED-SEX SYNDROME

The partners in a circumcised relationship may try to communicate their likes and dislikes in the bedroom scene, but they're not sure what they really want. One or both may know that something seems wrong or lacking, but they can't quite put their finger on it. The bells and whistles become increasingly out of tune. She seems to think that he's the cause of the problem, but he seems to think it's her. Neither can realistically verbalize what the problem is because they've known only the circumcised-sex experience. They wish they knew. The marriage needs rejuvenation, revitalization—and more love.

With the passage of time, the partners may experience increasing dissatisfaction with their mate and a strange sense of alienation. They may desire their sex partner less and less often, and one or both may seek out extramarital partners or turn to masturbation as an alternative. They may feel that their partner lacks a sense of genuine affection for them, or doesn't desire them for their sexuality, but instead desires sex only to satisfy his or her own basic sexual needs. In this respect, sex becomes more of a "me" experience instead of what it should be—a sharing "we" experience.

This is all part of what I call "the aging circumcised-sex syndrome." How soon you and your partner begin to experience it will depend on the age you began having intercourse, the frequency and length of time usually spent during intercourse, the tightness of the male's circumcision, variations in positions and thrusting techniques, and factors related to individual biochemical makeup. Depending on the above, you may already be experiencing it to a greater or lesser degree. Some couples may begin to experience it in their late twenties or early thirties, while for others, it may not begin to manifest itself until sometime later.

Maybe you've sensed all along that something wasn't quite right about your sexual relationship with your mate. Maybe you're just beginning to realize it. Whichever—by now you know what I'm going to say—all you need is the right equipment and you can discover the delights of natural intercourse and the beneficial effects it will have on your overall relationship. Through foreskin restoration, both sexual partners will come to discover what has been missing in their love life, allowing them to see their mate with new eyes of appreciation. Finally, the bells and whistles will be in tune.

7

Women Tell Their Personal Stories

Many of the questions in the survey asked respondents for comments. Some women commented extensively and talked about their life experiences. In each of the twelve narratives that follow, I took the composite comments (and some answers to survey questions) of each woman and strung them into a story format. Some editing was necessary to make the story flow, but the thoughts were not changed.

It is important to note that, in the introduction to the survey, I instructed the reader that I would use the term *natural* when referring to the uncircumcised penis. This was done to prevent confusion between the two terms, *circumcised* and *uncircumcised*, since the question format was comparative, going back and forth between the two types of penises. Many respondents picked up on this term—natural—and used it in their comments. They also picked up on the terms *natural intercourse, circumcised intercourse, bang and pound away*, and other words used in the questionnaire.

Story # 1

I really had deep feelings for my circumcised lover. He treated me fantastically and said he adored me, but I began to dread sex with him because it was so frustrating. His penis took longer to become erect, seemed drier, and was more difficult to thrust in and out. He had to work very hard to bring himself to orgasm, and he sometimes worried about pain on his penis. It took away from the spontaneity. He had a strong sex drive and sometimes

I felt used. I just did it because I liked his company.

My current natural husband is a sweet and wonderful lover. I'm very lucky to have him. I think the natural penis is more alive. My natural husband seems to get an erection easier, can maintain it longer, and I think his orgasms are stronger. I love the subtle feel of his foreskin as it moves along the shaft of his penis as we're making love, it's kind of like a massage. You're right about the natural penis jiggling in short strokes bringing more pleasure to the clitoris—I never thought about that before! What a realization. My natural partner and I actually joke about his "wiggling."

My fantasies are always about natural men. My first lover was natural. The foreskin can be lots of fun to play with. Our son is also natural. Although I was afraid of going against the "norm," I think he will someday thank me.

Story # 2

I have had a lot of different partners, but it was many years ago and my memories are rather faint. However, overall I did prefer the natural penis, and I would have liked to have married a natural man—but nobody asked me.

Twelve years ago when I had my natural experience, I did achieve my personal record of having intercourse nine times in a night. I could feel the skin moving freely over the penis and also enjoyed the lubrication.

I do enjoy sex with my circumcised husband, mostly because he concentrates a lot on my pleasure, but as soon as the penetration starts, the fun part is over for me. When our son was born, I insisted that he *not* be circumcised. I was thinking of his future wife!

Story # 3

I can't argue with the assumption that a natural man makes the best lover. I have had intercourse with 38 circumcised men.

I discovered how to bring myself to orgasm during intercourse with circumcised men. Then I slept with a natural man and had superb vaginal orgasms. I went back and slept with three circumcised men, then I went back to get more *amazing* natural sex.

In my experience, the natural man moves with a consistent rhythm that I find pleasing, whereas the circumcised man's movements are not in harmony with what I like. With the natural man, I emit more juices, but with circumcised men, I often had to make use of artificial lubricants.

Although foreplay was equally arousing with both types, with circumcised intercourse, too many times it was just two sets of genitals banging away at each other, detached. With my natural partner, I am a much more active participant. My natural man feels much more satisfying. His thrusts stimulate the inside *and outside* of my vagina [vulva]. I have vaginal orgasms every time we have sex. I have never had as many orgasms with a circumcised man as I do with my natural man—mind-blowing orgasms—which I never experienced with a circumcised man. Besides, my natural partner just physically feels better.

My sexual experience with my natural partner has been erotic and fulfilling. He is just more sensitive to my needs. To me a natural penis is a work of art, solid and erotic. My natural man is a much better lover than any other man I've ever had. He's yummy. We enjoy long, luscious, passionate lovemaking—but that may, of course, just be him. [*Author's Note*: This last statement points up the quandary some survey respondents had about attributing their good sexual success to the penis itself. Considering that this woman had intercourse with 38 circumcised men and only one natural man, what are the odds that out of 39 men, she found only one man to be superior and he just happened to be natural?]

On your survey question about natural men using shorter thrusts that gently grind against the woman's clitoral area and the circumcised man using long thrusts that result in less physical contact—very true. I thought I was the only one who felt that way.

Story # 4

My husband is circumcised and we have been married 14 years. He believes he has lost much of his sensitivity and I can tell. He often needs to work pretty hard to reach ejaculation. Fortunately, we still have a satisfying sex life because he's very in tune with my feelings, physically and emotionally, and is careful not to hurt me, but I know other women who have problems with men thrusting too hard. I suspect that circumcised men experience a loss of sensitivity in their penis and perhaps this is what causes their need to pound away. This reduced sensitivity makes them have to concentrate more on their own penis and how it feels, sometimes forgetting their lover.

Natural men seem less likely to do that. I've made love with only two natural men and both were very sensuous, their thrusting very loving and gentle. Never did those men pound away like some circumcised men. I enjoyed the feel of the natural penis. With one natural man, I believe I could feel his foreskin moving inside me. I seemed to be wetter too.

Interestingly, one of the natural men I had sex with had a rather small penis, so size proved to be unimportant to me. However, the fact that he was *not* circumcised did make a difference. It's been a long time since I've had a natural man, but I still remember the difference, and I like that feeling.

Story # 5

A good love life including sexual intercourse is a very important part of my life. One of the reasons I divorced my circumcised husband was my unhappiness with our sex life. He was totally engrossed in satisfying his own sexual needs and seemed preoccupied and frustrated, which frustrated me. He pounded and banged as if he were having intercourse with a non-feeling person.

It was so rare to have intercourse that lasted with my circumcised husband. I felt a deep sadness because I was usually just getting interested and he was finished. He would tell me to roll over and go to sleep, and I would quietly cry myself to sleep lacking sexual satisfaction. I never remember feeling like a whole woman during our marriage.

He was very interested in pornographic magazines, reading them almost daily during the last years of our marriage. At the beginning of our marriage, we had intercourse about once a week. It gradually came to the point where we had it once a month.

With my current natural husband, I've finally found a man who enjoys lovemaking and intercourse as much as I do, and as we get longer into the sex act, I get more and more into it. He truly satisfies me and makes me feel like a whole woman.

The natural men I've known have been more patient and affectionate and have spent more time and effort to enable me to have an orgasm. My other two natural partners were both from Europe. My Russian partner was the most gentle man. Intercourse was so rhythmic—it was like dancing gracefully together. We were so in tune with one another, I felt like we became one. I experienced a titillating feeling in my whole body—a pleasant, satisfying experience that I had only dreamed of before.

Story # 6

Natural intercourse is better. There is no comparison. When I am in the mood, I have no trouble becoming aroused with either, but none of my 14 circumcised partners lasted long enough so I was usually left hanging, which angered and frustrated me, and I suppose this ultimately affected my ability to derive any pleasure from subsequent sessions. My natural lover (I am presently having an affair) has the ability to "hold back" (most of the time) for as long as it takes me to reach orgasm.

My husband, who is circumcised, seems oblivious to my feelings, and this causes a great deal of anger and resentment on my part and creates a distance between us. He makes me feel like a prostitute, and I often tell him to leave my money on the bureau when he is through. Sometimes I talk on the phone or watch TV while my husband is having sex with me. He laughs at this but plows ahead nonetheless. I tell him how cheap and used he makes me feel and how selfish he is, but he never reacts to this, which makes me even angrier. This has been an ongoing issue in my marriage for the past four years and caused many arguments, hurt feelings, etc. The stress I have experienced from this situation also carried over into all other areas of my life as well. It has destroyed what little self-esteem I had and has caused me to seek gratification elsewhere.

With my natural partner, I feel happy, and loved. I would attribute this to the fact that my natural partner takes his time and is very gentle and loving. He does not act as if he's in a race or as though he is an animal in heat like my circumcised partners. I can only enjoy sex if I feel comfortable and relaxed. He makes me feel like I am important, whereas the others made me feel dirty. I experience no pain with natural; it is always pleasurable. With circumcised, I often experienced discomfort.

Story # 7

My first experience was with a natural man. He was a wonderful lover, slow and easy. There is a big difference, which I didn't find out until later when I went from him to four circumcised men and then to my husband who is half circumcised, but I would put him in with a circumcised man's status.

What I've found out about the circumcised men I've been with is that they have no motivation when it comes to sex. Sad, isn't it? I think when they cut off the foreskin, they cut away important sex nerves, so maybe sex isn't really fulfilling for a circumcised man, so he rushes to end it.

Natural is longer lasting and more pleasurable. The whole lovemaking experience is more intense. I honestly feel a natural man is more confident about lovemaking and himself. He knows how to please a woman and wants to make her happy not only for his pleasure but for hers too. There isn't this intense feeling to have it end as there is with circumcised men, who seem to want to end it quick.

Circumcised sex is not fulfilling unless you have foreplay. But with a natural man, I didn't need much, or even any, foreplay to feel wonderful when making love. I look back and wish I could go back to my natural lover of ten years ago, even for a moment. The feeling with him was like going to heaven. With circumcised sex, I feel cheated. I don't vaginally orgasm with my husband. I have never felt fully complete with any circumcised man. My husband is a good man and I love him, but his lovemaking has to be improved upon. Too bad his parents just didn't leave his penis alone.

Story # 8

I am 40 years old. I have had intercourse with more than 10 circumcised men and 3 natural.

All my circumcised relationships were short-term, lasting only a few months at the most. I went through several circumcised partners before achieving my first vaginal orgasm, and even though I am capable of achieving orgasm with a circumcised partner, I find I must work harder to bring it about.

As I've noted by my responses on your survey, I've found circumcised thrusting actions to be rougher and tougher than natural. Circumcised men always, at some point, seem to need to work really hard at thrusting. *They back way up and get into these long detached strokes that pound away at my vagina, causing it to tense up.* As intercourse progresses, I've noticed that my vagina loses lubrication and becomes dry, sore, and irritated. This is when sex becomes uncomfortable, boring, and unproductive, and I start to totally lose interest.

But during natural intercourse, the penis always felt so sensuous and comfortable. Our sex organs seemed to swoon passionately and blend into one another. The natural penis thrusting actions were gentle and tender. With my natural partners, my vaginal lubrication increased and I never had vaginal dryness or irritation no matter how long intercourse lasted. I never had a natural man separate his groin from mine for the purpose of thrusting; intercourse always stayed very connected genitally. One of the differences I noticed with the natural penis is a feeling of more tissue. The foreskin backs up and applies additional pressure to the vaginal opening, which I loved.

I think that circumcised men are more detached from their penis—as if their penis were a separate "thing" that they use and abuse, rather than it being an integrated part of their total body.

Of the three natural men, one was my ex-husband, which wasn't a good sexual relationship. This had nothing to do with his natural state but with his sexuality in general. The other two natural lovers were very gentle with their penis—the way they fondled it when urinating or dressing, etc. Their penis seemed to be an extension of their overall psyche—and they were quite loving and gentle to this body part that they respected and appreciated. The sexual experiences with these men were extraordinary in the gentleness, sensuality, and mutuality of the experience. As I mentioned a couple of times, I was very in love with these two natural lovers in ways I had not been with other men before.

Before taking your survey, I had never given any thought to the differences in the two types of intercourse. But as I progressed through it checking off my responses, I was continually amazed at the dramatic differences the two kinds of experiences brought me. I do think you are on to something here. Your analysis of the style of intercourse with the natural penis was so "right on" it made me feel like my experiences were under observation! I find it all so fascinating and very thought-provoking. I am currently partnerless and am doing the personals—God, do I have to request only non-circumcised men respond? I don't think I could go back to circumcised sex again. [*Author's note*: Fortunately for her and the other men and women in America, the foreskin restoration revolution has begun.]

Story # 9

The first time I ever had sex was when I was a teenager. It wasn't anything special, but it was memorable because it helps to show the difference between circumcised and natural.

It was during the summer, and I was spending most of my time at the beach. Every day I would sit out in the sun in my bikini, and every day this boy would sit down next to me doing the same. One day he asked me if it would be okay to remove his pants and get some sun in that area. I didn't see anything wrong with it, so I agreed. Upon removing his pants, he showed me what was to become my first exposure to a circumcised penis. From my memory, the head was very clearly delineated from the shaft, almost like it was manicured or something. He began to masturbate in front of me. I was horrified at first but very curious. He then said I could touch it, and I did. It seemed very coarse. He asked me if I had ever had sex. I said no, but that I might like to try it.

Without any hesitation, he ripped off my bikini and literally jumped my bones. Ramming me harder and harder, I felt like I was being pummeled with a jackhammer and at times as if sandpaper was attached. After he came off, I laid there feeling almost dead, feeling severely violated. It took me a while to recover.

A year later, I experienced sex with a natural boy. I can remember quite fondly the entire experience. I was spending the summer at a country farm. Every day we would get up early, milk the cows, feed the chickens, clean the house, and after a hard day's work, we all used to go skinny-dipping in a nearby lake. One day, when the other kids had gone home, I was sitting with a boy and we were talking for a while. He kissed me and began running his hands gently over my body. I returned the favor. The moment I felt his cock a smile came over my face. The skin moved up and down in perfect rhythm over the head and it was pleasantly soft. The conversation turned to sex and I was becoming very aroused. Then, in a very relaxed tone, he asked me if I would like to be the one on top. I accepted and lowered myself onto him. Moving my hips in rhythm, my face became flushed and all of a sudden this earth-shattering feeling overtook me. I came! The boy beneath me still hadn't come, so I kept going, and almost twenty minutes later I was coming again and again until finally we came as one. It was the best experience of my life and probably his as well.

Later in my teens, I had a circumcised lover for one year. Every time we had sex, I had to put some K-Y jelly on him or wet him with oral sex; otherwise there was always vaginal discomfort during intercourse. The aftermath of sex was worse. I always had to take a bath in some mineral salts because my vagina had a painful throbbing feel to it. But later, whenever I had sex with a natural boy, we never had to use a lubricant or anything else. And after intercourse, I would feel all warm and giggly, almost too happy. My whole body felt a warm tingling sensation, and I wanted to just lie beside him.

To me, circumcised and natural sex are quite different. Circumcised men not only pound away but they do it in long thrusts. By being far away, they always seem more distant. For me, there is never any contact when I am on the bottom, and when I am on top they usually want to control the movement of my buttocks with their hands, so contact, again, is not apparent. They usually want to have sex in the missionary position with my legs in the air or from behind. And when they start pounding, my breasts start banging me in the face and my whole stomach begins to go into convulsions. Even when I am on top and am able to have an orgasm, there is pain before the pleasure and the pleasure only happens once. The natural man, on the other hand, is more relaxed, confident, playful, and more experimental with your needs. They take their time. They move with your rhythm. In my experience, the number one thing the foreskin does is to make the man very sensitive so he moves more slowly and is much more gentle. The natural penis does not feel at all abrasive.

A natural man always seems to be in contact with my body. And when I am riding him or when he is doing most of the thrusting, I can always feel his constant grinding against my clitoris which either brings on multiple orgasms or makes me feel that another is imminent. Natural intercourse leaves me completely satisfied.

Story # 10

I remember growing up in the late 1940s when there was only one position—the missionary position. A girl was just expected to let the man take her as she laid on her back.

But in the '60s, I experimented with different sexual positions. I remember the first time I was on top. I was with a natural man, and I still remember the feeling I had in my vagina. It was quite intense. As I rocked back and forth, and all around, the foreskin moved with my rhythm. It was a natural stimulator in its own right. I couldn't help but to orgasm again and again. With the circumcised penis, this natural stimulator is gone so I don't get that tremendous feeling. In fact, I never want to be on top with a circumcised man because it does nothing for me.

I find when I'm riding a natural man's penis, for some reason, the flexible skin—or something—makes you crave it more. The penis feels like it belongs inside of you. I've never experienced discomfort from natural intercourse. After natural sex, I always feel happy—fresh and alive, like a little girl.

I've found with natural men, there is less anxiety. You can be on top for a while, then switch to other positions. And he seems to care more about your pleasure than his own. When I'm making love with my natural partner, I feel like we are one!

With circumcised men, my experience has been that they often come so quick you rarely get a chance to come yourself. Circumcised men have to be in control or on top because they need to control themselves as best they can, and they pump too hard. In the past, I learned to just be passive and let the circumcised man do his thing. During circumcised intercourse, I feel very little in orgasmic build-up, and afterwards, my vagina is red and sore. Sometimes, I even have to fondle my clitoris with ice cubes. With circumcised men, I feel totally violated, like I'm being used. I'm so glad that I'm now married to a natural partner who fulfills all my sexual needs and fantasies.

Story # 11

Throughout my early sexual years, all my partners, except one, were natural because in Europe very few men are circumcised.

In my late 20s, I came to the United States, met my husband, who is circumcised, and got married. At first, I couldn't figure out why I didn't really like to have intercourse with him that much. Finally, I realized that it had to do with his circumcision. My husband, however, does not believe me that there is a difference between a circumcised and natural penis, other than the way it looks.

We have been married for almost five years now. Intercourse with my circumcised husband is all right, but I know it could be much nicer if he had not been circumcised. I can't change that about my husband. I sometimes feel sad for him not having the chance to experience sex and intercourse with a natural penis. He does not see a problem with it. And I don't want to hurt his feelings by telling him that I really wish he was not circumcised so sex would be much better for both of us. He will never know the difference.

During my very first intercourse with a circumcised man, I noticed it was different right from the beginning. Foreplay is great and I am always excited at the beginning, but intercourse is not much fun with a circumcised man. With a natural man, even if I wasn't in the mood for sex, when I felt that sensuous penis inside me, I would get swept away with passion.

A circumcised penis is very dry. But when a natural man gets an erection, glands produce a silky fluid and that fluid makes it easy to move the foreskin layer back and forth, which makes the penis feel very smooth when it moves inside me.

Natural intercourse creates more fluids and that makes intercourse more comfortable. I have only had a few experiences where intercourse with a circumcised man lasted longer than 6-8 minutes, and I did not like it that much because I got so dry inside. Also, a circumcised penis feels harder during intercourse. Sex with a circumcised man is not nearly as good as with a natural man. The natural penis is a much nicer feeling for a woman!

INTRODUCTION TO STORY # 12

The thesis of this book is that nature equips every male with a foreskin to enhance the sexual pleasure and satisfaction of both partners, and that most women who have experienced both natural and circumcised intercourse can discern several differences between the two types.

The concepts presented in this book are disruptive to the status quo and, initially, some people may not want to hear its message. Consequently, this book may generate more than its fair share of critics, who may try to discredit its information by claiming that only a person educated in sexology is qualified to make the claims I make for the natural penis, and then only after conducting scientifically documented clinical studies.

In response to the above, I offer the following story, written by my very first survey respondent. When I wrote the survey, I knew that I could discern several differences between the two types of penises and the overall intercourse experience, but I wasn't sure other women would notice these differences and be able to express them in words. When I received this woman's survey back, I was amazed—she hit the nail right on the head.

This woman, of simple education, was able to figure out on her own, without a doctorate in sexology and a staff of researchers, that intercourse with a natural penis is more satisfying to a woman than a circumcised penis, and she was able to describe the differences with sincere simplicity.

Story # 12

My opinion of circumcised sex is that it is not very satisfying to me. Circumcised men try so hard to come, and the stroke of their penis feels so dry and undesirable it sometimes starts to feel like instruments that are used in a pelvic exam, unlubricated. I feel very threatened when they try too hard, and it gets painful.

Some of my experience was with a long-lasting relationship partner, but it didn't feel like it. Sometimes it seemed like a one-night stand.

About 70 percent of my circumcised men had problems keeping their erections. I used to think it was because of me, until I learned better.

I never had an orgasm with my circumcised partners. I used to get aggravated with circumcised men. And it made me feel so mad because 98 percent of the time it was no type of excitement at all for me, just something we would do and he gets all the pleasure, and I just lie there with my legs open.

Sex with my natural man is very satisfying and enjoyable. His penis seems rounder and fuller, plus it's more gentle. Circumcised men have a tendency to be really rough and unpleasurable, but the natural is really smooth and pleasurable when making love. I never had a vaginal orgasm until I met my natural man, and it was so satisfying that I've been with him ever since. But I can't just finger one thing that makes me aroused because there are so many ways.

I like a long-lasting, satisfying love session and the foreskin gives long-lasting pleasure. My natural man lets me have at least three intense orgasms and sometimes I'll have four orgasms during a 45-minute love session—that's when the pleasure is so good it sends chills up my spine. I feel so soothed and relaxed that my heavy, but quiet, ooh, oohs, turn my man on even more. When I had sex with a circumcised man, I felt a desire to hurt him for not being satisfied. But with my natural man, I feel a desire to kiss and caress him throughout the session. My opinion is that when me and my natural man have sex, it's so satisfying to the both of us there are no complaints afterwards.

I always praise my natural man on the way he makes love to me. And I always express the sensation and pleasure about the natural man to my friends. The foreskin feels so good and pure, and just the feeling of it going in nice and easy is a very pleasurable experience to a woman. But you can't really explain it. It's something I think every woman should try, just to see that the natural man is really worth the while and the time. I'm really glad that you want to share these feelings with the world, because I really thought I was the only one in the world who felt this way.

Author's comment: Bear in mind that these women had the vantage point of having had sex with both types of men; therefore, their comments may appear more critical than one might expect from the average American woman who has only experienced circumcised sex. This is also true of the comments from women appearing throughout the book. Once one has experienced the difference, one becomes more discerning and may therefore be less tolerant of the circumcised experience.

At some point in the book, it might strike you that circumcised sex couldn't be as bad as women's comments reflect. But keep in mind that our attitudes are influenced by the plethora of magazine articles, splashed weekly in the headlines at the grocery checkout stand, portraying women as insatiable sex kittens, perpetuating the myth that all is well and that the only problem is, we can't get enough of it. But truth be told, in the dark and quiet of America's bedrooms, women are secretly dissatisfied with circumcised sex, but just don't know what's wrong.

8 (Part A)

The Normal Thrusting Rhythm of the Natural Penis

vs.

The Abnormal Thrusting Rhythm of the Circumcised Penis

What is a "normal" thrusting rhythm, and what is an "abnormal" thrusting rhythm? That is the question. Can it dare be said that there is indeed such a thing as a normal thrusting rhythm? Does a man with a foreskin have a different thrusting rhythm from a man without a foreskin? And what effect does a man's rhythm have on a woman's pleasure during intercourse? What effect does it have on her ability to have a vaginal orgasm?

Nature endowed us with the potential to achieve orgasm and provided our sex organs with physiological mechanisms that are designed to bring on orgasm in ourselves, and in our partner, just from the interaction of the genitals and body contact during intercourse. In effect, then, it could be said that nature intended the sex organs of each partner to help bring the other to orgasm. And men usually have no problem achieving orgasm from the vagina during intercourse. So why should so many American women have trouble with the penis bringing them to orgasm? Rhythm! The secret is in the rhythm of a man's thrusting movements. Here are two survey respondents' comments:

"In general, the circumcised man either goes too fast or too slow. In my experience, the natural man is easier to fall into a *mutually rewarding constant rhythm*. To me, the natural penis is erotic and responds to the inner rhythm of my sexuality." (Emphasis added)

"With my natural partner, intercourse was so rhythmic, it was like dancing gracefully together. We were so in tune with one another. I felt like I was melting into him."

The lyrics of a popular song put it crudely but succinctly, "It ain't the meat, it's the motion." Many women would probably agree that the size of the penis in itself has little to do with the pleasure a woman experiences during intercourse. However, I think virtually all women would agree that motion* has everything to do with it. In her best-selling book, *How To Have An Orgasm...As Often As You Want*, Rachel Swift says, "Of the scores of women I have spoken to, all agree that a consistent rhythm in the buildup to orgasm is critical" (1).

This chapter adduces that the presence or absence of a foreskin makes a definite and discernible difference in the movements of the penis during intercourse. A man with a foreskin thrusts his penis more gently, using strokes that are lighter in pressure, shorter in length (while deep within the vagina), and *more consistently regular in rhythm*. Since the natural penis tends to stay more deeply embedded in the vagina using short strokes, it brings the

---

* Motion, in this instance, means the kind of action, stroking, thrusting, etc., a man puts into his sexual movements. Throughout this chapter, I refer to a man's thrusting movements during true-to-life intercourse. This implies the interactive participation of both partners. The thrusting movements shown in adult sex videos usually do not represent a man's true thrusting movements during real-life intercourse because the sexual activity is performed expressly for the camera, showing men and women in "unnatural" positions contrived for visual effect and camera angle, with little or no participation on the woman's part. However, though adult sex movies usually do not give an accurate representation of a man's true thrusting movements, they can be instructive for some of the points of this and the next chapter.

man's pubic area in frequent contact with the woman's clitoral mound, allowing her clitoris to be pressure-pleasured more often, and *at a consistent rhythmical rate throughout much of the intercourse experience.* Further, the woman's pleasure is often enhanced when his short strokes quicken into a rapid, exciting rhythm that can best be described as jiggling or diddling.

In contrast, the circumcised man thrusts his penis harder, using strokes that are more forceful in pressure, longer in length, and he often uses a thrusting *rhythm that is discordantly irregular.* His elongated strokes cause his pubic mound to make less frequent contact with the woman's clitoral mound. And when he does make contact, especially when he quickens the tempo of his long, hard thrusts, he often bangs his pubic mound and pelvic area against the woman's genital region. Here are what some survey respondents had to say:

> **"Circumcised man is too forceful with his thrusting. I lose all sense of feeling and I no longer desire to reach an orgasm.... When he is natural, he seems to be more gentle during intercourse and it really excites me."**

> **"Natural men thrust more sensuously, more gently."**

> **"A natural man has a gentler technique—more enjoyable. I noticed a difference after my first encounter with my next circumcised man after being with the natural."**

> **"The natural man was far more aware of my experience as well as his. Also, his thrusting was of a more sensitive/sensual motion—whereas the circumcised man tends to need more of a rougher stimulus to achieve orgasm."**

> **"Most circumcised men would or needed to bang away to get off."**

The thrusting techniques and rhythms of the natural and circumcised penis are determined by these major factors: 1) the location of the primary pleasure zone, 2) the kind of stimulation the pleasure receptors receive, and 3) how far the penis travels outside the vagina during its outward motion. These, as well as other factors, are influenced by the presence or absence of a foreskin.

The two types of penises have different *primary* pleasure zones. The primary pleasure zone is the area of the penis where a man experiences most of his pleasure *during intercourse*. For the natural penis, this area is in the upper area of the penis; for the circumcised penis, it is in the middle and base area of the penis.

Although the entire penis is sexually sensitive during intercourse, nature intended the male to derive most of his sexual pleasure and orgasmic build-up from the upper part of the penis. That's why nature densely packed this area with supersensitive nerves and then covered them with the outer foreskin to protect them from stimulation until sex takes place. *By concentrating most of the penis's sexual firepower into this localized area at the forefront of the penis and making this the primary area of activity, it minimizes the distance the penis has to travel during its inward and outward strokes to induce and sustain a high level of pleasure.* This is one of the reasons why the natural penis thrusts with shorter strokes. Much to the delight of the participating woman, because as stated, **the movement of these shorter strokes, thrusting while the penis abides deeply within the vagina, allows the man's pubic mound to make frequent pressuring contact with the woman's clitoral mound, which is her primary pleasure zone.** This rhythmic frequency of contact excites her sexually throughout the act and helps her achieve a vaginal orgasm—an orgasm induced by the movements of intercourse.

One survey respondent explained it this way:

> **My natural partner kept more constant contact and pressure on my whole genital area during intercourse. I felt like he was in sync with me, and with pleasuring me. During natural intercourse, I had more time to relax, and I would always orgasm before it was over, so afterwards I felt content.**

In contrast, for the circumcised penis, the upper penis nerves are not the primary source of pleasurable sensations. Circumcision significantly damages the functioning of this area. Consequently, the nerves of the upper penis cannot generate enough pleasure sensations to satisfy the pleasure centers of the brain. *The circumcised penis finds it can derive greater pleasure by stimulating its middle and lower area against the vaginal opening. To stimulate this longer area, the circumcised man thrusts with an elongated stroke that pulls more of his penis out of the vagina on the outward stroke.* This reduces the amount of time the penis stays deep within the vagina. *These elongated strokes cause the male's pubic mound to make considerably less contact with the female's clitoral mound* and at the wrong rhythmic frequency, which hampers her ability to achieve an orgasm from the movements of intercourse.* The survey respondent last quoted had this further comment:

> **In circumcised, I was aware of a lack of body contact and the absence of the nice constant pressure that I got with natural intercourse. It seemed that my circumcised partner wasn't paying attention to me.**

---

* The clitoral mound (the entire area surrounding the clitoris—the outer vulvar lips, the female pubic mound, and the clitoris itself) is sexually excited through body contact and pressuring by the male pubic mound during intercourse. Although the female pubic mound and vulvar lips are erogenous in themselves, importantly, they serve to transmit cushioned pressure to the female clitoris during intercourse. In effect, this entire area works as a unit to build up sexual excitement during intercourse, combined with penile stimulation of the vagina.

or my pleasure and was just banging away at my vagina. I often felt he was not in sync with my thrusts.

Both types of penises fall into a thrusting rhythm pattern that feels right for them, and both derive various amounts of pleasure from their thrusting strokes. Even though the two penises have different thrusting techniques, each man thinks his penis is using the right thrusting rhythm because, to him, it just feels "right." However, keep in mind that the woman is on the receiving end of the penis and, for her, the two thrusting techniques feel quite different and affect her *overall* appreciation of the experience. The following are four women's comments:

> "With circumcised men their bodies never seem close enough. There's not much stimulation during intercourse unless I use hand stimulation. Most don't pay any attention to know if I had an orgasm or not."

> "Natural men are more sexually satisfying—the sensations are more intense and pleasurable. I find I can attain orgasm more easily with a natural man."

> "Natural is more relaxing! I love to make love to a natural penis! With my natural partner's penis, I feel totally satisfied. After sex with my circumcised partners, I felt unfulfilled, painful, and very lonely."

> "Achieving vaginal orgasm with a natural man is much easier.... Vaginal orgasm is possible with a circumcised man but more difficult to achieve."

Nature designed the female sex organ to experience a certain thrusting rhythm (i.e., frequency and consistency of pressuring contact on the clitoral mound) in order to enhance a woman's pleasure and build her up to orgasm. When a man's thrusting rhythm feels naturally "right" for the woman, and at the same time feels naturally "right" for him, they have found nature's ideal thrusting rhythm. Since nature designed the male sex organ with specialized anatomical parts (like the foreskin) to bring about this compatible rhythm, and also designed the female sex organ with specialized anatomical parts (like the clitoris) to pick up on the man's gentle rhythmic pressuring, then this compatible, ideal rhythm must be nature's natural or "normal" sexual thrusting rhythm.

Excision of the foreskin causes the penis to thrust with an unnatural, elongated stroke and an inconsistent, irregular rhythm, which put the man's and woman's movements out of sync with one another. Thus, it must be concluded that the circumcised penis thrusts with an abnormal thrusting rhythm. (This will be further explained later.)

Why does a man thrust during intercourse anyway? Why doesn't he just rest his penis inside the vagina and bask in the delight of the vagina's warmth and softness? He thrusts in order to stimulate nerves on and within his penis, which in turn "fire off" sensations of pleasure. After these pleasure nerves have fired off, they require a split-second rest from stimulation in order to recharge themselves for the next firing. We will learn that thrusting not only stimulates, but also serves to give sexual nerves a chance to *rest* from stimulation. That is, the nerves stimulated on the inward thrust rest during the outward stroke, and vice versa.

To better understand the rest requirement of nerves, try this little experiment. Take your finger and run it lightly and slowly in a wide, circular motion around the underside of your wrist. Notice the pleasurable sensations. This is an erogenous zone. The touch of your finger excites nerves on your wrist to fire off sensations of pleasure. Now, move your finger around the underside of your wrist again, slowly and lightly at first, but gradually increase the speed until you are going quite fast.

You will notice that the pleasure sensations are strong at first, but as you speed up your finger rhythm, the pleasure sensors in your wrist seem to go numb. This is because the nerves need a certain amount of time to recharge themselves before they can refire, and if your finger stimulates them before they recharge, they yield little or no sensation.

This same principle applies to the penis, which finds that varying the tempo of its thrusts affects how strong a feeling its nerves give off and how quickly they flow in succession through the nervous system. By moving about (thrusting) inside the vagina, the penis is seeking to find the right motion and rhythm that will send a high level of continuous pleasurable sensations to the brain. It is important to understand that during intercourse, it is the penis that controls its thrusting motions. It automatically seeks out the best pleasure sensations and moves accordingly. The conscious mind doesn't even have to think about it, *for the conscious mind yields its control completely to the penis's quest for pleasure.* In effect, **a man's thrusting technique and rhythm are controlled by the penis, not by the man's conscious mind**.

This is an essential concept to understand, because after foreplay, it is the penis that sexes the woman, not the man, and as I've contended, the kind of sexing the penis gives a woman has a positive or negative effect on her attitude toward the man as an overall person, impacting the overall relationship.

IS IT THE MAN OR THE PENIS?

The vast majority of surveyed women noticed that their natural lovemaking experiences were more sexually and emotionally satisfying, but some were reluctant to attribute this directly to the penis. Instead, some explained that sex and the relationship were better because the man was more emotionally sensitive, more caring, and a more wonderful person. In effect, they wanted to say that it was the man, not the penis.

Likewise, if they found their circumcised experiences unsatisfactory, they were also reluctant to attribute this directly to the penis. Instead, they would explain that the sex and the relationship weren't as good because the man was a less considerate lover, or he was less sensitive emotionally, or they weren't really in love with him, etc. In effect, again, they wanted to attribute the unsatisfactory sexual and emotional relationship to the man, not the penis. Here are a few quotes representing the quandary some women had in this regard:

> **"Many of my negative feelings following intercourse with circumcised men had much more to do with the relationship with the man rather than the mechanics of the experience itself."**

> **"I'm not sure the difference was due to circumcised or natural. More likely the difference was due to the physical and emotional makeup of the man."**

> **"I think many of my answers are more positive toward the natural man because I care more about him than any of the circumcised men in my life. That has a lot to do with my answers. He treats me like no other man ever treated me...overall he makes me happy, satisfies me, and appreciates me. I'm in love, and when we make love it is very special. With circumcised guys, I used sex to fulfill my need for sex, just like the guys were doing, but I WASN'T satisfied!!"**

> **"With my natural partner, for some reason, it feels more like 'making love' than 'having sex.' It doesn't seem as rough. We are always happy afterwards and I feel so in touch with my lover because we both seem to enjoy it immensely. I'm not sure if I feel**

that way because I'm really 'in love' and the sex is great or what!"

In general, if a woman had wonderful lovemaking experiences with a man, she tended to speak glowingly of him and the relationship. On the other hand, if the sexual relationship was unsatisfactory, unfulfilling, and frustrating, she tended to be critical of the man and attributed their unhappy relationship to his faults. *But perhaps, in many cases, it is actually the other way around. Perhaps the dissatisfying, displeasurable sex caused her to be much less tolerant of the man's faults and nitpick him for things she might otherwise overlook if he were pleasing her in bed.*

Let me give you an example of the subtleties of this. In a situation where the husband lets his appearance slide on the weekend, a woman in a bad sexual relationship might say: "When you don't shave, you really look terrible." A woman in a good relationship might phrase it this way: "You look so much more handsome when you shave." In another example, the man gives his wife a little pinch on the bottom in company when no one is looking. In a good relationship, the woman might say, "You're acting like a teenager, but I love it." A woman in a bad relationship might say, "You're so immature. I wish you'd grow up."

The influence of the penis can be so subtle it can often go unrecognized. As noted in Chapter 2, Drs. Phyllis & Eberhard Kronhausen addressed this ***transference effect*** in their book, *The Sexually Responsive Woman*:

> One should not...be surprised to hear that failure to achieve sexual happiness is likely to have an adverse effect on the woman's total relationship with her partner and may lead to the breakdown of their relationship.
>
> *This does not mean that such a couple would themselves be aware of the sexual roots of their problem.... In many cases, the couple do not quarrel at all about their sex life, but may violently disagree on a variety of irrelevant matters* (2). (Emphasis added)

Some women had had numerous circumcised relationships, but when they "found" a man with a natural penis, they characterized him as being more gentle, more caring, more emotionally sensitive, a better lover, etc. For some reason this man was not only a better lover but had more of the qualities they were looking for in a partner. Is this just coincidental? How much of it was the man, and how much of it was the penis? How much does the lovemaking ability of the penis influence a woman's overall attitude toward the man in general? Let us consider this concept in the next comment.

> **The one natural penis I experienced belonged to a very wonderful, gentle person, therefore, his penis was gentler and smoother than the others [*the other 28 circumcised penises she experienced*].** [*Author's note:* This woman's comment is a clear example of how some women tended to entwine the personality of the man and the sexual experience he offered. In actuality, his personality couldn't really affect the physiology of intercourse, making his penis feel gentler and smoother. The penis simply felt gentler and smoother in and of itself. Could the physical appeal of the gentler, smoother penis cause her to look upon the man as a more wonderful, gentle person?]

Certainly, non-sexual factors enter into a woman's overall appreciation of a man—looks, personality, financial security, etc. But if all things were equal, and it were possible to have two men with equally pleasing looks and character traits, etc., the man who is the better lover would win out over the man who displeases a woman in the bedroom—every time. Moreover, if we were to find repeatedly that this better lover was a man with a natural penis, then we begin to see how important a role the type of penis plays.

The type of penis a man has controls its thrusting movements in the bedroom, and this affects a woman's appreciation for the sex act and influences her attitude toward the man as an overall person. After a Sunday morning of sex, she may either want to throw a shoe at him to vent her frustration or make him breakfast in bed to show her appreciation. She may then carry one of these attitudes with her throughout the next day or week of the relationship.

As you read the rest of this chapter and the next chapter, ask yourself from time to time: Is it the man or the penis? Then ask yourself at the end: Which of these two combinations would give a woman greater overall satisfaction: a wonderful guy with a circumcised penis or a wonderful guy with a natural penis? I addressed this in the survey with the following question:

> You have been shipwrecked and washed ashore onto a deserted paradise island in the Pacific. Your rescue ship won't be by to pick you up for five years. On this island is only one other person—a man—a very attractive man, who is interesting to be with and very likeable. Because you are in paradise, you will be having sex fairly often. When you begin your first lovemaking encounter and you are slowly undoing his belt and pants, would you be hoping that he is...
>
> Please circle: Circumcised   Natural

In response to the above, the overwhelming majority of women (89%) chose the natural penis. The comments from one survey respondent below clearly show what I am trying to say about the question, "Is it the man or the penis"?

> **I didn't realize sex could be anything different until I met my natural husband, who was my last sexual partner [after 10 circumcised partners]. During**

intercourse, he seemed closer to me and pelvic contact was greater. In fact, the first time I slept with him, I had a vaginal orgasm. The only other man I had a vaginal orgasm with was after many months of intercourse, and only when I was on top. I absolutely agree that a natural man uses shorter strokes and gently grinds the clitoral area. *I had thought that it was my husband's technique that resulted in greater pleasure for me. I never considered that it was due to his natural status.* (Emphasis added)

THE NORMAL THRUSTING RHYTHM OF THE NATURAL PENIS

The primary pleasure zones of the natural penis are located in the upper penis—the area that includes the penis head, the foreskin's inner lining, and the frenulum (the hinge of skin that connects the foreskin to the glans). As discussed, when the penis is flaccid, these highly erogenous areas are covered over by the foreskin's outer layer, but upon erection, both foreskin layers unfold onto the upper penile shaft, leaving the frenulum, glans, and inner lining exposed in readiness for sexual activity.

During intercourse, the exquisitely sensitive nerves of this area excite the man's sexual feelings and control the rhythm of the penis's thrusts. The pleasure sensations they send out tell the penis when to start and stop its inward thrust, and when to start and stop its outward stroke (just as the pleasure sensations that your wrist sent out told you at what rhythm to move your finger to derive the most feeling). The explanation below details how the foreskin's actions regulate the firing off and resting of these nerves and cause the natural penis to thrust with shortened strokes compared to the circumcised penis.

When the natural penis thrusts inward, the vaginal walls brush against the erotically sensitive nerves of the glans, foreskin's inner lining, and frenulum, causing these nerves to fire off sensations of pleasure. The inward thrust of the penis keeps these pleasure sensations ongoing, but after these nerves have fired off, the penis senses a reduction in pleasurable feelings, so it stops its inward thrust and begins its outward stroke in search of stronger sensations.

During the outward stroke, the foreskin's outer layer slides forward to cloak the nerves of its inner lining, while the inner lining itself covers the frenulum. Once covered, these nerves are allowed to rest from stimulation until the next inward thrust. As the foreskin moves forward on the shaft, it bunches up behind the coronal ridge, and may sometimes roll forward over the corona, depending upon the length of the stroke. This applies pressure to the interior tissue of the corona and coronal ridge, where nerves that are excited by pressure send a wave of sexual excitement throughout the upper penis. Once these nerves have fired off, the penis stops its outward stroke and returns to its inward thrust in search of stronger sensations, giving these pressure-sensitive nerves a chance to rest until the next outward stroke.

In effect, the natural penis receives pleasure sensations from one set of sensory nerves on the inward thrust and a different set of nerves on the outward stroke. And by moving from one set to the other at the right tempo, it can maintain a continuous stream of erotic sensations.

Because this area is so localized, the penis only has to travel a short distance to excite one set of nerves or the other. Once it has finished its inward thrust, it doesn't have to withdraw very far to receive pleasure on the outward stroke. This allows it to stay deep within the vagina, thereby keeping the man's pubic mound in close and frequent contact with the woman's clitoral mound, which receives pleasure whenever these two areas press together.

There are other erogenous nerves located elsewhere on and in the penis, but the pleasure sensations coming from the upper area are so intense they dominate the brain's attention. In the nervous system, stronger sensations override lesser sensations. For example, if you were suffering from a toothache and were to accidentally bang your thumb with a hammer, you would notice that the pain in your thumb could be so strong you'd lose awareness of the pain in your tooth. In much the same way, the upper area of the natural penis dominates the brain's attention so strongly it becomes the primary focus of sexual pleasure.

There is, however, a secondary area of pleasure located at the base of the penis and in the adjoining tissue of the pubic mound, and it contains many pressure-sensitive nerves that become aroused when the man's pubic area is pressed against the woman's genitals/clitoral mound.* The pressuring of these two areas against one another becomes more frequent as intercourse progresses because the woman instinctively draws the man in closer in order to satisfy her innate desire for the penis to remain deep within her and to pick up more stimulation against her clitoral mound. The man also draws his pubic area in closer because the act of pressing his pubic mound/pelvic area against her pubic mound/pelvic area and genitalia enhances his pleasure since it augments excitation to the pressure-activated nerves in this region. Eventually, their pubic mounds/genitals are pressing and pressure-pleasuring each other in either a rapid, rhythmic touching or gentle, grinding motion.

---

* The appearance of pubic hair at puberty is an indication that nature intended the pubic mounds of a man and woman to be in close proximity, and to press and grind each other during intercourse. Pubic hair cushions the contact and facilitates the sliding of the pubic mounds during intercourse, so that chafing of the genital area is minimized. I think its presence indicates that nature did *not* intend for the man to use the elongated strokes, characteristic of circumcised sex, that detach the male's pubic mound from the female's clitoral mound.

Various books on hygiene propose that pubic hair is a defense against germs because it provides pockets of air that allow moisture to evaporate, thereby discouraging germs from breeding. While it may be true that pubic hair has a hygienic function, keep in mind that young boys and girls are exposed to similar germ hazards and they don't have pubic hair. I think pubic hair appears at puberty because its primary function is sexual. It allows a man and woman to press their pubic mounds/genitals together comfortably, minimizing friction, and augmenting the pleasures of natural intercourse.

The genitally intact (natural) man tends to maintain a short thrusting stroke because, as intercourse progresses, the rhythmic actions taking place in the upper penis area have generated such a high level of pleasure intensity, the penis must use short strokes in order to not overstimulate its upper area nerves into climaxing before the man wants to. Shorter strokes give the upper penis nerves a respite from stimulation because the inner lining and frenulum get covered more often, and because some parts of the inner lining and frenulum may not get uncovered at all.

While the man is deriving pleasure from these rhythmic thrusting movements, the woman, of course, derives pleasure too. For her, the thrusts of a natural man produce frequent rhythmic contact with her clitoral mound, and they are gentle in pressure and often consistent in tempo. It is this type of gentle, smooth, rhythmic pressuring that her clitoral mound craves, indeed needs, to help bring her to orgasm.

One survey respondent described this rhythm of natural lovemaking beautifully:

> **Sex with a natural partner has been to me like the gentle rhythm of a peaceful but powerful ocean—waves build, then subside and soothe. It felt so natural, as if it were filling a deep need within me, not necessarily for the act of sex, but more in order to experience the rhythm of a man and woman as they were created to respond to each other. I didn't want the rhythm to stop.**

Continued as Chapter 8 (Part B)

8 (Part B)

The Male Clitoris: Its Discovery, Pleasurement, and How It Affects the Thrusting Rhythm

How can we be sure that nature intended the upper penis to be the most important area of excitability on the natural penis? Because it was designed to be covered over all the time and exposed only during sexual activity. Think about that for a moment. The anatomical design and sensory nerves of the penis head, frenulum, and foreskin inner lining are there for only one purpose—to create sexual excitement; and the outer foreskin is there to protect them from unwanted stimulation until sex takes place.

Another indication that nature intended the upper penis to be the focus of sexual excitement is new scientific evidence which attests that embedded interiorly within the glans' coronal area is *the male equivalent of the female clitoris.*

NEW SCIENTIFIC EVIDENCE IDENTIFIES
THE MALE CLITORIS

In her book, *Eve's Secrets,* sexual researcher Josephine Lowndes Sevely reports on the findings of a seven-year Harvard-approved study detailing the similarities of male and female genital anatomy. She presents intricate physiological evidence showing that highly erogenous tissue, in the core of the penis, beneath the corona/ coronal ridge area, is equivalent in makeup and response to what is commonly called the female clitoris, generally recognized as the woman's primary pleasure zone, essential to her arousal, pleasure, and orgasmic response.

I say "what is commonly called the female clitoris" because, as Ms. Sevely so eloquently explains through illustrations and text, the so-called female clitoris is really *only the tip*—although the most responsive part—of the complete clitoris, a much larger structure that extends deep into the pelvic region. In her words, "Many people may be surprised to learn that the female clitoris has deeper structures under the skin. These deeper structures are the organ's two leglike parts that run along the lower part of the pubic bones at either side of the lower vagina between the inner thighs" (1). She sums up her comparative evidence in the following statement:

> The new theory advanced here proposes that the [female] clitoral *tip* and...the *tip* of a male structure *inside* the penis [behind the glans are]...true counterparts (2). (Emphasis added)

(Essentially, this means that the *interior* corona/coronal ridge area of the penis is as sexually responsive as the female clitoris. We will soon learn how this interior tissue of the penis— identified below as the tip of the male clitoris—is pleasured during intercourse.)

Sevely further explains that the highly excitable tip of this male internal structure is actually only the apex of its larger structure (as described above for the female) that runs down the entire length of the penis and into the pelvic region. (This accounts for why the entire shaft of the penis is sexually excitable, though not as excitable as the interior tip behind the coronal ridge area.) She calls this entire structure the **male clitoris,** and she calls its tip the Lowndes crown.* (See Figure 8-1.) Here is her statement:

> [E]veryone knows that the penis gets erect because it fills with blood...[T]he part into which the blood flows [called the corpora cavernosa]...I now identify as—the male clitoris (3).

*A reprint of Sevely's "Lowndes Crowns Theory" appears in Appendix D.

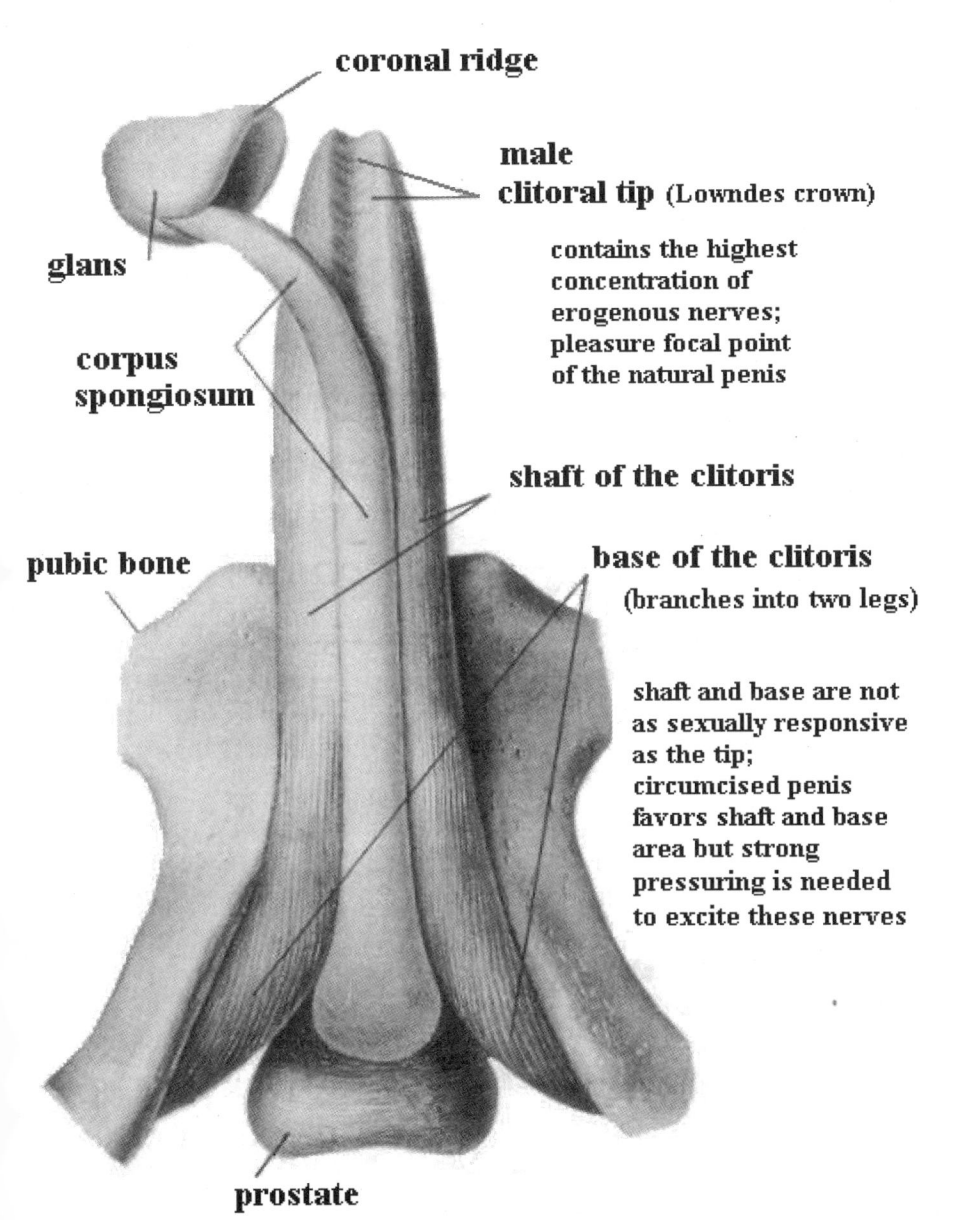

The Male Clitoris: Its Discovery,
Pleasurement, and How It Affects the Thrusting Rhythm

- **coronal ridge**
- **glans**
- **corpus spongiosum**
- **pubic bone**
- **male clitoral tip** (Lowndes crown) — contains the highest concentration of erogenous nerves; pleasure focal point of the natural penis
- **shaft of the clitoris**
- **base of the clitoris** (branches into two legs) — shaft and base are not as sexually responsive as the tip; circumcised penis favors shaft and base area but strong pressuring is needed to excite these nerves
- **prostate**

Figure 8-1. Visualize the **male clitoris** (corpora cavernosa) as a body composed largely of muscle tissue. From its tip, located *interiorly* beneath the glans, it extends down the length of the penis shaft and into the pubic mound, where it branches and continues into the pelvis and onto the pelvic bone, to which it is attached (4). (Adapted from Sobotta's drawing in *Eve's Secrets*.)

smooth-muscle meshwork of the male clitoris

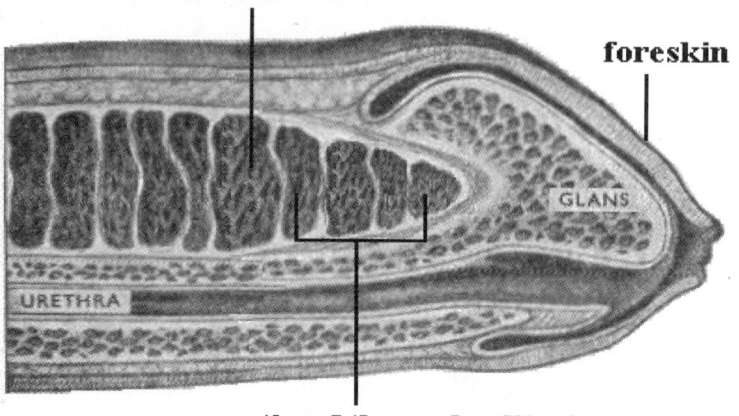

foreskin

GLANS

URETHRA

tip of the male clitoris

Figure 8-2. Cross-sectional view of the penis showing the meshwork of smooth-muscle tissue in the male clitoris. (Adapted from *The Illustrated Encyclopedia of Sex* by Drs. Willy, Vander, Fisher.)

The male clitoris is largely composed of smooth-muscle tissue— thin sheets of cells formed in a meshwork that is analogous to a fisherman's net. (See Figure 8-2.) The spaces of the meshwork are called sinusoids. When the penis is flaccid, the smooth-muscle fibers are shortened and the sinusoids are small, leaving little room for blood. Elongation of the fibers causes the spaces to enlarge during erection. The following describes how the smooth-muscle fibers control the erection process.

    Sexual desire and sensory stimulation trigger the release of chemicals (nitric oxide and histamine) in the genitalia that cause the smooth-muscle fibers in the male clitoris (corpora cavernosa) to elongate (stretch). This leads to increased blood flow into the enlarging sinusoids. Continued elongation of the smooth-muscle results in the flattening (or pinching off) of the exit veins that normally drain the clitoris of blood. Thus, the blood becomes trapped in the sinusoids, and the engorged penis swells into an erection. Upon orgasm, the smooth-muscle fibers shorten, the exit veins renew their function, blood is allowed to exit the sinusoids, and the penis becomes flaccid.

A survey respondent commented, "I envision the natural penis as being as sensitive as my own clitoris." Sevely affirms that,

> The female and male clitoris are composed of basically the same erectile substance (5) ...the male is [totally] internal, but [it too is] highly responsive nonetheless to indirect touch, or rather *pressure* (6). (Emphasis added)

The entire male clitoral musculature (muscle tissue) abounds with nerves that are sexually excited by pressure, but its tip contains the greatest density of these nerves (7) and is, therefore, the most sexually responsive part, just as the tip of the complete female clitoral structure is its most responsive part.

Like the tip of the female clitoris, the tip of the male clitoris enjoys playful indirect tickling and pressure—the kind it receives from **the massaging actions of the glans upon it, and the movements of the foreskin.**

GLANS' STIMULATION OF THE MALE CLITORAL TIP IS DIFFERENT FOR THE TWO TYPES OF PENISES

This section is one of the most important parts of the book, but unfortunately, it could not be brought up until now.

Sevely points out that because the penile glans and male clitoral tip are in close proximity to each other,

> Touch or press upon the glans, especially its ridge...and you excite the Lowndes crown [male clitoral tip] as well (8).

As explained in Chapter 6, the natural penis head has a spongy giveability, even when erect, that allows it to bend and flex as the penis thrusts the vagina. On the inward thrust, when the penis meets the slight resistance of the vaginal walls, *the glans is pushed inward and applies gentle pressure to the clitoral tip located interiorly* beneath the flexible glans. Then, on the outward stroke, the bunched-up foreskin butting against the coronal ridge *also causes the glans to apply gentle pressure to the clitoral tip.* These *kneading* actions on the male clitoral tip create magnificent sensations of pleasure in the upper penis area.

***** A SIMPLE EXPERIMENT GIVES PROOF *****

Male readers should try this important experiment. Hold your flaccid penis with one hand—or better still, your semi-erect penis.

Then, with your other hand, place your fingertips all around the coronal rim of your penis head. Next, holding this area securely, rock the glans left to right a few times, then forward and back several times. Notice that this produces sexual excitement to the interior tissue underneath the glans. This interior tissue—*the male clitoral tip*—is massaged during intercourse by the actions of the glans exerting pressure upon it.

****

Essentially, a major purpose of the glans is to apply a massaging-type pressure to the interior clitoral tip during thrusting. The clitoral tip is much too sensitive to be touched directly. It prefers and needs indirect, cushioned pressure.

The massaging stimulation by the glans on the clitoral tip is a major player in why the natural penis favors stimulation of its upper area with short strokes. Short strokes intensify the sensuous massaging movements of the glans against the clitoral tip, and the man is instinctively drawn to repeat them again and again, enraptured by the wondrous, pleasurable effects. All to the delight of his female partner, whose clitoral mound is softly pressured and greatly excited by the gentle, rhythmic actions of this vibrating type of (jiggling/diddling) stroke.

However, for the circumcised penis, the glans stimulation of the clitoral tip is dramatically and adversely affected. As you will recall, the circumcised penis is missing 12-15 square inches of shaft skin. *Upon erection, the skin of the shaft can get stretched so tightly it pulls down on the skin of the glans, compacting the glans' tissue and pushing it against the clitoral tip with unrelenting, continuous pressure. This compression reduces, or may entirely eliminate, the glans' massaging capabilities on the clitoral tip.* Essentially, the tissue of the glans gets compressed so tightly against the clitoral tip, the glans' massaging movements over the clitoral tip are severely restricted. Additionally, the tissue of the clitoral tip itself is abnormally compressed because the overly tightened shaft skin has compacted the overall penis. Consequently, the clitoral tip is denied the massaging effects nature intended. By analogy, this would be like someone hardening the muscle of their bicep (making a muscle), then asking a masseur to massage it.

If the penis is very tightly circumcised (which is a common complaint of circumcised men), a man may actually experience numbness or even pain in his clitoral tip. Remember the experiment you did in Chapter 6 (page 95) where you applied constant pressure with your thumb against the coronal ridge area and experienced a discomforting sensation? If you had continued applying this sustained pressure, it would ultimately result in a desensitization of the area. (In effect, the tightly compacted circumcised penis experiences constant pressure to its internal tissue and is thus desensitized.) Sevely attests to the desensitizing effects of overstimulation in the following:

> [P]rolonged stimulation in the exact same spot of either the male glans or the female clitoral tip can cause a numbing effect (9).

Masters and Johnson reported this observation:

> [For] those women who manipulate the clitoris directly.... A relative degree of local anesthesia may develop if too much manipulative pressure is applied to any one area (10).

In regard to the above (now that we realize the homologousness of the female and male clitoris), consider the following quotes taken from a national survey of men who are aware that circumcision affects their penis's sensitivity and sexual performance (11). (Keep in mind that because the glans and clitoral tip are in close proximity, and since these men were not knowledgeable of the clitoris's existence, when they say glans, they might mean glans/clitoral tip.)

> "Takes too long to orgasm due to desensitizing of head."

> "Glans is callused and numb to subtle sensations."

> "Constant, continual chafing and desensitization of glans."

> "I enjoy no sensations on my glans; orgasm requires painful thrusting."

> "I have to be at the point of abuse and pain to my penis to reach orgasm, it is so desensitized from circumcision."

The conditions described above could all be a result of continuous pressure by the tightly compacted glans on the clitoral tip.

This reduced or deprived pleasure in the upper penis encourages the circumcised man to favor stimulation of the middle and lower areas of the penis.

RESTORATION RENEWS THE GLANS' MASSAGING EFFECTS ON THE TIP OF THE MALE CLITORIS

One of the most important sexual benefits of restoration—perhaps the most important—is that after restoration (when the shaft has the skin it needs and the penis's internal tissue is no longer abnormally compacted), the massaging actions of the glans on the tip of the male clitoris—the penis's most responsive part during intercourse—is essentially completely restored. This important factor is one of the major reasons why restored men report that intercourse is exceedingly more pleasurable after restoration. This benefit, as well as 18 others, are presented in the Table of Sexual Benefits (of restoration) immediately following Chapter 12.

STIMULATION OF THE MALE CLITORIS
BY THE FORESKIN (AND ITS RIDGED BAND)
CREATES SEXUAL PLEASURE AND
MUSCLE CONTRACTIONS LEADING TO ORGASM

The foreskin's gliding and bunching actions over the upper penis shaft and corona sexually excite the upper area of the male clitoris (including its tip).

These stimulatory movements are further augmented by an elastic-like band of mucosal tissue at the tip of the foreskin's inner lining. The erotic characteristics of this specialized mucosa were only recently discovered by Dr. John Taylor (12). He calls this zone of tightly pleated, highly innervated tissue, the *ridged band* (Figures 8-3, 8-4), revised from his original term, "frenar band."

When the penis is flaccid, elastic fibers in the muscle tissue associated with the ridged band serve to constrict the foreskin opening like the drawstring of a duffel bag. This gives the tip of the foreskin a cone-shaped, sometimes puckered, appearance. (See Figure 8-3.)

During erection, the emergence of the penis head causes the ridged band to stretch open, slide back past the glans, and position itself on the upper shaft, where the inner and outer foreskin meet (called the mucocutaneous junction). During intercourse, as the penis thrusts, the ridged (elastic-like) band rolls up and down the upper shaft and coronal area. This rolling action stimulates the erogenous nerves of the ridged band to fire off sensations of pleasure as it rolls and stretches (when it encounters narrower and then wider parts of the penile shaft), and butts against the coronal ridge.

Additionally, as it rolls up and down the shaft, the ridged band applies gentle pressure all along the upper clitoris, exciting its pressure-sensitive nerves. This titillating and rolling/pressuring by the ridged band, along with the glans' massaging actions on the interior clitoral tip, create wonderful pleasure sensations in

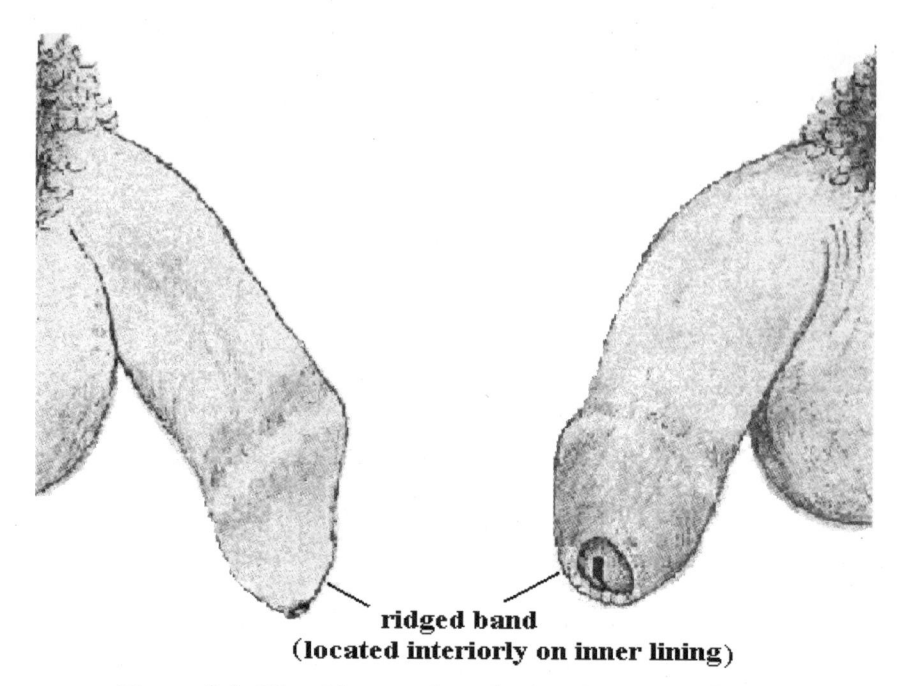

ridged band
(located interiorly on inner lining)

Figure 8-3. Flaccid natural penis showing approximate location of the *ridged band, a tightly pleated zone of mucous membrane densely concentrated with highly erogenous nerves* (13).

ridged band

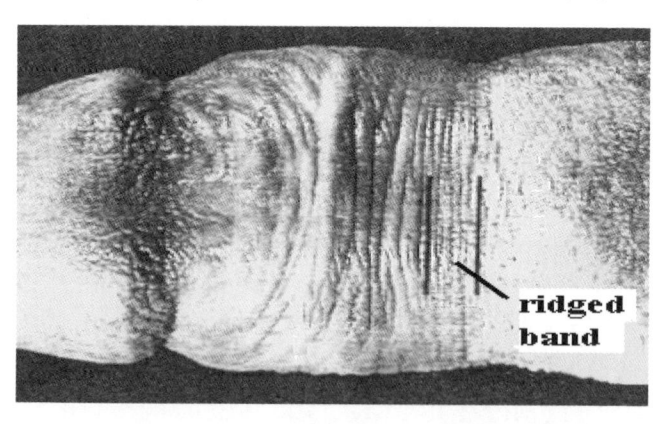

Figure 8-4. The *ridged band* rolls up and down the penis and excites the erogenous nerves of the male clitoris and of the ridged band itself. (Adapted from postmortem medical specimen photo, *British Journal of Urology*, vol. 77, 1996, p. 292.)

the male clitoris, but it does something more: it creates tiny spasms in the muscle cells that make up the clitoris. These spasms (minute muscle contractions) play an essential role in the penis's build-up to orgasm.

To nature, the object of sexual stimulation in the male isn't simply to generate pleasure sensations. Additionally, the objective is to build up contractions in the genital musculature, because it is these muscular contractions that bring on orgasm and the ejaculation of spermatozoa. When the genital musculature becomes excited by sexual activity and alternately contracts (tenses) and then relaxes over and over rhythmically, this alternating tensing and untensing action can ultimately lead to orgasm.

It is important to understand how muscular contractions can bring on orgasm because the intact (natural) man and the circumcised man induce them differently in their genital and pelvic regions, and the means they use to create these contractions affect their thrusting movements and rhythms.

The design of the natural penis evinces that nature intended for pleasure and orgasm to be induced by actions taking place mainly in the upper area of the penis. However, for the circumcised penis, the upper penis mechanisms and responses have been drastically altered and do not function the way nature intended. Consequently, the circumcised male is left to improvise alternative or supplementary means to attain orgasm. It is his use of these odd varieties of orgasm-building (pleasure-seeking) techniques that causes him to thrust much differently from the intact man, and which his female partner finds frustrating and disrupting to her pleasuring needs.

HOW EXCITEMENT IS BROUGHT ABOUT IN THE NATURAL PENIS

During intercourse, the upper area of the **natural** penis is titillated by several different kinds of actions that all work to bring on orgasm. There are 1) *mechanical* actions, like the bunching and unbunching of the foreskin, the massaging of the clitoris by the glans, the rolling/pressuring and stretching of the ridged band, and the excitatory stretching of the frenulum; 2) *electrical* actions involving the firing off and recharging of nerves; and, as we shall see in Chapter 10, 3) *chemical* actions, like histamine, released from the glans in response to pressure applied by the foreskin.

These actions bring on orgasm in gradual stages by first inducing tiny muscular spasms (contractions) in the tip of the clitoral musculature, which cause it to quiver with excitement. Second, these tiny spasms vibrate down from the tip and induce subsequent contractions in the rest of the clitoris. Third, rhythmic vibrations (quivers) in the clitoral musculature induce contractions in other muscles, in the pelvic region, in the thighs, buttocks, etc., and eventually induce contractions throughout other body muscles. Recurrent titillation of the clitoris, especially its tip, causes the contractions in this musculature and in associated pelvic muscles to build with ever-increasing intensity and frequency. As these contractions become more incessant, it eventually leads to orgasm. Orgasm occurs when the recovery time between contractions becomes so short that the muscles virtually seize up into one long, continuous contraction. It is the seizing up of many muscles all at once that produces the body's rigid posture during orgasm.

If you think of an orgasm as being much like a sneeze— a comparison that is often made—you can better understand *how the foreskin works to initiate orgasm*. A sneeze is such a powerful, explosive response it is hard to believe that it can be brought on by something so delicate as the light tickling of the nose by a feather. But it can, and similarly, the foreskin's feather-like tickling actions in the upper penis result in the explosive response of orgasm.

A feather works its magic by mechanically applying touch stimuli and light pressure to the nostrils, activating the release of histamine from the nose, which causes the muscles of the nose to twitch (contract). These contractions in the nose muscles soon radiate into the face and neck muscles, then into the chest and abdominal muscles. Continued tickling by the feather makes the slight contractions become stronger and more frequent, and ultimately many muscles in the body seize up and propel the person forward in a sneeze.

Similarly, like the feather, *the foreskin's mechanical movements and tickling actions generate electrical responses and chemical actions (like the release of histamine from the glans), which titillate the tip of the clitoral musculature into producing contractions.* These contractions radiate down the entire clitoris and into other muscles of the pelvic region and, eventually, many muscles of the body seize up into orgasm. The wonderful pleasure sensations of sex are provided by nature as a seductive diversion to keep the mind occupied while it subtly manipulates the body's muscles into orgasmic contraction, for it is, of course, through orgasm and ejaculation that the species is perpetuated. The foreskin's method of arousing sexual tension has some very special advantages.

First, most of the stimulation the intact man needs for arousal of his clitoral musculature and sexual pleasure can be generated in the localized area of the upper penis. This area is the prime focus of his attention and keeps his mind captivated. It's sort of like the old story about the country farmer who visits New York City by train and gets off at Grand Central Station. When he returns home, everyone asks him, "What was the big city like?" He explains, "There was so much happening at the depot, I never got to see the city." Similarly, for the intact man, there is so much pleasure going on in the upper penis, he has little incentive to wander away from this super-erogenous zone. (For the circumcised penis, however, this area loses much of its attraction as a generator of pleasure, so the penis must rely more heavily on other erogenous areas for pleasure and stimulates those instead.)

Second, since the intact man focuses his attention primarily on stimulating this localized upper area, he tends to use a thrusting motion that ideally pleasures this one area, and, in general, tends to stay with a regular, predictable thrusting pattern throughout much of the intercourse act. As a result, the natural penis falls into a consistent, predictable rhythm that is smooth, harmonious, engaging, and hypnotic, capable of inducing a trance-like state in both lovers.

A third advantage of the foreskin's method of arousal is that the penis's short-traveling strokes require less "work" from the man, so he can maintain a consistent thrusting rhythm longer without tiring. This is especially beneficial to the woman because she desires a sustained, consistent rhythm to build up to orgasm.

A fourth advantage of the foreskin's mode of arousal, the one mentioned most often by survey respondents, is that it results in a much gentler intercourse experience.

HOW THE NATURAL AND CIRCUMCISED PENIS ARE AROUSED DIFFERENTLY AND WHY IT'S IMPORTANT

We must understand nature's clever, delicate mode of using the foreskin's action (and the massaging effects it enables) to titillate the tip of the male clitoris into building up pleasure sensations and muscular orgasmic tension because it contrasts so dramatically with the circumcised penis's mode of arousal. The circumcised penis, rather than focusing on titillating the upper penis area, relies on strong pressuring to its middle and lower and base/pelvic area to induce feelings of pleasure and (male) clitoral musculature contractions. One woman, who said she hadn't really given any thought as to why the natural penis should be more gentle until filling out the survey, made this brilliantly insightful comment:

The circumcised penis can't feel, so it bangs harder

to try to get more vibrations. But with the natural, vibrations and energies are evoked naturally just by the delicate movements of the foreskin. [No banging thrusts are needed.]

The natural penis's arousal method is very indirect. Analogously, it works like a farmer who gets the muscles of a resting donkey moving by tickling his nose and whetting his appetite with a carrot on a stick. On the other hand, the circumcised penis's mode of action is more like a farmer who pushes and bumps against the donkey to rouse him and get his muscles moving. The strong-pressuring thrusts of the circumcised penis cause the woman to perceive intercourse as rougher and tougher. The following comments are representative of those received in the survey:

> "YES! YES! YES! Circumcised men are rougher and they tend to pound away."

> "Sometimes circumcised men just thrust too hard."

> "Circumcised men do have a tendency to be really rough and unpleasurable, whereas the natural is really smooth and pleasurable when making love."

> "The natural intercourse experience is softer...the man doesn't have to pump so hard.... Circumcised men pump very hard like they're trying to come but are having trouble feeling anything."

CIRCUMCISION DRASTICALLY ALTERS THE STRUCTURE AND FUNCTION OF THE PENIS

Circumcision dramatically modifies the structure of the penis and the layout of its erogenous zones. When the foreskin is surgically removed, all of the erogenous zones in the upper penis are affected by its elimination. Consider the impact of this loss for a moment.

Gone are the numerous sensory receptors of the inner foreskin and ridged band, which come alive upon sexual arousal. Gone is the foreskin's rolling and bunching-up action with its alternating pressure-pleasuring of the corona and coronal ridge. Gone (or significantly reduced) is the massaging actions of the glans on the internal clitoral tip. Gone is much or nearly all of the frenulum, which (according to many natural men I've spoken with) is the most erogenous tissue of the entire penis. Gone is the thin, moist, delicate layer of membrane on the penis head, which allows its nerves to fully experience the ecstasy of intercourse. These are major losses when you consider that just about all of the sexual receptivity of the natural penis takes place in these upper erogenous zones.

Removal of the foreskin devastates the ability of the upper penis pleasure zones to function: 1) The penis head is dramatically reduced in sensitivity because the unprotected circumcised glans becomes dried out and desensitized by many layers of keratinized, unfeeling skin which smother the penis head's nerve endings. 2) The glans' massaging actions to the clitoris are impaired. 3) The highly erogenous frenulum, as stated, may be partially or completely eliminated. 4) The corona and coronal ridge have no foreskin to roll over them, giving their nerves alternating periods of rest. And 5) There is no outer foreskin to roll over the nerves of the inner foreskin lining, giving them time to rest from stimulation.

Instead of a rest period, the circumcised upper penis gets continuous direct stimulation. *It receives no intermittent periods of rest.* Remember what happened on your wrist when you applied too much stimulation? It made it difficult for you to discern the pleasure sensations because the nerves on your wrist seemed to go numb. Similarly, this is what happens to the upper penis pleasure nerves when the foreskin is missing. Because they are continually stimulated, they don't get a chance to rest and recharge, so the pleasure sensations they fire off are greatly reduced in both quantity and intensity. Essentially, during intercourse, the upper part of the circumcised penis, which already suffers from a dramatic reduction in sensitivity, becomes further numbed out due to overstimulation.

WHY DOES THE CIRCUMCISED PENIS UPPER AREA GO NUMB BUT THE NATURAL PENIS DOES NOT?

The concept that the upper area of the circumcised penis can go numb from being overstimulated by continuous, uninterrupted contact with the vaginal walls is usually grasped by most people I've talked to. But they have difficulty understanding why the natural penis doesn't also go numb. After all, they reason, when you visualize either type of penis thrusting inside the vagina, it would seem that they both receive the same amount of direct stimulation from the vaginal walls. But I propose that this is not the case. In actuality, each type of penis undergoes a different experience in the upper penis area. In the two types of penises, touch-sensitive (fine-touch) nerves and pressure-sensitive nerves are affected differently, and this difference accounts for why the natural penis derives such a high degree of pleasure from its upper area while the circumcised penis does not.

During intercourse, the *touch-sensitive* nerves of the circumcised penis's upper area are always exposed, always in direct contact with the vaginal walls, and therefore receive continuous stimulation. But in the natural penis's upper area (more precisely, the foreskin's inner lining, frenulum, and coronal area), the touch-sensitive nerves are *alternately covered* by the foreskin and are thus intermittently shielded from continuous, direct vaginal stimulation. In effect, the foreskin acts as an intermediary—a mediator—between the upper area's nerves and stimulation by the vaginal walls. The foreskin's cloaking action gives the touch-sensitive nerves time to recharge so they are able to send out strong pleasure sensations, as explained.

In contrast, *the touch-sensitive nerves of the circumcised penis* —more precisely, the upper shaft skin forward of the circumcision scar (which is what remains of the foreskin's inner lining*), any remnant of the frenulum, and the coronal area— *are denied rest, so they tire out from overstimulation and consequently send out weak sensations, or they go numb.*

At the same time, the two types of penises undergo a different experience in the *pressure-sensitive* nerves of the upper penis. Keep in mind, while reading the explanation below, that pressure-sensitive nerves are not located on the surface skin but are instead located beneath the surface, where they may be found randomly dispersed or densely packed throughout the interior tissue *at various levels of depth*. When light pressure is applied, the nerves nearest the surface will fire off. Applying greater pressure will cause additional nerves, located at deeper levels, to fire off. In effect, *different degrees of pressure excite nerves at various levels of depth.*

When a pressure-sensitive nerve receives pressure, it fires off. When pressure is released, the nerve rests and recharges. When pressured again, it will fire off another sensation of pleasure. The objective (similar to the wrist experiment) is to alternate pressure stimulation with sufficient rest so that the nerves can fire off a strong sensation. On the natural penis, the foreskin works to assure that pressure-sensitive nerves at different depth levels receive the right amount of stimulation, *alternated with the right amount of recharge time*, so that they keep firing off strong sensations of pleasure.

The foreskin works to regulate the firing off of pressure-sensitive nerves as follows: On the outward stroke, while the penis shaft is in the process of retracting, the ridged band slides up and *progressively* applies a light pressuring all along the shallow nerves of the upper shaft. This elastic-like band continues moving upward until it encounters the coronal ridge area. Here it applies a light pressuring as well. The ridged band, impeded by the coronal ridge, causes the rest of the foreskin to bunch up

---

* Although the circumcised penis has some inner lining, this area, externally exposed like the glans, has lost most of its sensibility because it is dried out and keratinized.

and this applies a second, *stronger* wave of pressure to the upper shaft and coronal ridge. (The ridged band may then roll forward onto the corona itself, to pressure-pleasure this area.) Then, on the inward thrust, when the penis shaft moves forward, the foreskin unbunches and *gradually releases* its pressure. The ridged band slides back down the shaft and *progressively* re-applies its light pressuring.

The ridged band and the foreskin's bunching-up action work in tandem to assure that pressure-sensitive nerves at different depths receive gradually varying amounts of pressure, and release from pressure, all along the upper penis. If you try the thumb experiment described in Chapter 6, page 88 again, or if you have someone give you a body massage, you will notice that varying pressure/release action is perceived as much more enjoyable than continuous, constant pressure. It is the alternating gradations of pressure and release that excite the sexual nerves into firing off their most pleasurable sensations.

The above described the natural penis. But the circumcised penis, divested of its foreskin, does not experience these alternating gradations of pressure/release in its upper area. Instead, it receives continuous, unvarying pressure throughout the inward thrust. And on the outward stroke, it also receives continuous, unvarying pressure, especially as the coronal ridge scrapes against the vaginal walls. Too much continuous, unvarying pressure overstimulates its pressure-sensitive nerves, giving them essentially no recharge time. Consequently, they fire off weak (numb-like) sensations of pleasure.

THE CIRCUMCISED PENIS SEEKS TO DERIVE PLEASURE BY USING AN ELONGATED STROKE, AND THIS ABNORMALIZES ITS THRUSTING RHYTHM

Because of circumcision's devastation to the upper penis, the circumcised penis looks to its middle and lower area for pleasure and finds that by stroking this area *directly against the constriction of the vaginal opening*, it can compensate for some of the pleasure it isn't receiving from its upper area.

To stimulate this longer area, the circumcised penis uses an elongated stroke, as discussed. This elongated stroke creates pleasure for the man by stimulating more of the penis against the *vaginal opening*. This increased pleasure is augmented further because the nerves of the middle and lower penis are exposed to a longer rest period during an elongated, outward stroke when the penis withdraws far outside the vagina.

Elongated strokes feel "right" to the circumcised man because they increase his pleasure. But unfortunately, they are not sexually satisfying for his female partner because they cause the man's pubic mound to make less frequent contact with her clitoral mound; his pubic mound is detached from her genital area for an elongated time.

When women of the survey were asked if circumcised men tend to thrust with longer strokes, an overwhelming percentage agreed that they do. Here are four representative comments:

> "It's like they don't get close enough. Too distant."

> "YES. YES. He ain't anywhere near me. However, when I'm on top, I use short, rubbing, jiggling movements like you describe. My circumcised husband doesn't find this satisfying and keeps trying to do longer strokes."

> "I've noticed a big difference with the closeness of our bodies. Circumcised men don't feel close. They are too busy moving in and out, instead of staying in and moving around."

> "I get aggravated because the circumcised man always pulls his body away from my clitoris. I keep trying to pull him closer, but he keeps pulling away. It's really annoying, like being in a wrestling match. However, I do not have this problem with my natural

partner, who always stays in close to my genitals, giving me the consistent pressure I need to attain orgasm."

If a woman doesn't receive the right frequency of rhythmic pressuring to her clitoral mound, she may not be able to have an orgasm. From the woman's point of view, the abnormal thrusting rhythm of the circumcised penis is out of sync with the rhythm she desires. Its elongated thrusts do not give her clitoral mound the right rhythmic pressuring it needs, *not only for orgasm, but also for her overall pleasure throughout the intercourse experience. Her clitoris, the center of her sensual focus, simply does not get enough physical contact.*

This is why the woman may often say: "faster, faster." Faster thrusting will pleasure her clitoral mound more often. But with circumcised sex, faster *elongated* strokes will still not pleasure her clitoral mound at the frequency she desires because the long distance the penis travels when it withdraws far out of the vagina prevents the right frequency of contact. *What the woman actually yearns for is not faster thrusting, but shorter strokes*, which effectually pleasure her clitoral mound more frequently. Consider the following hypothetical example: Suppose the intact man uses a 2-inch stroke, and the circumcised man uses a 4-inch stroke (the approximate length of the penile shaft). Accordingly, the intact man's pubic mound would pressure-pleasure the female clitoral mound twice as often, without thrusting any faster.

THE CIRCUMCISED PENIS SEEKS TO DERIVE MORE PLEASURE BY APPLYING GREATER PRESSURE AGAINST THE VAGINAL WALLS AND OPENING

Another thing the circumcised penis discovers as it seeks to derive more pleasure from its middle/lower area is that it can generate pleasurable feelings by pressing itself hard against the sides of the vaginal walls and opening. This hard-pressing action serves to stimulate the penis with greater pressure and sparks the pressure-sensitive nerves deeper within to fire off. Pressing hard also serves to induce contractions in the clitoral musculature, which help to maintain erection and build up tension toward orgasm.

The circumcised man feels an arousing response in his penis from pressing the shaft against the vaginal opening, so he instinctively *bears down harder* on his thrusts to elicit stronger sensations. In order to bear down harder, he tightens up his abdominal muscles into a hardened mass to brace the penis's thrusts. Also, his elongated strokes cause him to put more driving force behind his hard-pressing thrusts. Upon moving the penis forward into the vagina (when using this technique), he may often come in at an angle to press the penis more firmly against the side of the vaginal opening.

To the woman, the combined effect of an abnormally stiff, unyielding erection (backed up by hardened abdominal muscles) driving against her genital area with an elongated hard-pressuring stroke delivered at a slanted angle is an experience characterized best by the word "jammed." Webster's defines the verb "jam" as, "to press into a close position; to thrust or apply with force or suddenness." ***The natural penis gently strokes the vagina. The circumcised penis jams it.*** Below are the comments of three survey respondents.

> "Circumcised intercourse is like being poked. I don't like that feeling of being poked."

> "Circumcised thrusting seems to be...hard and fast, therefore eliminating any pleasure I might feel in my clitoris."

> "My circumcised partners required greater contact pressure to reach orgasm, resulting in rougher

thrusting, which sometimes caused me pain, preventing the continuation of any pleasure I was experiencing."

THE JOLTING ACTION OF THE CIRCUMCISED PENIS FURTHER DISRUPTS ITS RHYTHM

The above jamming technique, with its hard-pressuring angled stroke, creates another problem for the woman: a "jolting action." The circumcised man may not use a hard-pressuring angled stroke on every stroke but when he does, it jolts her physically and mentally. Webster's defines the verb "jolt" as, "to shake with sudden jerks...to shock or surprise." This jolting action is very interruptive to any kind of regular, measured rhythm, and the woman finds it disconcerting and unproductive to creating any kind of relaxing, blissful, trance-inducing state. Below is an analogy, which attempts to describe the irregular rhythm and jolting action of the circumcised penis.

Imagine you and your lover riding in the back of a limousine. You're sitting back comfortably, enjoying the smooth, relaxing ride and looking lovingly into each other's eyes as you sip champagne. Suddenly, the limousine hits a speed bump in the road while moving at 30 miles an hour. Boom! You're jolted right out of your seat. You bump your head on the front head rest and spill champagne all over your party outfit. But then the limo quickly returns to its smooth, comfortable ride, so you settle back into your seat and pour another glass of champagne. Eyeing each other again romantically, you lean in toward each other for a kiss. Boom! The car hits another speed bump and jolts you again, and this time you hit your head on the limo roof. But because this is an expensive automobile, it quickly settles into its original, smooth ride. You and your lover gather your composure, but this time you move forward toward the edge of the seat. You nervously pick up the wine bottle and begin to cautiously pour another glass of champagne, when suddenly—Boom!—you hit another speed bump. This time you're thrown back and bounced off the back of the seat and the wine bottle bangs against one of the glasses and breaks it. The limo ride quickly smoothes out again and attempts to lull you back into security. Only this time you're not going to be fooled. You are *on alert* now, awaiting the next jolt. You can't relax knowing that any minute it could happen again.

For the woman, the actions of the circumcised penis aren't consistently smooth and harmonious; instead, there are occasional or numerous interruptive jolts, which can disrupt her ascent to orgasm. In *How To Have An Orgasm...As Often As You Want*, Rachel Swift emphasizes that, "A man's failure to maintain a consistent and acceptable rhythm is one of the chief causes of a woman's failure to climax.... [A] consistent rhythm...is critical. If the pace is broken, so is the ascent to orgasm" (14).

9

Why Does the Circumcised Man Thrust Hard or Bang and Pound Away?

> **My circumcised husband was totally engrossed in satisfying his own sexual needs; therefore, he pounded and banged as if he were having intercourse with a non-feeling person.**
>
> —A.J., survey respondent

Bang-away thrusting is evidently a familiar scene in many American bedrooms. Naura Hayden, author of the multi-million-selling book, *How to Satisfy a Woman Every Time*, refers to it as "The Big Bang" and describes it this way:

> He got her excited with foreplay. She's burning up with desire, and as soon as he enters her and starts pumping, she's turned off. That wonderful, excited feeling, that glow all over her body, that tingling in her sex organs, vanishes. Why? Because he's doing his BIG BANG number. In and out, in and out—Bang Bang. He doesn't realize it doesn't feel good to her. It doesn't always hurt at first, but it sure doesn't feel terrific. And after a while of being 'banged,' it does hurt, and she wishes he would get it over with fast!
>
> If you men would just try this experiment, you'd

understand exactly what it feels like. Put your left arm out and with your right fist hit your left arm for about thirty seconds (the longer you do it, the more it hurts). I did this on several TV shows to show the male hosts what 'banging' feels like, and they were amazed. They had no idea that that's what happens when a man enters a woman and starts pumping (1).

When the base of the penis [pubic mound] rams against the clitoris, the woman initially feels pain (which makes her tense up), then her whole sexual area loses all feeling.... At first it hurts, then it gets sort of numb and loses feeling (2). ...[T]he woman, not knowing what he's doing wrong (but absolutely knowing it's all wrong!), pretends finally to have an orgasm because she knows that the way he's doing it she'll *never* have one, and she wants to get the whole thing over with to end the boredom and/or pain (3). ...[S]he's [left feeling]...*very* frustrated, unhappy, and unsatisfied...(4). ...[N]ever dreaming it could possibly be...[the] man's ineptness, these women all think they are, or thought they were, 'frigid' (5).

When women of the *Sex As Nature Intended It* survey were asked about the thrusting action of circumcised men, 72% agreed that "they tend to pound and bang away." Below are some representative comments:

> **"Circumcised men are rough and they tend to 'pound away' at me."**
>
> **"With circumcised intercourse, too many times it was just two sets of genitals banging away at each other detached."**
>
> **"With circumcised men, I wanted to get it over with. Especially with a new guy or a short relationship, it sometimes felt like just 'banging' away."**

"After circumcised thrusting, I'm exhausted from the prolonged, pounding thrusts."

"ALRIGHT! Thank you, yes. Absolutely. I'd never thought about this configuration of experiences, but I do have to agree. Banging is the word. Awful. I agree with all of it."

This banging action of the circumcised penis is obvious in adult sex videos. During these videos, if you watch the woman's breasts closely as she is being sexed, the rippling waves and movement of her breasts register the shock of every jarring thrust.

Why would circumcision cause a man to bang away during intercourse? The following explanations may provide some insight into this problem.

THE ABSENCE OF THE FRENULUM

The bang-away thrusting motions of the circumcised penis are related, in part, to its missing frenulum.

> I am a 30-year-old engineer...in India, and I am a Hindu [uncircumcised].... I became obsessed with looking at circumcised penises.... In recent years of world travel, I have been to practically all countries of the world and observed hundreds of penises from every race. I have seen the results of various circumcision methods, but only in the United States do I see penises which have been entirely stripped of the frenulum (6).

Dorland's Illustrated Medical Dictionary defines the word "frenulum" as "...a small fold of integument [skin]...that *checks, curbs, or limits the movements of an organ or part.*" (Emphasis added)

On the natural penis, the foreskin and penis head are connected by the frenulum's stretchable hinge of skin. (See Figure 4-1, p.55.) *The frenulum serves to make the man's thrusts more gentle by "telling" the penis not to thrust forward with a hard, forceful action, because if the ultrasensitive frenulum is jerked on forcefully, it overstretches, creating a discomforting pulling sensation.* Try this experiment. Thrust your tongue fully forward quickly and forcefully. This will give you an idea of the feeling, because the tongue, too, has a frenulum that attaches it to the bottom of the mouth. In much the same way, the frenulum of the foreskin acts to discourage the intact man from putting too much force behind his forward thrust, making him a gentler lover. One survey respondent stated it this way: **"The natural penis has a softer, smoother feel. Less hard thrusts are necessary. He seemed a gentler man."**

In contrast, most circumcised penises don't have a frenulum because it is usually removed during the circumcision surgery. Even if some remnant of the frenulum is left, *it will lack the frenulum's tugging alert feature* because it is no longer hinged to the foreskin. Because the circumcised penis lacks this mechanism to regulate its forward thrust, it allows the circumcised man to pile drive his penis into the vagina and bang his base/pubic mound/pelvic area against the woman's genitals, pubic mound/pelvic area with unrestrained force. (Again, watching a few adult videos makes this bang-away action of the circumcised penis obvious.)

WHY THE CIRCUMCISED MAN FINDS BANGING PLEASURABLE

> [One sexual] researcher noted...that several of these men masturbated in an odd manner...(as in one case)...getting...pleasure by striking the shaft of...[the] penis forcefully with the heel of the hand... (7).

Why does the circumcised penis find this pounding and banging pleasurable? Because it activates pleasurable sensations in the pressure-sensitive nerves, found in abundance interspersed amongst the muscle cells of the clitoral tissue of the penis base/pubic mound/pelvic area (the region where the musculature branches into two tracts). (See Figure 8-1, page 135.)

In this lower region of the clitoral musculature, the pressure of rhythmic pounding creates sexual excitement and brings on contractions in the genital musculature that ultimately induce orgasm. Contractions that should, however, be brought about by the foreskin's titillation of the *tip* of the clitoral musculature.

Essentially, the circumcised penis bangs its base area against the woman's genital region to make up for the pleasuring it isn't experiencing in its upper area due to its missing foreskin. It finds forceful banging pleasurable for two reasons: 1) banging causes many nerves to fire off simultaneously; 2) many nerves in the base area are deeply set, so strong, forceful pressuring is required to incite them. *The circumcised penis's use of an elongated stroke adds greater force to its banging action* because of the momentum it builds up by withdrawing far out of the vagina and then pile-driving itself inward. Below is a letter I received from a man circumcised *in adulthood*:

> **Since I had my penis circumcised: 1) I have lost about 80% of my penis's sensitivity. 2) I have no response to my wife's vaginal movements. 3) I take so long to reach orgasm that I irritate my wife's vagina, even though we use lots of lubricant. 4) She complains that my penis often feels hard and painful now that it lacks the soft skin folds of the foreskin. 5) My wife can only reach orgasm now with her own hand stimulating her clitoris.**
>
> **I will add just a bit more, since I'm making such a full confession. In reading over the survey questionnaire you sent to my wife, I can see the probable truth in some of the statements. *You are***

quite right in saying that in sexual intercourse, circumcised men are more rough and tend to pound or bang away, using long thrusts. I have found this ever increasingly true about my style, since being circumcised. This is because I now have so little sensitivity and thus no build-up of feeling or response during intercourse that I just pound harder and faster in a desperate hope of reaching orgasm. (Emphasis added)

Every circumcised male may not always need to bang or pound away at his partner's genital region to derive pleasure and reach orgasm (this will depend on several factors, including the tightness of his circumcision and how much frenulum tissue remains). But in theory, virtually every circumcised male prefers strong, hard pressuring against his middle/lower shaft and pubic/pelvic area. To apply this hard pressuring, they tense up the muscles in their abdomen and thighs and then drive forward. When they do, the woman can feel the difference in power even though the penis only travels a few inches. It may seem difficult to believe that the muscle force driving a thrusting penis could make that much of a difference to a woman, but think about this for a moment. In boxing, an uppercut punch travels about the same distance no matter who delivers it, yet whose uppercut would you rather be on the receiving end of, Pee Wee Herman's or Mike Tyson's?

A FURTHER CLARIFICATION OF THE DIFFERENCE BETWEEN NATURE'S WAY OF SEXUALLY EXCITING THE PENIS AND CIRCUMCISION'S WAY

The penises of intact and circumcised men share the same common objectives of creating pleasure sensations for the brain and inducing contractions in the clitoral musculature, which bring on orgasm, but they go about it in different ways and at different locations on the penis.

Here is a comparative example showing how the two kinds of sexing work.

For the moment, imagine that your penis is a leg, with your foot being the upper area of the penis and your leg being the middle-shaft and lower-base area. If someone tickled the bottom of your foot (upper penis), you would feel sensations in your foot, and soon your leg muscle (penis's clitoral musculature) would tighten up (contract). In this case, contraction of the muscle would be brought about by titillating stimuli, and the focal point of stimulation and feeling would be in your foot (the upper penis). This is how nature's method works to sexually excite the clitoral musculature. The mechanical actions of the foreskin create pleasurable sensations in the upper penis while simultaneously producing chemical and electrical actions, which titillate the clitoral muscle cells into contracting. Like the tickling of your foot, the natural penis's method of bringing about muscle contractions and arousal is indirect, subtle, and gentle.

If, on the other hand, someone were to bang a fist repeatedly against your leg muscle (middle shaft/lower base of the penis), here again, your leg muscle would tighten up (contract). But in this case, the contractions would be brought about by forceful pressuring, and the focal point of stimulation and feeling would be in your leg (penis shaft/base). Circumcised thrusting works in a similar manner. It uses strong, hard pressuring (by jamming the penis shaft against the vaginal walls and opening, and/or banging the penis base/pelvic region against the woman's genitals and genital region) to induce sexual sensations and rhythmic contractions in the clitoral muscle cells. In comparison to natural thrusting, circumcised thrusting isn't indirect, subtle, or gentle at all, but is instead blunt, direct, and forceful.

For the woman on the receiving end, the experience described above can range from mildly discomforting, to rough to the point of being violent. Many women in the survey were able to notice these characteristic traits of circumcised thrusting when they commented on the differences between natural and circumcised sex:

> "Natural men can be more gentle and sensitive. Circumcised intercourse seems to have a more aggressive pattern."

> "My husband is circumcised. He's careful not to hurt me, but I know other women have problems with men thrusting too hard. I've made love with only two natural men and both were very sensuous, their thrusting very loving and gentle. I like that feeling."

> "The natural man has more intense feelings at the head of his penis, and he tends not to 'cram' and 'bang,' which makes the woman's experience much better also."

> "The natural man tends to be more sensitive. It was a gentler, more sensuous overall experience. He was far more aware of my experience as well as his. Also his thrusting was of a more sensitive/sensual motion, whereas the circumcised man tends to need more of a rougher stimulus to achieve orgasm."

> "My ex-boyfriend, who was circumcised, seemed desperate to achieve orgasm and would thrust quite violently, occasionally making me bleed. He always felt bad about it, but it would happen again."

Could all this rough, tough thrusting, and banging and pounding, cause some circumcised men to think of the woman's body as little more than a masturbating object, since the sex act loses its significance as a soft, gentle intermingling of two organs joined together in a blissful state of sensuous sexual union? Could it cause some men to view their female sex partners as insensitive, "harder" physical specimens, thus causing them to lose regard for how softly delicate the female body really is? Could it cause some circumcised men to make an association between hitting and pleasure, between violence and sexual stimulation? I will leave this for others to debate, but I am sure of this: Circumcised sex does not promote the same communion of warmth and love between a couple that natural sex does. This is evidenced by the following composite of survey comments from one woman, which answers, in such a beautiful way, the question: Could the presence or absence of a foreskin have an influence on how a woman feels emotionally about a man during and after their lovemaking experience?

> **My natural man arrived after being with circumcised men. I have had no relations with circumcised men since I met my current natural lover, but the difference is very obvious to me.**
>
> **All my circumcised men seemed too anxious to reach their own orgasms and too caught up in getting their own pleasure. And they often left me unsatisfied leaving me irritable, aggravated, and frustrated as hell.**
>
> **Circumcised men are more rough and they tend to 'pound away' at me. With them, I seldom achieved orgasm. During circumcised intercourse, it always felt like there were two sexual experiences going on—his and mine. It was never making love—it was only 'fucking.' I often felt used—leaving me feeling blue.**
>
> **My natural man is very tender, passionate, and loving. Sex is more relaxed, mellow, and gentle with him than with circumcised men. My natural man takes more time. I could make love with him for hours (and sometimes do). He is softer and gentler than circumcised ones were. *With circumcised intercourse, my noises and utterings sounded painful because it was close to painful at times!* With a natural lover, it is more cooing, purring, and sounds of contentment that come from inside one.**

> My natural partner is more sensitive, but I tend to think it is because he has a natural penis—hence he is more delicate—he is more in touch with his penis, and his penis is more in touch with his heart.
>
> When my natural man is inside me, he moves more smoothly, more gently, which is what I need. Also, a natural penis feels more filling and seems to have an extra gliding sensation inside me. My current natural lover is usually in close physical contact with me, adding to the feeling of intimacy.
>
> I usually have multiple orgasms with my natural partner but not with circumcised partners. My natural man gives me more frequent, powerful, all-encompassing orgasms. On a scale of 1-10, my natural orgasms rate a 12. With my natural partner, I can relax and enjoy, knowing it will lead to orgasm.
>
> After intercourse with my natural partner, I am much more relaxed, peaceful, fulfilled—brimming over with contentment. Bedtime sex often leaves me purring in my sleep and needing an early morning quickie before we get up. The afterglow can last for most of the day, making me horny for him that night. (Emphasis added)

This woman was obviously sexually happier with her natural partner than with her previous circumcised partners. And we can reasonably assume that she was experiencing immeasurably more emotional fulfillment too, and that this played a role in causing her to look upon him with more "loving eyes." This woman's comments illustrate what I was trying to say in Chapters 3 and 8A: If a woman is receiving "good loving," she will tend to be far more appreciative of the man and look upon him more favorably, in general. She will be more inclined to overlook his little faults, confirming the old adage that "love is blind." In this regard, happiness and compatibility in the bedroom tend to lead to a happier relationship overall.

THE GENTLENESS OF NATURAL INTERCOURSE

Women of the survey consistently remarked that when the man had a natural penis, intercourse was a much gentler experience. Below are several typical comments:

> "Natural intercourse was a gentler, more sensuous overall experience."

> "Natural intercourse is gentler sex, nicer thrusting."

> "Enjoyment for the natural man is concentrated in the frenulum, according to my lover. I think that the slow, easy movements enjoyed with natural men are wonderful and that circumcised men, who had this removed, need that hard, 'used as a masturbating object' kind of movement to reach orgasm."

> "With natural men the sensation is gentler and simply more erotic. Gentler entry, gentler thrusting, gentler movements altogether. It is a *comforting* movement...also a richer, more erotic experience evoking greater pleasure in me." (Emphasis added)

The magical effects of the foreskin cause a woman to perceive intercourse as gentler for several reasons. It is gentler because the foreskin is a delicate and sensitive tissue; thus it favors gentler intercourse movements. Also, the other erogenous zones in the upper area are so exquisitely sensitive, they only need easy motions to excite them. Further, it is gentler because the penis uses shorter strokes, which require less muscle force behind them. And it is gentler because of the foreskin's cushioning effect. These and other reasons have been previously explained. However, one important factor, which has not yet been mentioned, is how the natural man uses his body to thrust his penis more gently.

I have observed repeatedly in adult videos that the intact man typically thrusts his penis by using the muscles in his legs, primarily his thigh muscles, rather than his hips. He tends to keep his hips straight in line with his back and legs; then he rocks his body gently back and forth from the joints of his knees. *This results in a straight-on, gentler stroke for the vagina.*

In contrast, adult videos show that the circumcised man typically thrusts his penis by pulling his hips back with his buttocks and then swinging them forward abruptly. He pulls back smoothly, but he rams forward with a jolting action that angles the penis upward instead of straight on. He uses this technique to increase *his* pleasure, because it applies quick, intense pressure to the deeply set pressure-sensitive nerves of the lower clitoris, located at the base of the penis where the clitoris branches into two tracts (Figure 8-1, page 135). If you watch a few adult videos yourself, this characteristic of circumcised sex will become obvious. Here are three representative comments from the survey:

> **"Most circumcised men slam hard and women respond hard."**

> **"Circumcised man uses hard thrusts, like a battering ram, which desensitize my clitoris."**

> **"It's important not to make them [circumcised men] feel inadequate. Some men can compensate for a lack of a foreskin by being caring, affectionate, sensitive—and by being patient during intercourse and doing what they can to limit *their need for fast, hard pumping.*"** (Emphasis added)

In order to swing his hips forward with a quick, forceful movement, the circumcised man tightens up his abdominal muscles into a hardened mass, and when he swings his pelvic area forward forcefully against her pubic area, it is not a pleasant experience for the woman.

In contrast, when the intact man thrusts, he keeps his abdominal muscles relatively relaxed and rocks his body from his knee joints, using primarily his leg muscles. It is much easier and more relaxing to rock the body from the knees than it is to jerk the hips back and forth, as does the circumcised man. The intact man's rocking thrusts need very little muscle force behind them, resulting in an infinitely gentler experience for the woman.

IT ALL ADDS UP TO TWO DIFFERENT EXPERIENCES FOR THE WOMAN

Adding it up from this and the preceding chapter, it comes to this: The circumcised man's upper penis erogenous zones just don't fire off enough pleasure sensations to excite him sufficiently. As a result, his attention shifts to the middle/lower penis area, where he derives more pleasure, especially when he applies strong, hard pressuring directly to the penis shaft by pressing against the vaginal opening. He thrusts with elongated strokes in order to give the sensory nerves of his middle/lower penis a longer rest/recharge time. These elongated strokes cause his pubic mound to make less frequent contact with the woman's clitoral mound, and she finds them out of sync with the stroking rhythm she desires. In effect, the "instinctive" thrusting rhythm of the circumcised penis that feels "right" for the man, feels "unnatural" to the woman. Moreover, when his pubic mound does make contact with her clitoral mound, it often does so with a slamming pound, or bang, due to its missing frenulum and the male's desire to use strong pressure to incite the lower clitoral musculature into contractions that build up to orgasm. As a result, the woman's clitoral area does not get the "natural," gentle pressuring it wants and needs, and too often the woman is jolted out of whatever relaxing, pleasant feelings she might be experiencing.

The natural penis, on the other hand, derives its pleasure primarily from one erogenous zone—the upper penis—and it thrusts in a consistent pattern that rhythmically stimulates this area using a gentle, smooth, rocking motion that rhythmically mesmerizes both partners into a trance-like state of sexual ecstasy. *Since this rocking motion is so easy to maintain, the man can keep it going without tiring, and this leaves both partners free to relax and float on the waves of pleasurable feelings it creates.* This mutually shared rhythm puts the bodies, minds, and emotions of both lovers on the same wavelength, and they perceive sex as a shared experience. The high level of physical pleasure and heartfelt emotion created in the bodies and minds of both partners wells up inside them as a feeling of love. And it is this feeling of love and closeness that helps to bond them together as one. Below are some typical comments from survey respondents:

> "I have *never* been more connected on physical, mental, and emotional levels than I was with this natural partner."

> "I am now in a relationship with a natural man and we are getting married in two months. He is overall wonderful, but I base a lot of my emotions about him on our lovemaking. We have a fabulous sex life. Lovemaking with him is more pleasurable than any of my circumcised experiences. I was married for 10 years to a circumcised man and never enjoyed sex."

> "All of my experiences with the natural man were positive. He was so in sync with my body, his penis actually seems connected to my inner being."

> "The natural man seems more 'like me' in the way his body functions sexually—there's more *synchronicity* in the stages of arousal and completion with one of these men. Definitely a different experience."

> "Natural lovemaking is a complete experience—physically, emotionally, psychologically, sexually...I feel more connected to an uncircumcised man."

> "After sex with my natural partner, I find the afterglow is very pleasant. I feel a mild, warm, sensual awareness and even days later I will remember the experience and refeel that same afterglow for a few moments."

"DAMMIT!" YOU CURSE

If you are a circumcised man, you may have, by now, reluctantly resigned yourself to accepting the idea that your circumcision is a problem for your female partner, even though you may not think it is a problem for yourself—or you might still want to deny it. You might confront your wife or lover and insist that she tell you that nothing is wrong with your lovemaking. You are angry. And understandably so.

When you confront her, she is afraid to tell you the truth, afraid to tell you that sex isn't all it's cracked up to be for her and that it may even be discomforting—she doesn't want to hurt your feelings. Besides, she's never had sex with a man with a natural penis, so she doesn't really know what "real" sex is all about. When you confront her, she may tell you that everything's okay, because she doesn't want to jeopardize the relationship, the marriage, the kids. She is a little (or a lot) afraid of how you'll react. She doesn't want to admit to you, or herself, that anything is wrong. She looks at you and says it's silly, it's stupid, of course you're a wonderful lover. But she's only kidding herself, and somewhere in the back of her mind she knows it. And somewhere in the back of your mind, your subconscious tells you that you know it too.

You aren't really happy with the tone of the answers she's giving you. Dammit!—you're going to take her to bed right now!

You're going to prove to her that you are the sexual man of her dreams. She Ooos, she Ahhs (or rather, she Aghhs in a guttural tone and volume that reflects pain and pleasure combined, not like the soothing, soulful, lustful, low-pitched, relaxed moans of natural sex). But by now you can sense it—something is missing. She's not really and truly getting off on your sexing, and you're not really and truly getting off on her response. You become aggravated and more angry. Something *is* missing. "Dammit!" you curse, "What a fucking bummer! Why the fuck was my foreskin ever cut off in the first place?"

There is nothing I could ever say that could console you right now. As a woman, I can never know the emotional pain you are experiencing and may continue to experience until you have come to terms with this dreadful truth, and come to the realization that restoration is the only solution. But, if it is any consolation, remember, millions of men will be going through this with you.

10

It's Over in a Flash!
But What If It Lasts?
And Desire Deficiency: Hers, His

> I was born and raised in France. It is not common over there to circumcise little boys. All of my early sexual experiences were with natural men, but when I was twenty, I did have one boyfriend who was American and circumcised. Sex was okay, but intercourse never lasted very long. He wanted to have sex all the time, but only 'quickies.' At that time, I believed that his way of making love was a personality thing and not a matter of being circumcised or not.
>
> About 8 years later, I came to the United States, met my husband, who is also circumcised, and got married.... I have had very few experiences where intercourse with a circumcised man lasts longer than 5 minutes. But even when intercourse lasts...I often just don't get excited. Intercourse seems to be not much fun with a circumcised man. With a natural man, even if I didn't feel like sex, I often would get right into it when I felt that sensuous penis inside me.
>
> — M.T., survey respondent

Could circumcision be a contributing factor in premature ejaculation, and if so, why? Conversely, could it cause a man to take excessively long to reach orgasm, discomforting his partner?

Could the circumcised penis cause a woman to want to shorten the length of time a man spends in active coital thrusting? Could it have a negative effect on how frequently a woman, or man, desires intercourse?

One of the startling discoveries that came out of the survey was that premature ejaculation was significantly more common among circumcised men. Surveyed women were asked to indicate the number of men who usually (50-100% of the time) had their orgasm within 2-3 minutes after insertion. A much higher percentage of circumcised men fell into this category than natural. This was surprising because the circumcised penis lacks the erogenous sensitivity of the natural penis, as discussed. (See Appendix B for my suggestion on how to minimize or eliminate premature ejaculation, and the "tap me" secret to prolonging intercourse.)

The survey's statistics for both types of penises are detailed in Chapter 13, but for now, let us consider the reasons why circumcision might contribute to premature ejaculation. (The following detailed discussion about premature ejaculation may not interest all readers. Some may want to skip to the section entitled, A SHORT INTERCOURSE MAY LEAVE A WOMAN LONGING FOR MORE, BUT IF SHE WERE TO GET PROLONGED CIRCUMCISED INTERCOURSE, WOULD SHE FIND IT DESIRABLE?, page 181.

CIRCUMCISED MEN MAY BE MORE PRONE TO
PREMATURE EJACULATION
DUE TO HISTAMINE RELEASE

Circumcised intercourse may often be over in a 2-3 minute "flash" because the penis head receives too much direct stimulation, which causes it to release too much histamine too soon.

The release of histamine into the bloodstream during sexual excitation is essential for bringing about orgasm.

Histamine causes smooth-muscle tissue (as found in the penile clitoral and ejaculatory muscles) to contract, and these contractions lead to orgasm. Histamine is evidenced during sexual excitation by the red flushing (blushing) it often produces in the face, neck, shoulders, chest, etc. (1)(2).

In the 1970s, Carl Pfeiffer, Ph.D., M.D., along with scientists at the Princeton Bio Center in Princeton, New Jersey, discovered that cells in the penis head test high in stored histamine (3). Dr. Pfeiffer states in his book, *Mental and Elemental Nutrients*:

> [T]he ability to attain orgasm or ejaculation with sex or masturbation is directly correlated with the level of blood histamine and perhaps with the level of tissue histamine.
>
> Microscopic examination of the penis from autopsy specimens discloses mast cells containing histamine are concentrated in the glans but not in the skin of the shaft or the foreskin of the penis. A collection of objective reports from twenty-eight male...patients shows that the quickness of ejaculation is significantly correlated with the blood histamine level.
>
> This indicates that ejaculation may be a local reflex which is activated by the disruption of mast cells [in which histamine is stored] and liberation of histamine.... With excess histamine, the clinical phenomenon known as 'premature ejaculation' may occur (4).

The rubbing action that the circumcised penis head receives from scraping against the corrugated ribbings of the vaginal walls during intercourse causes histamine to be released from the penis head *in overabundance and too quickly*. This could be why many circumcised men ejaculate prematurely.

But for the **natural** penis, during the outward stroke, the foreskin bunches up behind the coronal ridge, or rolls over onto the penis head, and applies a soft, cushioned pressure against the more pliable glans, which activates a *moderate* release of histamine. In contrast, as the unprotected corona/coronal ridge of the **circumcised** penis scrapes against the wavy ridges of the vaginal walls, it receives *strong* pressuring, which activates a greater release of histamine.

Squeezing or rubbing any body tissue that is high in stored histamine will activate its release. Like the penis head, the nose is also high in stored histamine. If you were to repeatedly squeeze or rub your nose (like when you have a cold), it would turn red, an indication that histamine has been released. Hard, vigorous rubbing causes more histamine to be released than light, gentle rubbing.

Friction irritation is an indication that vigorous rubbing has taken place. Surveyed women commented on the discomfort of friction build-up experienced during circumcised intercourse.

> "Circumcised intercourse feels like a friction burn—sometimes even with heavy lubrication."

> "With my circumcised partners, I experienced irritation of the vagina because of the friction when sex was too dry."

> "With natural, I didn't get sore—there was no friction against me."

Friction triggers the release of histamine. Histamine has chemical actions that induce rhythmic contractions in the smooth (pubococcygeal) muscles that control the ejaculatory reflex. If too much histamine is released too quickly in the circumcised penis, the ejaculatory muscles may be hurried into ejaculating prematurely.

Intact men are not, of course, exempt from the possibility of having premature ejaculations. As Dr. Pfeiffer states, any man whose penis head tests high in stored histamine can be prone to premature ejaculation. But I suspect that this problem can be a consequence of not only high levels of stored histamine, but also too rapid release of even moderate levels of stored histamine, which I surmise is the case during circumcised thrusting. Since the survey results indicate that premature ejaculation occurs significantly more often among circumcised men, I suspect it occurs *not* because they all have higher levels of stored histamine than intact men, but because the circumcised penis lacks the foreskin's mediating actions, which work to administer a more gradual release of histamine, thus permitting the intact man to better pace his build-up to orgasm.

OVER-RELIANCE ON STIMULATING PRESSURE-SENSITIVE NERVES AS A POSSIBLE CAUSE FOR WHY PREMATURE EJACULATION IS MORE COMMON WITH THE CIRCUMCISED PENIS

The circumcised penis over-relies on exciting pressure-sensitive nerves to generate pleasurable feelings. During coital thrusting, the natural and circumcised penis both generate pleasurable feelings, but the source of these feelings comes from essentially two different kinds of tactile nerves.

Scientists have established that there are different types of touch-sensitive nerves. These nerves differ in their cellular structure and in their response to tactile stimulation (5). Tactile nerves can be grouped into two major categories, either conveying 1) *touch* sensations or 2) *pressure* sensations—*the distinction being that sustained touch (and/or bearing down) is considered pressure.*

Tactile nerves of the touch-sensation category are found on the skin or immediately beneath the skin. Try this simple experiment. Run a moistened finger *lightly* over your lower lip. Feel the erogenous sensations. Your lip abounds with touch-sensitive nerves. Now *press* your finger down on your lower lip. Notice that there is an absence of feeling. Your lower lip is deficient in pressure-sensitive nerves.

Try an inverse experiment. Run your finger lightly on the

inside of your cheek. Notice the lack of feeling. This surface is devoid of touch-sensitive nerves. However, if you push your finger hard against your inner cheek, you can feel that it does contain pressure-sensitive nerves.

The erogenous nerves of the foreskin's inner lining and frenulum are of this touch-sensitive category (not the pressure-sensitive category) and are designed to perceive light touch. These nerves are also discriminative, having the ability to recognize the precise point where the body is touched. This is one of the reasons why the intact man senses that most of his pleasure sensations come from the localized area of the upper penis.

The foreskin and frenulum are composed of specialized flexible connective tissue. A study published by the Mayo Clinic, "Erogenous Zones: Their Nerve Supply and Its Significance," found that on skin areas where erotic sensations registered high (like the ridged band, the lips, nipples, fingertips, and tip of the tongue) "...the rete ridges [i.e., the connective meshwork that comprises this flexible tissue] are well formed, and more of the organized nerve tissue rises higher [i.e., closer to the skin's surface] than in other skin-type regions" (6). Also in the erogenous connective skin, there is a preponderance of touch-sensitive nerves, especially a type called Meissner's corpuscles, (7) "which respond in a fraction of a second to contact with light objects that bring about deformation of their capsules" (8). *Most of the erogenous sensations felt in the foreskin, ridged band, and frenulum originate with these touch-sensitive nerves (especially Meissner's corpuscles) (9). The natural penis derives significant pleasure by thrusting to stimulate these touch-sensitive nerves.*

In comparison, the circumcised penis is missing the touch-type nerves of the foreskin and frenulum. Therefore, it thrusts primarily to stimulate pleasure sensations from pressure-responsive nerves, called Pacinian corpuscles, which are located in the deeper tissues of the penis (10)—within the penile clitoral musculature and other muscles of the pelvic region. Pressure-sensitive nerves have weak discriminative ability, and this is one of the reasons why the circumcised man thrusts to stimulate the entire penis rather than a localized area. Pressure-sensitive nerves, also, are poor at registering subtle changes in tactile force; this is why he bears down more forcefully on his strokes.

In physiology, there is a characteristic of muscles known as Trousseau's phenomenon, which states that "spasmodic contractions occur in muscles when pressure is applied to the nerves which go to them" (11). In other words, *when pressure is applied to a pressure-sensitive nerve in a muscle, it leads directly to spasmodic contractions in that muscle.*

In light of this phenomenon, it makes sense that the stimulation of many pressure-responsive nerves of a muscle will lead to many contractions in that muscle. As discussed in previous chapters, low-level, but frequent, contractions in the genital musculature help to bring on orgasm. I deduce that during the beginning phase of intercourse, when the nerves and muscles are fresh and fully-primed, the circumcised penis's propensity for using a strong-pressing, elongated stroke to elicit pleasure sensations from its pressure-responsive nerves causes a rapid build-up in muscle contractions. Once involuntary contractions begin accelerating in a muscle, they are difficult to stop (as anyone who has ever had a leg cramp knows). Exciting many pressure-sensitive nerves in the genital musculature can quickly accelerate contractions to the point where the man cannot stop them. And because pressure-sensitive nerves lack the ability to register subtle changes, the man doesn't realize until it's too late that he has gone over the edge into premature ejaculation.

In contrast, for the natural penis, the nerves of the frenulum and foreskin are not pressure-sensitive nerves but, instead, are touch-sensitive (primarily Meissner's corpuscles). Stimulating these touch-responsive nerves causes them to send out feelings of pleasure, *but exciting them does not simultaneously lead to a quick build-up of muscle contractions.* Certainly, over a sustained period of stimulation, exciting these nerves will cause contractions in the tip of the (male) clitoral muscle, but the mode of action is more indirect (as previously explained) and works on a different principle than the muscle contractions of pressure-sensitive nerves in the lower genital region. Consequently, the natural penis experiences an intense degree of pleasure when the upper penis nerves are stimulated, but muscle contractions in the genital/pelvic region build up more slowly. *In essence, the natural penis experiences a higher ratio of pleasure sensations to subsequent muscle contractions; whereas, when the circumcised man attempts to approach these same levels of feeling by stimulating the pressure-sensitive nerves in the middle and lower penis/pubic mound/pelvic area with a hard-pressuring, elongated stroke, the accompanying muscle contractions accelerate too quickly, rushing him uncontrollably into a speedy ejaculation.*

THE EXPOSED FRENULUM THEORY

Another possible explanation for premature ejaculation may be related to remnants of the frenulum left permanently exposed. Although the frenulum is removed during most American-style circumcisions, for some circumcised men, part of it may remain. For those men, this ultra-sensitive frenulum remnant is permanently exposed during coital thrusting, causing the penis to become overexcited too quickly, resulting in premature ejaculation. (During natural intercourse, the frenulum is covered over by the foreskin during the penis's outward stroke.)

A SHORT INTERCOURSE MAY LEAVE A WOMAN LONGING FOR MORE, BUT IF SHE WERE TO GET PROLONGED CIRCUMCISED INTERCOURSE, WOULD SHE FIND IT DESIRABLE?

Like a man, a woman, too, desires the relief of orgasm, but 2-3 minutes of intercourse is usually not enough time for her to achieve one. An abbreviated intercourse may leave her feeling unsatisfied, with a craving for additional sexual stimulation. Of course, not all circumcised men ejaculate prematurely; some are capable of lasting for a considerable time. One would think that when the man can last, the woman would like this. But one of the astonishing revelations of the survey was that when women actually did get extended circumcised thrusting, they began wishing "to just get it over with."

Women were asked the following question:

Of your CIRCUMCISED experiences, where the time of ACTUAL intercourse lasted for 8-10 minutes or more, as intercourse progressed,

Did you OFTEN start wishing to just get it over with?   Yes No

— OR —

Did you OFTEN really get into it and want it to continue? Yes No

An astounding 70% of surveyed women indicated that *for circumcised*, they *OFTEN wished to just get it over with*.

In contrast, when this same question was asked of their *natural* experiences, the opposite was true; the vast majority of them, **91%**, *indicated that they really get into it and want it to continue*.

We can deduce from the above that there must be something about circumcised intercourse that interferes with the wonderful experience nature intended, causing a woman to want to get it over with, even though the man may be capable of prolonged intercourse.

The following comment is from a woman who speaks from a unique vantage point because her husband underwent foreskin restoration. She had the opportunity to compare, not *different* men, but the *same* man, before and after his restoration, and here is what she noticed:

> **My husband acquired Jim Bigelow's book [*The Joy of Uncircumcising!*] and completed an uncircumcising procedure [foreskin restoration].... We both appreciate the control and staying power his more abundant foreskin gives him. What I was totally unprepared for was the physical difference I experienced. I began to notice that I no longer experienced any soreness, even with prolonged intercourse. This was something I had lived with all of my adult life, although I used lubricants...(12).**

Essentially, for many women, circumcised intercourse is a let-down from two perspectives: Too often it is over before the woman has a chance to get into it, and even when it does last, she often finds it displeasurable or unarousing, and she may even find it discomforting or painful. This dilemma was stated best by the woman from France, whose story begins this chapter:

> **I have had very few experiences where intercourse with a circumcised man lasts longer than 5 minutes. But even when intercourse lasts...I often just don't get excited.**

And as another survey respondent commented:

> **I often experienced discomfort with my circumcised husband, at which point I would usually try to hurry him along, first physically and if that didn't work, verbally.**

A woman may innately desire a prolonged intercourse (at least 8-10 minutes or more of thrusting), but apparently this leads to a problem during circumcised sex. For when she is in the process of getting it, her vagina simultaneously tells her that she is no longer enjoying the circumcised penis's thrusts because of the various displeasureable or discomforting factors discussed in previous chapters. A woman may be dissatisfied with the 2- to 3-minute man, but on the other hand, when she does receive prolonged circumcised thrusting, she often begins wishing to "just get it over with." With circumcised sex, it seems to be a case of "damned when you don't get enough, and damned when you do."

PARADOXICALLY, THE CIRCUMCISED PENIS MAY TAKE TOO LONG TO REACH ORGASM

Forty-two percent (42%) of the survey respondents indicated that their circumcised partners had to work too hard at achieving orgasm. Below is a typical comment:

> **All I know is that with circumcised men, it's generally harder to bring them to climax, which can take the joy and closeness from the encounter, leaving me feeling frustrated and unsatisfied.**

Previous chapters touched on the idea that some circumcised men have considerable difficulty achieving orgasm and that it takes them too long. (*Be sure to check out my suggestion in Appendix C on how to hasten the man's orgasm, when desired.*)

The many reasons for the above have been discussed throughout the book, involving the desensitization of the penis and the resultant abnormalization of the sex act. When the circumcised man can't come when he wants to, and thrusting becomes too prolonged, it can be stressful. And as intercourse progresses, one or both partners may find it discomforting, or even painful.

Granted, the concept that one is taking too long to achieve orgasm is relative. But perhaps the thought arises because one or both partners aren't really enjoying themselves during circumcised sex. If they were, instead, experiencing the pure comfort and blissful sensuousness of natural thrusting, they might not perceive the sex act as taking too long at all. They'd be more inclined to get absorbed in it and swept away in passionate eroticism. During natural intercourse, the male may purposefully delay his orgasm to prolong the copulatory pleasure of both partners.

THE CIRCUMCISED PENIS MAY CAUSE DESIRE DEFICIENCY DISORDER

A lack of sexual desire in one's self or one's partner is reportedly the most common complaint that brings people to seek the help of a sex therapist (13). Doctors Knopf and Seiler point out in their book, *Inhibited Sexual Desire:*

> [A] lack of interest in sex, or an inability to feel sexual or get sexually aroused or...desire discrepancies [between partners]...are...very common....
>
> Most sex therapists...will tell you that they see far more patients with...[the above] disorders than any other type of sexual disorder and that these conditions are clearly on the rise nationwide. According to recent research and surveys of the general population, as many as half of all married or cohabiting adults (both male and female) mention their own or their partners' lack of sexual interest when asked about difficulties in their sex lives or relationships (14).

In the countless hours spent in couples counseling, I wonder if anyone has ever thought to question the role that the surgically altered penis may play in desire deficiency disorder (DDD). Considering how extensively it denatures the sex act, how could it not have a detrimental influence on a woman's interest in sexual relations—and a negative impact on a man's interest as well? DDD may be more widespread than we realize because neither men nor women want to publicly acknowledge or personally admit to themselves that they suffer from a lack of sexual desire.

In my own personal experience and that of my husband's, we found that circumcision played a definite role in lessening our sex drive. Before his restoration, we had sex about once a month, but since his restoration, we have it at least once or twice a week, and we are both in our late fifties. Although it is well known that libido diminishes with age, we now have sex about 4 times more frequently than when we were in our 30s. Indeed, before his restoration, both of us had more or less lost interest in intercourse, and sex was almost a chore. But now, sex is infinitely more satisfying and pleasurable for both of us, and we both look forward to our sexual sessions with eager anticipation. And while we're making love, we can't seem to get enough of each other. We both agree that our sex life is better now than when we were first married, more than 25 years ago.

Circumcised sex can create a paradoxical conflict in a person's sexual desire in the following way. Most people eventually find someone to love and settle down with. Since love and sex go together like a hand and glove, over a period of time they have hundreds and hundreds of intercourse experiences with this person. The conscious mind craves sexual stimulation and intimate closeness to one's lover, and it innately expects to find intercourse ecstatically pleasurable and joyfully sensuous. But the circumcised sexual experience doesn't fulfill these conscious desires. Instead, it leaves one hungering for something more—something just out of reach—and it may even be displeasurable.

Over a period of time, the frustration, discomfort, and shortcomings of circumcised sex leave their marks on the conscious and subconscious, and when the primal sex drive sets in and says, "Tonight's the night," something in the back of your mind says, "Why don't we make it tomorrow night or next week instead." The way I see it, sexual desire falls victim to a conflict between the primal sex drive and the disheartening memories the mind has stored from prior unsatisfactory circumcised experiences. Over time, repeated exposures to circumcised intercourse take its toll, manifesting itself in decreased desire for one's partner.

In general, the younger you are, the more successful the conscious mind will be in ignoring the deeply set thoughts of the subconscious. When you are young, your youthful sex hormones are bubbling over with excitement, and you will jump on practically anyone's bones when your sex drive gets strong enough. (I cannot stress enough the importance of age—experience—as a factor in the correlation between DDD and circumcised sex.) Couples in their 20s and 30s may think their sex life is "just fine." They are driven to it—good or bad—by their innate drive for sexual stimulation. But I contend that as time goes on and they subject themselves to repeated circumcised intercourse experiences, their conscious and subconscious minds become more and more aware of the discomfort, frustration, and incompleteness of the act, and they will find themselves desiring sex less and less often.

We must keep in mind that the purpose of sex, besides procreation, is to bond the man and woman together with love. Sex is what connects you back to loving life, and loving and appreciating your partner. Infrequent sex will have a detrimental effect on the love bond.

Since we usually think of *desire deficiency* as a disorder affecting primarily females (the popular myth being that men are always ready, willing, and able), let us consider the woman's perspective. When a woman finds her sexual desire for her partner coming less and less often, she may begin to secretly wonder if something is wrong with her: Is she frigid or something? And yet, if she turns to masturbation, she finds herself capable of sexual arousal and usually has no trouble achieving orgasm, perhaps even two or three orgasms. It makes her wonder when she stops to think about it: Why should she have such a sexual appetite when she stimulates herself and yet have little or no desire for her mate? The circumcised penis could be at the root of the problem. For, with the passage of time, the female's conscious and subconscious register so much negative feedback from her prior exposures to circumcised intercourse, if she even contemplates having sex with her partner, she gets turned off before she can get turned on—"Not tonight, dear, I have a headache." The same thing, of course, may happen to a man, for men, too, suffer from DDD.

Perhaps the following anecdote (a true story) will bring home the point of what I'm trying to say.

At one time, I did a lot of trade shows in New York City and became casually friendly with a man who owned a company that was in direct competition with my company. We sometimes chatted about business and exchanged the usual "Hi, how are you today?" but we didn't really know each other that well. You can imagine my surprise when he came running up to me one morning and said (excitedly), "The most incredible thing happened to me last night! For the first time in our 12-year marriage, my wife and I achieved sexual compatibility." I was a bit taken aback by his open discussion of his private life, but I said, "That's wonderful, Marty, I'm really happy for you." Then he grinned and said, "Yeah, we both got a headache at the same time."

Paradoxically, circumcision may be a factor in causing a man to desire intercourse not less often, *but more often*. The following is another true story: A man *who was circumcised in adulthood* told me that he once masturbated about 25 times over a two-day period. His analysis of the situation was that he just couldn't achieve the same level of satisfaction with circumcised masturbation that he had formerly experienced with his natural penis. After each orgasm, he still felt sexually unsatisfied. He then tried to relieve this dissatisfaction with more masturbation. After 25 times, he still felt sexually unsatisfied but he gave it a rest.

When the foreskin is missing, sexual stimulation from intercourse, and even orgasm, can leave an incomplete message in the pleasure centers of the brain. The brain may then try to compensate for this incompleteness with an excessive desire for intercourse (and/or masturbatory) stimulation. *In this way, the brain attempts to use quantity as a substitute for the quality that it isn't receiving due to the foreskin's absence.* If a man desires intercourse too frequently, it can put a strain on a relationship if the woman does not have the same level of interest, resulting in a certain degree of sexual incompatibility.

An incident from one of Woody Allen's movies comes to mind. Woody is chatting with his psychiatrist and tells him that he and his girlfriend hardly ever have sex, "about two or three times a week." Meanwhile, his girlfriend is at a different psychiatrist telling him that Woody wants sex all the time, "about two or three times a week."

FORESKIN RESTORATION IS THE ONLY REAL SOLUTION

But it doesn't have to be like this for you and the person you love. You don't have to be worlds apart regarding your sexual compatibility. You don't have to live on the morning side of the mattress while your partner lives on the twilight side of the bed. For you, there is a "real" sexual future because The Foreskin Restoration Revolution is here at last, to obliterate the absurdity of what will surely soon be known as the past.

Yes, the "revolution" has already begun, and you can be part of it. Imagine that. In the wink of an eye, just like that, a revolution is about to take place. Right here in America, the good ole U.S. of A.—the land of the free, the home of the brave, and the birthplace of the NOCIRC movement.

If I were you, I'd be in a real hurry to get started on the road to your restoration. "Right away," you say. Good for you! Now you're talking. Soon you'll be hearing those bells and whistles ring.

11

My Personal Story

I grew up in the sexually repressed '50s when society dictated that a woman should save herself for the man she'd marry and be a virgin on her wedding night. It was considered trampy and morally wrong to have sex before marriage. And if you did—so you were told—the guy would immediately lose respect for you and talk to all the other guys about you behind your back. A girl really worried about getting a "bad reputation" in those days. Neighborhoods were more of a close-knit community back then, and if a girl slept with someone, she felt certain that everyone would know about it the next day. Gossip was the neighborhood pastime.

In the mid-'60s, "the pill" came onto the scene to free a woman from the fear of unwanted pregnancy. This kicked off the beginning of the sexual revolution, and sexual mores relaxed considerably. It was just about that time that I fell madly in love with Tom, a married man who was one of my co-workers. To make a long story short, we began an affair that lasted for three years, and lingered on intermittently for another 12.

In retrospect, I feel guilty for having intruded on another woman's territory. But at the time, I was young, naive, and much too much in love to comprehend the reprehensibility of my behavior. And this is not a justification, but if I hadn't had that affair, I wouldn't be writing this book, because Tom had a natural penis, and the men of any consequence who came into my life after him did not.

I saw Tom once a week, and during the time I was involved with him, I also got involved with another man named Mike.

Mike was circumcised. I was about 25 at the time, and like most women of that age, I was hoping to find a great guy to marry and settle down with. In the back of my mind, I realized that my relationship with Tom, the married man, was a dead-end street. I was hoping that Mike could fill his shoes.

Mike lived some distance away, so I only saw him on Wednesday nights and weekends. On average, I was having sex with Tom once a week and twice a week with Mike. It was probably because I was having sex with two different men within a short period of time that I was impacted by the vast difference in both the intercourse experience and my general attitude toward these two men.

With Tom, the natural man, sex was passionate, gentle, softly-smooth, and sensuous—all the wonderful things a woman dreams it should be. When we had sex, I truly wanted it to go on forever and would beg him for more, more, more. Too much was never enough. He knew the exact thrusting rhythms to use, bringing me to indescribable heights of passion and pleasure. Every cell of my body became filled with desire and ecstasy when we touched. I eagerly anticipated our next rendezvous and constantly daydreamed about his sweet, sexy, splendid lovemaking.

In comparison, sex with Mike, the circumcised man, was considerably less pleasurable. His penis felt much too hard and his thrusting actions were uncomfortably bang-away. Our sexual thrusting rhythms were completely out of sync and I always had to tell him, "Please don't do it that way—do it this way." This frustrated me to no end because he didn't seem to be able to get it right no matter how many times I mentioned it—what was naturally pleasing for him wasn't naturally pleasing for me. We were obviously having two separate experiences, his and mine. It definitely lacked a feeling of unison. Sex seemed to be narrowly focused in the genital area, and although my youthful hormones gave me a healthy sex drive, still, I was always glad to get the sexual session over with. I seemed to desire sex with him only to satisfy my own inner craving for sex itself, rather than a desire to experience *him*. Sex with him had a wide-awake, on-alert edge to it and an awareness of my genitals being completely separate from his. The one thing that stands out most in my mind about circumcised intercourse is its complete lack of connectedness—like I was just using his penis as a masturbating object without being emotionally and physically connected to the penis and the person on the other side of it. My vagina seemed to have the attitude, "Let's have our orgasms and get this over with."

But in contrast, when I had sex with Tom, the feeling was dreamy, ecstatically relaxed—both sets of genitals melted into one another—there was no feeling of separateness; I didn't know where my genitals ended and my partner's began—we were one—it was an experience of mutual pleasuring, each giving and receiving, receiving and giving, simultaneously.

My sexual attitude toward Tom was in sharp contrast to my attitude toward Mike. With Tom, I just couldn't get enough, absolutely couldn't get enough of him, but with Mike I seemed to be able to take it or leave it—driven only by my innate need for sex itself. There was no daydreaming of our next rendezvous. In fact, many times I said to myself, "I hope he doesn't want sex when I see him tonight." But if Tom could have miraculously appeared instead, it would have been just the opposite; I wouldn't have been able to get him into bed fast enough.

I was always very uninhibited when it came to sex—I had absolutely no hangups—I wanted to derive as much pleasure as possible. During natural sex, I would surrender myself completely to the pleasure of the moment. But during circumcised sex, I never felt like I totally surrendered to my partner. I was never truly enraptured. I was aware of pleasure and lack of pleasure simultaneously, never going over the edge, never able to truly abandon myself in unbounded passion.

At the time, I had no idea that the difference in my sexual attitude toward Mike was related to his surgically altered penis. I thought it was because I was in love with Tom, and not in love with Mike. It simply never occurred to me that it could be the penis, not the man. My relationship with Mike lasted about a year. During the next two years, I continued to see Tom on a once-a-week basis, while at the same time, I had several short-term involvements with mostly circumcised, but also two uncircumcised men.

At some point, I began to *vaguely* realize that I enjoyed sex much more with men who were natural, and I remember remarking to a female friend that I thought there was a difference. *But it didn't strike me, profoundly, on a conscious level*, that there was actually something about circumcised intercourse that I didn't quite like. At the time, being young and full of passion, I more or less thought I enjoyed myself during circumcised sex, and I'm sure my partners thought I did, but in retrospect, I found it simultaneously annoying—it had an unpleasant edge to it—even though I would have categorized it overall as pleasurable.

It's a very difficult thing to explain. Sex is so overpoweringly pleasurable it's hard to conceive that it could strike one as both pleasurable and bothersome at the same time. The following anecdote from an article that appeared in *Glamour* magazine may help me to make my point:

> Sharon, a 30-year-old concert violinist, fell in love with Kevin when she was 23. Wanting to please him, she read as many books as she could find about sexual technique. "I felt like everyone in the world knew what to do in bed except me," she says. "He was six years older and much more experienced than I was at the time—I thought he wouldn't consider me a good lover. Well, I made up for that! I must have suggested three different positions every night."
>
> Despite the athleticism of their lovemaking, Kevin suspected something was wrong, and over dinner one evening he asked Sharon point-blank if she enjoyed having sex with him. "I was embarrassed, even angry," she remembers, "but I surprised myself by saying, no, I didn't" (1).

I think that in the above scenario, if the truth were to be known, the circumcised penis is the real culprit behind Sharon's dissatisfaction. I've spoken with many women personally (women who have experienced only circumcised sex) and virtually all of them could identify with the concept that sex can be both pleasurable and simultaneously aggravating. As mentioned, however, some women may not consciously discern displeasure during the act, especially if a woman has never experienced natural intercourse as a comparison; the displeasures of circumcised sex may be below her level of conscious awareness. She may simply get caught up in whatever pleasure she is experiencing and make the best of it. Yet, in the back of her mind, she may be quite dissatisfied, like Sharon, in the above anecdote.

At the end of the third year of my affair with Tom, I met my future husband, Jeff. I was instantly attracted to his kind, gentle personality, his intelligence, and his philosophy of life. I had never met anyone quite as wonderful, warm, and genuine. I realized that if my relationship with Jeff was to ever get off the ground, I would have to stop seeing Tom, though I was still painfully in love with him. After a concerted effort, I was finally able to break away from Tom (who was no longer my co-worker), and Jeff and I began to see each other steadily. I developed a genuine, deep affection for him and wanted it to blossom into the kind of love I knew was possible. I grew to love him for the wonderful human being that he is, but I didn't fall as deeply *in love* with him as I had with Tom. I blamed it on the fact that I was still nursing the wounds of my previous love affair. I didn't realize that Jeff's surgically altered circumcised penis was a factor in the depth of our love relationship.

Sex with Jeff was good, and he was a caring, considerate lover, but it wasn't great. It didn't lift me to the overwhelming heights of passion and pleasure I had experienced with Tom. I enjoyed sex with Jeff, but I didn't swooningly love it the way I had with Tom. I continued to blame the difference on the fact that deep down I was still in love with my old flame. I was sure that with time I would fall more in love with Jeff and that that would bring new meaning to our sexual relationship.

About a year after Jeff and I met, we got an apartment together, and a year after that we got married in a simple, but beautiful, outdoor ceremony. It was the happiest day of my life. But something happened on our honeymoon that jolted me back to reality. We spent our honeymoon canoeing the Saco River in Maine, and at every bend of the river he wanted to have sex again. It suddenly struck me, profoundly, that I had just made a permanent commitment to him, and although he was the greatest person I had ever met, if I was going to be completely honest with myself, there was something about his sexing that I didn't quite like. It just wasn't the same as it had been with Tom—something was fundamentally wrong.

I tried to put it out of my mind. After all, I would never meet a more wonderful person, and sex with him wasn't *that* bad; it just wasn't quite right—it was somehow strangely frustrating even though I always achieved vaginal orgasm.

After the first year of marriage we settled into a twice-a-week schedule. Although sex with Jeff was enjoyable, and he was a kind, considerate lover who tried to please me in every way and did not "bang away" at my genitals like Mike, still, his penis felt too hard, I didn't like his long thrusts, and my vagina didn't "melt" and "purr" like it had with Tom. I must emphasize that I probably would not have had these thoughts, to such a degree, if my vagina hadn't been "spoiled" by the softly-stiff characteristics of the natural penis; I would have thought that the sex Jeff and I were having was "normal," not knowing any better.

Yet, I was never truly lifted to overwhelming heights of ecstasy and passion. It always seemed like we were having two separate experiences and that that feeling of sexual oneness was somewhere out of reach. It lacked a feeling of true connectedness, like I was taking, instead of giving and receiving simultaneously. *There was always a frenzied concentration toward achieving orgasm without being truly excited throughout the experience* because I had to simultaneously block out those aspects that the vagina considered bothersome and annoying. There was an unpleasant edge to it when he was actively thrusting. In order to enjoy it, I had to limit his long thrusts by pulling him in close with my legs. His instinct was to pull away and use long strokes. It was always a struggle.

Even though I usually achieved multiple vaginal orgasms using the face-to-face, side-by-side position (see Appendix A), they weren't *truly* satisfying. They had an edge of frustration to them in the build-up. They provided physical relief, but it was an "on-the-surface" relief, not deep, not connected to the depths of my inner being. It was more like a masturbatory experience rather than a union of pleasuring. And my mental attitude after sex seemed to be, "Well, we got that out of the way—that should hold me for a few days." **Yet I knew that my attitude really should have been**—"Boy, I can't wait until the next time we have sex." Why such a difference? It made me wonder.

As time went by and I began to comprehend the meaning of the word "forever"—that I was going to live the rest of my life with him—I began to resent, more and more, his inability to give me the kind of sexing I intensely craved and fantasized about. I became increasingly irritable toward him and started quarrels over little, meaningless things. I didn't realize that the frustration I was experiencing between the sheets, due to the inadequacies and displeasurements of circumcised sex, was being carried far beyond the bedroom door into our everyday relationship. His surgically altered penis was inhibiting us from developing a meaningful love bond.

A few years into the marriage, I began seeing Tom again. I couldn't help myself—I absolutely could not resist him. And I still hadn't resolved my love for him. He was a magnet, and I was steel.

I really wanted to remain faithful to my husband, and I wanted the marriage to work out, but the memories of the moments and hours I shared with Tom were irrepressible. I loved everything about him—the way he walked, the way he talked, his smile, his laugh, his moments of pensiveness, his very touch, his kiss. And the way the light sparkled in his eyes when he spoke—I swear I could hear the angels sing. But in actuality, was he really *that* great? How much power did the penis wield over my adorations—and how much of it was the man? In all honesty, a little of both, for this was truly an exceptional man. But would I have thought him so charming if he had been circumcised? I'm certain that I would not have. I would have been sexually dissatisfied with him and would be bitching and complaining about him, just like the other two men in this story. And the affair would have been short-lived. Instead, I remained head over heels in love with him.

After renewing our affair, we saw each other five or six times over a couple of years, then we drifted apart for a few years. But the memory of his lovemaking crowded my thoughts and filled my dreams.

Meanwhile, the relationship with my husband was strained, but for the most part civil. We got along, probably as well as most circumcised couples do, but our relationship was deficient in sexual love. I loved him for the good, gentle person that he is, and we enjoyed each other's company. But our love lacked depth—the kind of depth that exists when a couple has a deeply satisfying, exquisitely delicious, sensuous, sexual interconnectedness. Although we were still having sex about once a week, it was encumbered by the problems previously discussed. I learned to endure the way things were, but I longed for so much more.

About eight years into the marriage, Tom and I renewed our affair again, and we saw each other two or three times a year for a couple of years. Sex with him was always totally enrapturing— incredibly luscious—sensuously thrilling. Beyond description. No wonder I couldn't stay away from him. His natural lovemaking had me spellbound.

During our rendezvous, I couldn't help but notice that his penis felt much more sensuous inside me; it felt infinitely better, deliciously better, indescribably better. Entirely different from the sex I was experiencing with my husband Jeff.

In characterizing the differences, now that I have thought about this in-depth, I would say that the circumcised experience is like being *repeatedly penetrated* in an annoying way, even though simultaneously there is pleasure. And the penis feels too hard, almost foreign-like—you want it, but don't want it, at the same time, driven onward only in hopes of achieving orgasm, the sooner the better. Whereas with natural, the vagina totally surrenders to the soft sensuousness of lingering ecstasy, as it hungrily caresses and lovingly responds to the erotic movements of the softly-stiff penis, and the penis adores and gently strokes the vagina in return. Like two halves of a perfect whole, each organ swoons and sighs to a passionate intermingling and sexual connectedness—the way it was meant to be. With no holding back, lost in voluptuous abandon, you TOTALLY want it, you TOTALLY need it, and you TOTALLY love it.

At some point, I began to vaguely suspect that Jeff's circumcision might have something to do with why his penis felt completely different from Tom's, and that circumcision might have something to do with our waning sexual desire for one another (by this time we were having sex only once or twice a month). It was just starting to seep into my consciousness that circumcision was the culprit. Even though I had remarked to a female friend about ten years earlier that I thought there was a difference between the uncircumcised (having not yet thought of it as natural) and circumcised experience, I had somehow totally repressed it after that time. It was just beginning to strike me on a profound level that it was the penis itself.

About ten years into the marriage, I began to notice considerable vaginal discomfort after Jeff and I had sex. My vaginal cavity would ache with discomfort and pain for about an hour after intercourse, even though we used an artificial lubricant. (I was probably more cognizant of discomfort than the average woman is because we always had our sex in the morning or afternoon, whereas most couples usually have it at bedtime. I'm sure many women experience discomfort after sex, but because they fall off to sleep soon afterwards, they are not conscious that the sensation lingers, and by morning, it may be completely gone.)

Then, from out of nowhere, I developed vaginismus—a condition where the vaginal muscles clamp up tight, making penis entry virtually impossible. From that point on, every time Jeff and I would try to have sex my vagina would not cooperate, even though he would try to loosen up my vagina with circular motions of his inserted fingers. The vagina would accept his fingers, but would only accept his penis after 5-15 minutes of forced entry. After entry, intercourse was quite discomforting; I could only tolerate an extremely minimal amount of thrusting, and after sex was over my vaginal cavity would ache with pain for several hours. I began to increasingly sense that my condition was somehow related to his surgically altered circumcised penis.

Although various explanations have been proposed regarding the cause of vaginismus (molestation during childhood, rape experience, underdeveloped genitalia, anxiety, frigidity, etc.), I would like to propose a new explanation. I submit that many, perhaps most, cases of vaginismus are an involuntary vaginal reflex reaction related to repeated exposures to the circumcised penis, which traumatizes and assaults the woman's vaginal entrance and walls with its hardness, friction, and scraping action. With time, the *vagina* begins to recognize and "remember" the abuse it is receiving. Over time, it takes its toll, and the woman may suddenly develop spontaneous vaginismus. Although it seems to happen "overnight," it may actually develop gradually. Long before a woman has full-blown vaginismus, she may notice that her vagina feels abnormally tightened and tensed during intercourse. The vaginal muscles respond autonomically by recoiling and tensing up in response to the physical trauma it is receiving. As time goes by, the vaginal opening becomes tighter and more resistant to penetration. This condition should be considered mild vaginismus, or sub-clinical vaginismus. Eventually, it may develop into full-blown vaginismus, at which time the man will find penetration increasingly difficult, if not impossible. Even if full-blown vaginismus never develops, the abnormally tightened vaginal walls and entrance should not be considered a normal condition.

How quickly a woman develops full-blown vaginismus from sub-clinical vaginismus will depend on several factors—her age, how much exposure she has had to the circumcised intercourse experience, how frequently she has intercourse, how long intercourse lasts, the degree of lubrication, how tightly her partner is circumcised, and how vigorously he thrusts during intercourse.

After I developed vaginismus and suspected more and more that the circumcised penis was at fault, I became curious to see if the natural penis could "undo" my vaginismus. To check out my theory I called Tom, whom I hadn't seen for some time. A few days later we met for lunch and then went to a motel.

I told him nothing about my vaginismus, having decided that the best resolve was to simply let nature take its course. Much to my surprise and delight, when his penis head approached the vaginal opening, the vagina gave a split-second wince and then accepted his penis easily and willingly. Incredibly, the vaginal opening could somehow tell the difference between Tom's natural penis head and Jeff's circumcised penis head. We then proceeded to have a lengthy, heavenly intercourse. Afterward, there was no vaginal discomfort or pain; instead, there was a pleasantly pulsating afterglow throughout my entire genital area, just like I had experienced with him before. That experience was enough to convince me that the circumcised penis was the cause of my vaginismus. I mentioned to my husband, briefly, that I thought circumcision might be at the root of our sexual problems, but I didn't think there was a solution, so I didn't press the issue.

Not long after that, Jeff inadvertently came across an article on foreskin restoration. I was incredibly excited about it. We had a long talk about everything, including Tom, and I persuaded him to get surgically restored. I was certain that it would cure my vaginismus and make a 180-degree difference in our sex life, and that this in turn would add new depth to our love relationship.

After his operation healed, we attempted intercourse. My vagina did not instantly accept his restored penis, but each time we attempted intercourse, intromission got progressively easier and less discomforting. After about four months, we were able to have normal sexual relations—*totally fabulous, in fact*. I think the reason it took a while for things to normalize was because it required time for his penis head to gradually change from abnormally hard to softly stiff, as a result of the foreskin's moisturizing effects. As the vaginal opening gradually noticed the difference, it gradually became more accepting of his penis, and ultimately my vaginismus completely corrected itself.

(I must stress that for normal sexual relations, it is very important to the woman's pleasure that the restoring man achieve full coverage, whereby his foreskin extends beyond the glans. This insures that the necessary moisture to maintain the glans softly-stiff characteristics will be present.)

I am delighted to say that our love and sexual relationship is now everything I knew it should be—everything I've attributed to the natural penis throughout the book—because our relationship has been able to develop its sexual dimension. And we owe it all to the restored penis. After almost 30 years of marriage, we are now more in love than we have ever been, and I feel like a princess in a fairy tale who gets to live happily ever after with the love prince of her dreams. Not only is Jeff the most wonderful man I could ever hope to meet, but his magical, restored penis, with its splendorous lovemaking abilities, takes my breath away, making me fall more in love with him with every passing day, if that's possible. In my opinion, from the woman's sexual perspective, the restored penis is virtually equivalent to the natural penis in every respect.* For the circumcised man and his female partner, who are now caught "in between times," foreskin restoration truly offers a quantum leap in improved sexuality, allowing them to resurrect the sexuality that was stolen from them, and holds the promise for a love relationship to be "born anew."

---

* In actuality, I can only speak for the restored penis as reconstructed using Dr. Greer's surgical technique (see Jeff's story Chapter 12). However, women are reportedly very happy with the non-surgically restored penis.

IMPORTANT

Be sure to check out the Appendixes below.

The secrets they reveal are worth a thousand times the price of the book.

APPENDIX A:

HOW TO HAVE A VAGINAL ORGASM 99.99% OF THE TIME USING THE SIDE-BY-SIDE (FACE-TO-FACE) POSITION—THE MOST COMFORTABLE AND MOST SATISFYING POSITION OF ALL

APPENDIX B:

HOW TO MINIMIZE PREMATURE EJACULATION AND THE "TAP ME" SECRET TO PROLONGING INTERCOURSE

APPENDIX C:

A SOLUTION FOR THOSE CIRCUMCISED MEN WHO TAKE LONGER THAN THEY WANT TO REACH ORGASM

12

Joining the Foreskin Restoration Revolution
and
The Personal Stories
of
Two Men Who Restored

[As a result of being circumcised] I experienced continuous decline in sensitivity and sexual pleasure to the point of not being able to orgasm within a period of time comfortable for my wife. Fortunately, all this has been reversed by my foreskin recovery. I again have the sexual performance of a teenager.

— J.S., Colorado (1)

My husband is now undergoing non-surgical restoration of his foreskin and even though I have never been very interested in whether men were circumcised or uncircumcised, I find that I enjoy sex much more since he began his restoration.

— Survey respondent

I have been restored for two years. Coverage is wonderful and the sensations of my foreskin moving back and forth over my more sensitive head are great. No more tight, often sore, erections, no more dried out glans, and artificial lubrication is no longer needed.... My wife enjoys sex much more, too, and we owe it all to foreskin restoration. For the first time in my life I feel like a whole man.

— M.L., California (2)

> I think my wife enjoys my new foreskin as much as I do (she says she enjoys it more than me, but I don't think that's possible). She thought I was crazy when I told her what I wanted to do [restore] and even tried to talk me out of it. But I knew I had to be missing a lot. Now she thinks it's the best thing I ever did and is the best part of my body! The foreplay is just out of this world. We quit using all that lubrication that used to be necessary. That may be the reason she thinks she likes it more than I do, because sex is no longer dry and unpleasant like it was before restoration.
>
> — H.W., Wisconsin (3)

A GROWING NUMBER OF MEN ARE ANGRY OR UPSET THAT THEY WERE CIRCUMCISED

Every time the circumcision issue is raised in public—whether by television, radio, newspaper, or magazine—letters pour in from circumcised males in every part of the country, either to say some of the things they usually do not dare to say or to ask for advice.

Because many people feel uncomfortable talking about the sex organs and because of the hush-hush nature of circumcision, relatively little time is devoted to this topic by the media. If it were given the amount of national attention it deserves, hundreds of thousands of letters might result.

Many men may be having various problems with their penises, but they are unaware that these problems—uncomfortable erections, inability to maintain an erection, lack of sexual desire, discomforting intercourse, etc.—may be a consequence of their circumcision. As the subject of circumcision comes out of the closet, more and more of these men are speaking up. Other men may appear to be indifferent about their circumcision; they don't like to discuss anything about it or even hear the word. This suggests they may have psychological wounds that have not healed.

No one knows at this point how many circumcised men are unhappy or angered about their circumcision, but organizations such as NOCIRC, NOHARMM, and NORM (see Resources at back of book) have received thousands of letters from men who resent having been circumcised as infants without their consent, or from men who regret getting circumcised in adulthood. We are just beginning to see the tip of the iceberg.

Until now, there has been little public awareness that many men are secretly unhappy about being circumcised. Many men, approaching this subject with their doctors and requesting information about restoration/reconstruction, are typically answered with responses like these: (4)

> "He was shocked that anyone would want restoration and refused to discuss the subject."
>
> "...thought I was stupid."
>
> "He cut me off and talked about 'foreskin fanatics.'"
>
> "...told me I needed psychiatric counseling."
>
> "He laughed at me."

It is an objective of this book to give a strong and dignified voice to circumcised men who wish to restore or reconstruct their foreskin and become "whole" again. One man, born in 1952, wrote:

> I remember *more than one* birthday, before blowing out the candles on the cake, wishing that, if wishes were granted, I should become uncircumcised. I was brought up in a moral but unreligious family of Christian background. I was never instructed to pray but I do remember, skeptically but seriously, praying to God (if you exist) to please make me whole again (5).

The following statements were distilled by John A. Erickson (a pioneer in the anti-circumcision movement) from personal communications with circumcised men over several years.

> ...Circumcision—I hate the word. It makes me shudder.
>
> ...Adrenaline shoots through me when I hear the word 'circumcised'—I freeze.
>
> ...I couldn't even make myself *say* 'circumcised' until I was in my twenties.
>
> ...I think of myself and other circumcised men as amputees.
>
> ...I have nightmares about being circumcised by force.
>
> ...I was circumcised when I was five, seventy-five years ago. I felt rage then and I still feel rage now.
>
> ...I am always thinking: where is my foreskin?
>
> ...I think of myself as existing in two parts: my missing foreskin and the rest of me.
>
> ...When I was a child I prayed I would get my foreskin back in heaven.
>
> ...I have never been able to accept the fact that someone cut part of my penis off when I was a baby. Sometimes I think I'm beginning to make some sort of adjustment to it, but then I see an unmutilated man in a shower or magazine and I become overwhelmed by uncontrollable feelings of outrage and disbelief that I was made the victim for life of something so sick.

...I tried several times to ask my mother about what had been done to me. But when I opened my mouth to speak, the words stuck in my throat and no sound came out.

...I have wondered what it's like to have a foreskin all my life.

...I have always felt I was cut off from my foreskin, not vice versa.

...I never got used to being circumcised. I just learned to endure it.

...I pretended I didn't care.

...The head of my penis is just dead.

...I never let women see my penis because I think it's ugly.

...When I masturbate I always have the same fantasy: the image of my foreskin as it would look and feel now, had it not been cut off when I was born.

...I feel that my father betrayed me by letting my mother have me circumcised against his wishes, and I've always sensed that deep down he rejected me because he saw me as damaged.

...I have revenge fantasies about circumcision.

...My feelings about the doctor who circumcised me are too violent to describe.

> ...I asked a friend if he felt 'different' when he was the only uncircumcised man in the shower and he said, 'Yes, gloriously different.'

> ...I'm restoring my foreskin because I was born with one, and damn it, I'm going to die with one.

MEN CIRCUMCISED IN ADULTHOOD NOTICE IT AFFECTS THEIR SEXUALITY

The men above were obviously very emotionally scarred by circumcision, but how does it affect a man sexually? Below are three commentaries of men who were circumcised *in adulthood*.

> "...[S]ight without color would be a good analogy...only being able to see in black and white rather than seeing in full color would be like experiencing an orgasm with a foreskin and without. There are feelings you'll just never have without the foreskin" (6).

> "The greatest disadvantage of circumcision, in my view, is the awful loss of sensitivity and function when the foreskin is removed.... I was deprived of my foreskin when I was 26; I had ample experience in the sexual area, and I was quite happy (delirious, in fact) with what pleasure I could experience—beginning with foreplay and continuing—as an intact male. After my circumcision, that pleasure was utterly gone. Let me put it this way: On a scale of 10, the uncircumcised penis experiences pleasure that is at least 11 or 12; the circumcised penis is lucky to get to 3.... If American men who were circumcised at birth could know the deprivation of pleasure they would experience, they would storm the hospitals and not permit their sons to undergo this unnecessary

loss. But how can they know? You have to be circumcised as an adult, as I was, to realize what a terrible loss of pleasure results from this cruel operation" (7).

"After thirty years in the natural state, I allowed myself to be persuaded by a physician to have the foreskin removed—not because of any problems at the time, but because, in the physician's view, there might be some problems in the future. That was five years ago, and I am sorry I had it done now from my standpoint and from what my female sex partners have told me...the sensitivity in the glans has been reduced by at least 50%. There it is unprotected, constantly rubbing against the fabric of whatever I am wearing. In a sense, it has become callused. Intercourse is now (as we used to say about the older, heavier condoms) like washing your hands with gloves on.... I seem to have a relatively unresponsive stick where I once had a sexual organ" (8).

Granted, there are some men circumcised in adulthood who report that they are pleased they got circumcised. This puzzled me for quite some time, until I figured it out. For some intact men, circumcision may have corrected a medical problem that caused them to experience substandard function before the operation. For example, there is a disorder called *phimosis*, a condition where the foreskin cannot retract. For a man with phimosis, the penis area beneath the foreskin stays constantly covered and thus cannot make contact with the vaginal walls during intercourse.

If a man had phimosis and then got circumcised, he would think that circumcision gave his sex life a boost because it would allow the upper penis area to make contact with the vaginal walls. Although he notices an improvement after circumcision, the real question is: What if he could have achieved foreskin mobility and its accompanying sexual benefits without losing his foreskin? How much improvement in sexual pleasure would he notice then?

Wouldn't he be even more pleased? The challenge to the medical community is: Find the cause of phimosis (I suggest it may be due to chronic low levels of vitamin C and/or zinc, which do not allow the skin to develop its proper elasticity—see discussion on page 214). And until the cause of phimosis is found, investigate the documented medical techniques that can correct phimosis without circumcision or other forms of surgery. (Some non-surgical corrective approaches to phimosis are discussed in Chapter 17.)

Other men circumcised as adults, who may not have had a functional problem but who state that they experience no sexual deprivation after circumcision, may be deluding themselves, or unwilling to admit to family and friends that they made a mistake—it's too humiliating. *Considering the great loss of erogenous tissue and penile function, it flies in the face of logic to think that circumcision could improve a man's sexuality. And even though he may say he likes it, what about his female partner?*

Lastly, the circumcision debate is so full of emotional fanaticism and hardheadedness, it is conceivable that a circumcised man could step forward praising circumcision, stating that he was circumcised as an adult, when, in fact, he was actually circumcised in infancy, not adulthood. He speaks out to defend it and states untruths in order to cloud the issue because his emotional biases, sexual ego, (or religious precepts) compel him to do so.

MORE AND MORE MEN ARE REALIZING THEY WERE HARMED BY CIRCUMCISION

A national survey of men who are aware that they were harmed to some degree by *infant* circumcision (9) was conducted by NOHARMM (National Organization to Halt the Abuse and Routine Mutilation of Males). Here are a few of their comments:

> **...I am angry and bitter and depressed about being circumcised and I resent that it was done to me.**

...It hurts too much...from being cut so tight.

...I've been mutilated* and denied full functioning of my penis due to an unnecessary and ignorant procedure.

...My penis is unnatural this way!

...A deep longing to be complete and intact.

Perhaps you, like the men above, have been unhappy about your circumcision for a long time. Or perhaps it did not strike home until reading this book. Whatever situation, it is perfectly normal for you to feel angry and shortchanged and have a desire to get back what's rightfully yours—a functioning foreskin. The circumcised man who does not face up to the realization that he got "cheated" is the one acting inappropriately. These men may seem indifferent about their circumcision status and may say, "I'm circumcised and I'm fine," but in actuality, they are not. Eventually, as this information becomes common knowledge, they will have to confront their denial and concede that they were harmed. And that by delaying restoration, they are keeping themselves, and their sex partner, from experiencing the sexual pleasure they both deserve. You, on the other hand, by facing up to this situation now and beginning the process of restoration, will be well on your way to being restored.

---

* Some readers may object to the word *mutilation*, arguing that circumcision does not mutilate the penis. However, according to definitions found in various dictionaries, circumcision does qualify as mutilation. The following are examples.

Mutilate: to damage, injure, or otherwise make imperfect, especially by removing an essential part or parts. (*Webster's New Universal Unabridged Dictionary*, 2nd edition, 1983.)

Mutilate: Biology. Of an animal or plant: having some part, common to related forms, either absent or present only in an imperfect or modified state. *(The New Shorter Oxford English Dictionary*, 1993.)

Mutilation...implies the cutting off or removal of a part essential to completeness, not only of a person but also of a thing, and to his or its perfection, beauty, entirety, or fulfillment of function. (*Webster's Dictionary of Synonyms*, 1968.)

What can you expect from restoration?—*a rainbow of new sexual and physical sensations and sensuousness, and new feelings of wholeness.* There is no way to explain how wonderful it's going to be until you get there. Of course, restoration is not an exact replication of the original foreskin, still, the sexual benefits are so overwhelmingly awesome, my husband describes it as—"It's too beautiful for words."

A bonus benefit attributed to restoration, reports *www.norm-socal.org,* is an increase in the overall size of the penis. Many men have taken careful measurements before and after their restoration and noted increases in both penis length and girth. Penis enlargement evidently results because when the shaft has its full complement of skin, its tissue is free to expand to its full dimensions. Prior to restoration, if the penis is tightly circumcised, as many men are, penile tissue during erection can get pushed internally into the mons pubis, instead of expanding externally to full length. Regarding girth, keep in mind that insufficient shaft skin, stretched to its utmost limits, constricts the penile tissue. Restorative skin loosens this constrictive vise, enabling the penis to expand to greater fullness.

The foreskin has been successfully restored (reconstructed) using a revolutionary surgical technique developed by Dr. Donald Greer. Although this technique holds promise for the future, at the present time no one is performing it (see discussion later in this chapter). Other methods of surgical restoration, developed by other plastic surgeons, are not advised. Presently, non-surgical methods are the most tried and approved means of restoring the foreskin.

Non-surgical methods of restoration typically involve various stretching and taping techniques, whereby a man stretches his shaft skin and then tapes it in place to produce tension. When the penis shaft skin is regularly stretched in this manner, the body responds by growing new skin. This works on the same principle as a person whose skin expands when they gain weight. Stretching and taping the shaft skin will eventually grow into a substitute foreskin. (Visit website: *www.infocirc.org/rest-e.htm* for an overview of this topic.)

NEW TAPELESS TECHNIQUES

Taping techniques have been the principle method of restoration to date, but they may soon be superseded by an exciting, new tapeless technique that has recently been invented called the TugAhoy. Like taping techniques, this device also applies gentle tension to the penile shaft skin, causing it to expand and lengthen. But the inventor proclaims it has several advantages, principally, the extreme ease and speed of attaching and removing the device from the penis (less than a minute), and the fact that it leaves no sticky tape residues that have to be periodically removed by chemical means. Because of this, it allows for spontaneous sex. Men who have used this technique are very enthusiastic about it, and the restored foreskin photos at *www.tugahoy.com/ Foreskin_Photos.htm* display proof that the results can be remarkable.

Also, another tapeless device, that works on a similar principle as the TugAhoy, comes highly recommended. It's called the RECAP method. Email the inventor at *recap_ez@hotmail.com* for details.

These tapeless techniques have garnered high praise. But a few individuals have not been successful with them. And some men, who are very tightly circumcised, may need to use taping techniques to produce enough startup skin for these devices to attach onto, enabling them to work their magic. If you start with one of these two techniques and it does not work for you, try the other. And if neither technique works, there are other options. Don't give up. Surf *www.norm-socal.org* and its links for further information.

Men who have restored speak glowingly of the increased sexual pleasure and self-esteem they have derived from it. Nevertheless, restoration cannot reinstate the exact nerve structure and the exact functioning of your original foreskin—better if you had not been circumcised in the first place. But please do not let this freeze you with distress, because restoration can bring back many— nearly all—of the advantages of the natural penis.

Circumcision truly is a tragedy of the highest degree, yet today's circumcised men must now try to move beyond their sadness and anger, to that place where they can hear the water's lapping on a higher ground, through the hope and promise of restoration. Please take a few minutes to study the **Table of Sexual Benefits** on the two pages following the end of this chapter to see how closely the restored penis and natural penis compare.

Unfortunately, restoring the foreskin through various skin expansion techniques is not achieved overnight. Some men report full coverage of the glans in less than a year, but these represent exceptional success stories. Realistically, one should anticipate about 2 to 3 years to cover the glans completely using traditional taping techniques. TugAhoy and RECAP users may achieve results more quickly because application of these devices is easier so men are more inclined to stick with the routine, and many are able to use them 24/7, so restoration progress is accelerated.

It is important for restoring men to know that nutrients play an essential role in progressive skin expansion. Dr. Carl C. Pfeiffer in his book, *Mental and Elemental Nutrients: A Physician's Guide to Nutrition and Health Care* says,

> Both *zinc* and *copper* are needed for effective crosslinking of the elastin chains to make the perfect elastic tissue. ***When imperfect, any overstretching will cause long tears*** which appear as striae or stretchmarks.
>
> Elastin comes from...*lysine* [an amino acid] in a process furthered by lysyl oxidase-a copper-containing enzyme. This enzyme requires pyridoxal phosphate (***vitamin B-6***) to make either collagen or elastin...***Vitamin C*** is also necessary in this process to stabilize the easily oxidized...copper-containing enzyme). (Emphasis added)

Taking a high-potency multiple vitamin-mineral supplement daily (preferably a brand that is designed to be taken in divided doses after each meal) while you are restoring will help insure that you have sufficient amounts of the above nutrients in your body to make new skin. Supplementary lysine, available at healthfood stores, should also prove beneficial, as well as extra vitamin C. I recommend a type of vitamin C called Ester-C, since it is more absorbable, stays in your system longer, and will not upset your stomach the way some acidic formulations might. For all nutrients, simply follow the dosage recommendations on the label. Also, be aware that dietary protein, in general, is necessary for the generation of skin.*

In any event, restoration requires perseverance and fortitude. Encouragement and inspiration from men who have successfully restored, or are in the process of restoring, are essential for keeping your spirits up and your outlook optimistic. Support groups can be found on the Internet (see Resources section at back of book, under Foreskin Restoration, for one such group—"restore list"). And again, surf *www.norm-socal.org* and its links. Ultimately, as the revolution gains momentum, support groups will be found in your local area.

A detailed explanation of the various methods of restoration is a book in and of itself, and is unfortunately beyond the scope of this book. For a complete description and in-depth discussion of the techniques currently available, I recommend *The Joy of Uncircumcising!* by Jim Bigelow, Ph.D. Originally published in 1992, as of this writing Bigelow's book is being prepared for Internet publishing. Contact Jim Bigelow, POB 52138, Pacific Grove, CA 93950, for details on how to purchase.

As you will soon read in my husband's story, Jeff was surgically restored by Dr. Donald Greer, who developed a scrotal implant method whereby skin from the scrotum is grafted onto the penis. Scrotal skin is high in sensitivity. And it has the advantage of having muscle tissue, so when the penis is flaccid, the tip of the foreskin contracts like a drawn-in duffel bag, keeping the penis head protected and moist for maximum sensitivity. Also, this muscle tissue allows the man to experience the thrill of the s-t-r-e-t-c-h (described on page 300.)

---

* Requisite Disclaimer: The above is not intended as medical advice. Always consult a physician and/or qualified health-care professional before embarking on any program of nutrient supplementation.

Although reconstructive surgery does not replace the nerve tissue that was inherent in the original foreskin, still, my husband and I are very happy with the results of Greer's surgical solution, as are reportedly other men who have undergone his technique. But, as of this writing, no one is performing it. Greer discontinued reconstructive surgery in the mid-'80s when he moved his practice to a rural area in Wyoming far away from air transportation. His concern was that for those men who occasionally developed post-surgery complications to his two-step procedure, he was not accessible to deal with their problems in a timely manner. Dr. Greer recently retired from practice. However, other doctors may begin researching his technique, and it may one day become an eagerly sought out form of restoration because outstanding results can be obtained in a very short period of time.

I must stress that surgery of any type is something that should not be entered into lightly or hastily. There are a few doctors who have developed their own surgical restoration techniques, but I have no personal familiarity with the results. I would be wary of any technique requiring a large patch of donor skin from some part of your body. This skin, usually taken from the thigh or buttocks, will have little or no feeling and will leave an unsightly scar at the site from which the skin was taken. Keep in mind that your objective is not merely to cover your glans, but to improve your sexual feeling, while simultaneously acquiring functional benefits similar to the natural foreskin. With this in mind, surgical restorations using these types of skin grafts are not advised.

If surgical restoration is to offer a viable solution for circumcised men, the medical community must acknowledge the obligation it has to the millions of men who were surgically separated from their foreskins at birth without their consent, and address the vast demand that potentially exists for a surgical solution. Concerned doctors must come together in a symposium to discuss the merits and drawbacks of potential approaches—current and future. The media has a responsibility to make public the findings and recommendations of such a symposium and to present in-depth discussions on this topic.

In my judgment, once this topic is thoroughly investigated, I believe Dr. Greer's technique will emerge as the universal approach to surgical reconstruction. Greer's technique is documented in medical literature (10). But importantly, his articles do not reflect (to doctors who might research them) refinements he made to the procedure in subsequent years. Originally requiring four operations, he reduced it to two (one inpatient and one outpatient.) Although Greer is now retired, I expect that he will emerge to accept the challenge of updating his technique to reflect advancements in today's medical technology and to present the medical community with in-depth knowledge on his technique at the above-mentioned proposed symposium. If there is anything to report on the topic of surgical restoration, *www.ForeskinRestoration.org* will keep you advised.

Facing Up to the Inescapable Truth: Jeff's Story of What It's Like to be Circumcised and Later Restored

What is it like to live for 42 years without a foreskin and then have it reconstructed? Absolutely great!

I was born with a long foreskin. Why this should have been considered a problem, I'm not quite sure, but the doctor who delivered me told my mother that my foreskin was long and recommended circumcision. My father, who was natural, was not consulted because he was away on a World War II battleship.

For the first 42 years of my life, I didn't give my circumcision much conscious thought, but if anyone mentioned the word "circumcision," a feeling would run up and down my spine as if someone had just scraped their fingernails across a blackboard.

During my childhood, I never thought too much about my circumcised penis in terms of how I compared to other boys and men. I definitely noticed a distinct difference between my father's natural penis and my own. Obviously, his was bigger because of his bigger body size, but I wondered why the head of his penis was covered while mine was not. Yet, I never dwelled on it; I never felt shortchanged, envious, or castrated, and never asked him about it.

My younger brother had a natural penis. Perhaps my mother and father discussed the issue of his circumcision more thoughtfully, rather than just blindly accepting some doctor's recommendation. At about age 13, I examined my brother's semi-erect penis and was struck by the mobile skin that covered his penis head. I was fascinated by how easily it glided up and down and how moist and pink it was underneath (my penis head was grayish-white by comparison). Although intrigued with his penis, I did not become envious or angry, nor did I feel weird or odd because I was different from him. I was a pretty well-adjusted kid and I accepted my penis for what it was. Besides, my penis looked like most other boys in the shower room, so I didn't become concerned, though I did notice that a few boys had penises that looked like my father's and brother's.

During the first 42 years of my life, if someone had asked me if I was satisfied with my circumcised penis, I would have unthinkingly said, "Yes." But something happened at age 42 that dramatically changed my answer to a resounding, "NO." I came to the shocking realization that my circumcised penis was sexually abnormal.

In the mid-'80s, I read a magazine article that described a revolutionary surgical procedure that grafted skin from a man's scrotum onto his penis to make a restored foreskin. Developed by a plastic surgeon, Dr. Donald Greer, who at that time worked for the University of Texas Medical Center, it was a very new operation, and only 16 men had ever had it done. I became the 17th. The operation and aftercare went smoothly. The whole process was not much different from any other type of cosmetic surgery, and I became the happy owner of a wonderful new foreskin.

Having my foreskin restored so late in life gave me the rare opportunity to experience the differences between having a circumcised penis and having a penis with a foreskin. Now that I have experienced the difference a foreskin makes, I can better understand and describe the dissatisfactions I had with my circumcised penis.

Long before my reconstruction, I was unhappy about how my circumcised penis head always felt openly exposed, naked, and distinctly separate from the rest of my body, much like the feeling one gets when there's a hole in your sock and your big toe sticks out. You keep wishing the exposed toe were covered like the rest of your foot. Now that I have a foreskin, my penis feels like it's part of my whole body, and I don't think of it as being separate anymore.

When I used to be circumcised, I was dissatisfied with the unwanted tactile stimulation my upper penis was constantly getting from rubbing against my underpants, sticking to my skin, and brushing against my pubic hair, etc. I remember shifting it repeatedly from one side of my underpants to the other. It constantly intruded on my thoughts because it felt prickly, itchy, and uncomfortably sensitive. Now that I have a foreskin, my penis head is insulated and doesn't constantly intrude on my thoughts with feelings of discomfort, as my circumcised penis did. It is a joy. My penis head is now more sensitive, but the foreskin protects it, so I can save my sensitivity for the caresses of the vagina.

I really noticed circumcision's negative effects when I discovered my sexuality, although at the time I didn't realize they were a consequence of my circumcision. I thought the various discomforts I experienced were a normal part of having a penis.

When my circumcised penis became erect, it stretched the shaft skin very tightly (so tightly it caused my penis to curve upward). While most circumcised men might consider this "normal," to me it often felt uncomfortable, overstretched, and prickly hot, as if the shaft skin was working too hard to contain all the swollen tissue. Now that I have a foreskin, I have plenty of skin when my penis is erect and there is no strain on the shaft skin. My erections always feel comfortable.

When I first began to masturbate with my circumcised penis, if I ran my hand up and down the shaft, for even a short time, it would build up too much friction and burn. I learned that some guys lubricated their penises with cooking oil or Vaseline to make masturbation easier, but I found this too messy, too much work, and I still didn't like rubbing my whole shaft. It just wasn't comfortable.

I soon discovered that nearly all the pleasure in my penis was concentrated in a little dot of skin, not much bigger than a sesame seed, on the underside of my penis. That little dot of skin was frenulum tissue and was all that remained of my original frenulum and foreskin, but boy was it powered with pleasure. Just jiggling it, along with the area behind the coronal ridge, was enough to bring me to orgasm. Now, however, with my reconstructed foreskin, that dot of skin still gives me pleasure, but because my overall penis has been brought back to life, it is only another pleasure zone on my penis and not the central command center.

How is masturbation different now that I have a foreskin? My hand *glides* on the *mobile* shaft skin, and there is no friction build-up because my hand does not move frictionally along the penis shaft. Now, during natural masturbation, my hand and shaft skin act as one unit, gliding together over my inner shaft tissue. In addition, the glans is intermittently stimulated by the foreskin gliding over it, intensifying my pleasure.

Another irritating effect I experienced, once I engaged in circumcised sex, was an "aching" erection and soreness after intercourse. As I mentioned before, my shaft skin would become very tight as my erecting penis filled into it. During masturbation or intercourse, as I got increasingly excited, my circumcised penis would get even fuller, stiffer, and the skin would be drawn exceedingly tight. This would give me an "aching" erection— too stiff and too hard. It felt good and bad at the same time.

After moving it in and out of the vagina for a while, it would feel prickly, itchy, and would eventually get sore and chafed from the friction of sliding my overstretched thin skin in and out too many times. And often, the next day my penis would be red and sore, remaining prickly, itchy, and sensitive for up to two days. I remember vividly the day after a particularly lusty one-night stand spending my entire lunch hour in my car with my sore penis hanging out because it was so chafed I couldn't stand my underpants touching it.

Also, in retrospect, I sometimes thought that intercourse was deficient somehow, not fulfilling; that it was a bit of a let-down. It didn't seem to measure up to the "big deal" it was supposed to be. Too often, after it was over, I'd feel a strange sense of disappointment—a gnawing feeling that there should have been something more—like the experience didn't really connect the way it should have.

Although I was aware of various discomforts and negativities during and after my sexual activities, and even though the thought crossed my mind that sex was a bit of a let-down, it never occurred to me that these problems were related to my circumcision. Throughout my 20s and 30s, I maintained a fairly active sex life and considered myself a competent lover. I had read many sex manuals and incorporated their advice into my sexual technique. I was thoughtful and considerate of my sex partners before, during, and after sex. I had excellent control over my orgasmic timing and was capable of lasting a considerable length of time. Women were impressed with my staying power, but occasionally I would get complaints that my prolonged in and out thrusting made their vagina sore.

When I first began seeing Kristen, the author of this book, she was in the process of breaking up a long-standing love affair with a married man. He had a natural penis. Kristen and I dated for a year, lived together for a year, and then got married. Everything seemed fine during the first few years of our marriage, but as time went on, we became increasingly aware of our sexual incompatibility. Even though she praised me as a good lover, she began to suggest various ways to improve my thrusting techniques. Unfortunately, *I discovered that when I performed the way she wanted, it detracted from my enjoyment.* In order to please *her*, I had to give up what made *me* feel good.

After incorporating her suggestions, she showed a renewed interest in sex, but I didn't find her thrusting-technique suggestions sexually arousing enough and I lost interest. When I asserted my desires and performed in a way that pleased me, *she* lost interest. We sensed something wasn't right. We eventually realized we were sexually out of sync. It reminds me of a line from a song, "Just once, can we figure out what we keep doing wrong?"

Without my knowing, Kristen reunited with her previous natural lover and saw him intermittently. (As she later told me, they made love easily and naturally without any of the problems we were experiencing.) After that, she became much more insistent on making love her way in an effort to re-create the intercourse experience she'd had with her natural lover.

I worked hard to please her. We worked at entering very slowly and at a certain angle because her vagina was reluctant to accept my penis. After penetration, I kept my pubic mound close to hers and minimized my long in-and-out strokes. She liked my pubic mound to grind up against hers and continually pulled me in closer to restrict my thrusting movements. If I used long thrusting strokes, she would get frustrated and annoyed. When I used the short, close-in strokes she liked, I would lose my erection; I needed the long, hard, in-and-out strokes to excite my interest and keep my erection. We were travelling down two separate avenues for obtaining pleasure. In order for Kristen to achieve orgasm during intercourse, I had to give my full attention to pleasing her with the method *she* liked, and then I would achieve orgasm using the long-thrusting technique *I* liked.

In effect, we were each using the other's body to masturbate against, which is not the same as making love. Lovers totally abandon their individual egos, their individual awareness, and become a union of pleasuring.

It became more difficult for me to keep my mind on my sensations as I struggled to maintain a thrusting motion that felt unnatural to me, but was pleasing to her. Our sex organs were not mutually pleasuring each other in a compatible way. One night Kristen and I had a long talk and she told me she had gone back to re-experience her natural lover and concluded that our difficulties were related to my missing foreskin. I was shocked and humiliated, but deep down I suspected she was right.

By chance, not long after that, I came across a magazine article about Dr. Greer's surgical restoration procedure. I showed it to Kristen. She was very excited and called up right away to get all the details. I was reluctant to consider it. I shuddered at the thought of a cutting object near my penis. I thought—maybe the problem is Kristen. Maybe she's just too damn fussy. Maybe if I looked for a different sex partner, I could escape the problem. I was in conflict over this entire matter, but at the same time, I was coming to the realization that nature must have designed the foreskin for a sexual purpose. I began to consider that restoration might be my best option, because once I accepted the idea that circumcised sex wasn't anything like natural sex, I knew that even if I got myself another woman and was able to fool her for a while with various techniques that imitated the movements of natural thrusting, I would not be able to fool myself. My experience with my wife convinced me that circumcised sex was a second-rate experience for a woman, and I was not one for giving out second-rate anything. Moreover, my circumcision was causing me to miss out on one of life's supreme pleasures— wonderful, natural sex. An absurd social custom, the routine circumcision of infant boys, had cheated me out of the greatest gift nature can bestow on a man: a complete, intact, fully functioning penis.

Although I was still uncomfortable at the thought of being operated on, I felt more reassured when I spoke to John Strand, Dr. Greer's first restored patient. He was very supportive and talked glowingly about how wonderful it was to have his foreskin restored. After that, I booked myself for the earliest possible appointment.

The actual reconstruction operation was really no different from any other operation. The procedure was done in two stages, about four months apart. The first required anesthesia, the second did not. After the second procedure, it took another two months of healing before I could become sexually active again. But everything went smoothly, and although it was an adventurous undertaking, I am very happy I had it done and exceedingly pleased with the results.

With my foreskin restored, I feel like a whole person. Even if I never had sex again or never masturbated again for the rest of my life, I would still consider my restoration completely worthwhile because just having the foreskin covering my penis head is so protectively comforting. And the excitement of owning a foreskin isn't a feeling that goes away after a month or two, as is the case with most new toys. It's been about fourteen years since my restoration and not a day goes by that I don't think to myself or say to my wife, "I love having my 'foreskin' back. It's the best thing that I ever did for my body."

A foreskin makes you feel comforted, secure, and protected. It's like coming out of the water after a cool dip and wrapping yourself in a fluffy towel. It's like lying on the couch shivering and someone places a warm blanket over you. It's like walking in the hot sun and then sitting under a shady tree. It's like the feeling you get the day the doctor removes the cast from your leg that's been there for three months—you feel whole again and all your parts are working properly. It's a totally great feeling. I can't praise it enough.

One of the most enjoyable experiences of having a foreskin is getting an erection. How wonderful it feels as the head slowly emerges from under its protective cover. At the onset of arousal, the head slides its way along the inside of the foreskin, exciting the erotic nerves of both the inner lining and the head itself, especially the coronal area.. As it grows to fullness, the head stretches the opening at the foreskin's tip to make room for its emergence. My whole body tingles with anticipation. Suddenly, it bursts through the tip opening. And the foreskin then glides over the corona and down the penis shaft, stroking and titillating the nerves with its soft, slippery cover, very similar to the sensation of entering the vagina. When I first got my foreskin, I repeatedly got hard and then went soft and then hard, over and over, merely to delight in this sweet pleasure.

What is sex like after your foreskin is restored? Beyond your wildest imagination. Once restored, you are, for all intents and purposes, *functionally* restored back to a "natural" state. In your "natural" state, you are now equipped with everything you need to make lovemaking wonderful, so when you make love, you just do what comes naturally. You don't have to concentrate on technique. It's almost effortless; everything flows so easily. You just relax and drink in the pleasures. The vagina feels more deliciously soft, and you can feel it truly loving every stroke, as it loves you back with its sensuous caresses.

Everything you do seems to make the experience more wonderful for you and your partner. You feel like a natural-born lover. Together, almost as if you are one, you build yourselves to higher and higher plateaus of pleasure and ecstasy. You forget yourself, your problems, your technique—you just enjoy. And you don't have to wonder if it's good for her too, because you *know* it is. You feel very close to your partner. Very loving. Very grateful to be having such a wonderful time and participating in a shared experience that brings the two of you closer together in body and spirit. There's no anxiety about how you're performing, or that you might lose your erection, or that you might have trouble coming to orgasm, because these problems are now non-existent. No anxiety, no frustration, no hard work. It's mellow and relaxed—no tensed-up muscles.

And most importantly, your penis's upper shaft and head are alive with pleasure sensations you were never able to experience before. Some new sensations are intensely thrilling, while others are delicate and subtle, yet still superb. For example, one thrill, in particular, that I've become acutely aware of is the temperature-sensibility of the nerves in my upper penis.

In preparation for intercourse, when the penis is becoming erect, I sense the warm glans stirring inside its protective sheath. At full erection, with the foreskin retracted and the moist head exposed to the open air, I perceive a sensual cooling. Then, when the penis enters the vagina, the first touch of the 98.6^0 haven against the cooled glans feels like a trip to a tropical paradise. Upon deeper insertion, the penis head throbs with delight from the wondrous waves of warmth radiated by the hot, passionate vagina and the joyous returning to the temperature environment it was meant to live in—98.6^0—the temperature inside the vagina, the same temperature as inside the foreskin.

The increased pleasure from being restored is totally awesome. It's beyond totally awesome. There's no way to really describe how wonderful it is. And orgasm comes so much more easily and exquisitely (but you have complete control over when to have it).

Even though I used to think circumcised sex was enjoyable (although I'd find myself letting it lapse into infrequency, probably because it wasn't really *that* enjoyable), in retrospect, it is completely different from natural intercourse. There is no comparison. They're not even in the same league.

Natural sex is relaxing. The longer I partake, the more relaxed I feel. Circumcised sex, by comparison, was adrenalizing. I remember it as being a lot of work. And it seemed the longer I partook, the more I'd feel pumped up with tension.

My wife and I prefer to have our sex during the day. Often, after circumcised sex was over, even with the release of orgasm, I'd still feel pumped up physically, mentally, and emotionally. Though we'd cuddle for a few minutes afterward, and I might even dose off for a quick forty winks, when I finally got up I'd be set to do any activity—wash the car, watch a football game, paint the cellar stairs, whatever—right back to life as usual.

But with natural sex, I'm transported to a different world. Total escape. Life as usual is the furthest thing from my mind. Everyday concerns are far removed, as I am swept away in total surrender to the greatest physical joy in life. I am overcome with paradisal, blissful feelings of sensuosity, of peace and mellowness, and loving closeness to my partner. After cuddling and falling asleep after orgasm, I awaken, not to the usual way I feel, but to a feeling of freshness and rebirth that connects me back to the joy of being alive—a renewed love of life. And a knowing that natural sex, and the love it brings, is truly "nature's second sun."

And my wife and I relate to one another completely differently after natural sex than we did after circumcised sex. After natural sex, there is this wonderful feeling that we shared something extraordinarily special. We always comment on how lucky we are to have discovered the born again ecstasies of natural lovemaking, as we bask in the afterglow of supreme serenity and a renewing of our love for one another.

Whereas, after circumcised sex, we used to come away with "Well it wasn't what we had hoped for, but at least we got it out of the way." And arguments would sometimes develop.

As I said, circumcised sex was adrenalizing. By analogy, it's like driving in rush-hour traffic, it's tense, on alert, stop-and-go, working the traffic flow, checking your mirrors, inconsideration for the other driver, and subliminally irritating.

In contrast, natural sex is like a day off—no problems, relaxing in the warm sun while sitting on the soft grass of a peaceful river bank, a fishing pole in one hand, a refreshing drink in the other, and your dog sitting beside you, surrounded by the sounds of birds, the murmuring river, and jumping fish. In retrospect, if I were to rate sex before my restoration, I'd give it a two. Now that I'm restored, it's a ten. How sweet it is.

AN EXTRAORDINARY SEXUAL SECRET MAXIMIZES PLEASURE FOR THE RESTORED MAN

I also discovered something wonderfully important for men who restore.

Scientific research by Dr. John Taylor, et al., has proven that when circumcision cuts away the foreskin, thousands of highly erogenous nerves of the "ridged band" are removed and cannot be restored by present-day restoration methods. Disheartened circumcised men often fixate on this tragic loss and assert that with so much missing erogenous tissue, the restored man can never hope to approximate the experience of the genitally intact man. They wrongly conclude: Why bother to restore?

While it is true that restoration does not bring back the nerves of the ridged band, it does monumentally improve a man's sexual pleasure, as presented in the **Table of Sexual Benefits** following the end of the chapter.

But in addition, I have something more to add. Over time, after I became restored, I noticed that I was able to compensate for this loss in erogenous tissue by having my partner twiddle my nipples, intermittently, during intercourse.

As you will recall from Chapter 10, a Mayo Clinic study entitled, "The Erogenous Zones: Their Nerve Supply and Its Significance," evinces that *the ridged band of the foreskin and the skin of the nipples are comprised of the same specialized nerve tissue called "rete ridges."* Nipple skin abounds with Meissner's corpuscles (erotically responsive touch-sensitive nerves), like those found in the foreskin and frenulum.*

If you are a circumcised man, try this experiment. On your penis, locate the remnant of your excised frenulum. (On me, as mentioned, it is the size of a sesame seed, located at my circumcision scar, on the underside of my penis. Your remnant may be there too, or at the groove in your penis head, on the underside of the glans. You might want to refer back to page 55 where the frenulum is illustrated.)

Once located, caress it lightly and you'll notice how erogenously sensitive it is. Next, move your fingers to your nipples and stroke them gently. Notice that they, too, are erogenously sensitive.

---

* "The *specific* type of erogenous zone is found...in the genital regions, including the *prepuce [foreskin]*, penis, clitoris, and external genitalia of the female, and...lip, [and] *nipple*. It is the special anatomy of these regions that requires the use of the term 'specific' when one speaks of erotic sensations originating in the skin. This anatomy favors acute perception" (11). (Emphasis added)

Now go back and caress your frenulum remnant again, *first by itself, then caress it while simultaneously caressing your nipple.* Notice that when you caress only the frenulum remnant, you feel the pleasure sensations *only* in your penis. And that when you touch only your nipple, the pleasure sensations emanate *only* from there. *But when you caress them both together, the feelings are not localized to either area. Instead, you become aware of a general, overall feeling of heightened ecstasy.*

Keep in mind that the erotic nervous system of the body is interconnected. When you kiss a woman on the lips and caress her breasts at the same time, you will excite her more than if you do either act singularly.

When you have your partner twiddle your nipples during intercourse, combined with the increased pleasure experienced after restoration, I reckon that it heightens your sexual feelings to those experienced by the genitally intact man when his penis alone is stimulated during intercourse. **Essentially, the erogenous nerves of your nipples stand in for the departed sensory nerves of your foreskin and frenulum, allowing you to experience intercourse with your restored foreskin virtually as though you had a fully functioning intact penis.** I know it drives me to indescribable, overwhelming heights of pure ecstasy.

During this activity, the levels of ecstasy are so magnificent, I don't feel cheated in any way, even though I'm missing the nerves of the ridged band.

However, let me add that before restoration, this nipple-twiddling technique brought only minimal increased sensuosity, probably because of the many detractions in pleasure circumcision causes. Full appreciation of this technique can only be experienced after restoration.

And one final suggestion. As stated, this nipple-twiddling technique should be done intermittently because it's more pleasurable than constant twiddling. Therefore, whenever I want my partner to start or stop, I tap her lightly on the shoulder as a signal.

THE ULTIMATE ECSTASY: FRONT-DOOR TIPPING

Another awesome way I learned to compensate for the loss of the foreskin's erogenous nerves is through a technique I call "front-door tipping" (or "tipping", for short), where the tip of the penis gently kisses the tip of the vagina (the "front door"), repeatedly.

Front-door tipping utilizes our newfound knowledge of the male clitoris. If you had any doubts about the existence of the male clitoris, using this technique will allay them permanently.

Here's how it's done: Pull your penis out of the vagina until only its very tip is touching the vaginal entrance. Then, *while your partner twiddles your nipples,* slowly and gently move the penis forward about an inch or two (but no more) so that the penis head gets fully covered by the vagina. Then withdraw anew to the start position, where only the penis's tip touches the vaginal entrance. Pause briefly so stimulated nerves can recharge (this is the secret to why it works so well). Then move inward again.

I emphasize that your actions should be slow and methodical, allowing you time to savor each swooning caress against the vaginal opening. Each inward movement causes the male clitoral tip to be massaged internally and localizes all your sensations to this supremely erogenous area. Front-door tipping is only fully effective after restoration affords the upper-penis area relaxation of its inner tissue, due to the presence of sufficient shaft skin. Knowing about this technique is worth 1,000 times the price of the book and will bring you pleasure beyond your wildest dreams. Let me add this final point. *This technique is only attainable using the side-by-side position described in Appendix A* (because it allows you to completely relax and enables your partner to cross her hands and twiddle both your nipples simultaneously).

ONE MAN'S ACCOUNT OF RESTORING HIS FORESKIN USING *NON-SURGICAL* METHODS

I was born in Mississippi in 1949. My father was intact and saw no reason for routine infant circumcision. Luckily for me, my mother's obstetrician agreed, so I was left as God made me.

My brother was born a year later and he, too, was left intact. He and I were almost the only intact boys we knew. This didn't bother my brother, but it did concern me. So, at the age of 19, I elected to be circumcised. I soon realized what a great mistake I had made!

Prior to circumcision, the glans had been tender and moist, similar in texture to the inner surface of the mouth. The inner surface of the foreskin was smooth and tender as well, and very sensitive to erotic stimulation. The frenulum, also, was delicate and extremely sensitive to stimulation.

When I learned about masturbation from my (circumcised) peers, I first attempted to masturbate as I imagined they did—keeping the foreskin retracted with one hand, I tried rubbing the other hand up and down over the glans. Ouch! This was much too painful to be pleasurable at all. I soon learned the most common masturbation technique of intact men—holding the penis on the shaft and pulling the foreskin back and forth over the glans.

On each downstroke, the foreskin's delicate moist inner surface glided erotically over the glans, and the ridged band's gentle constriction slipped down the glans and "snapped" past the highly erogenous coronal ridge. When the foreskin was completely retracted, the frenulum gently pulled down on the underside of the glans (which I now know improves sensation to the glans during intercourse).

On each upstroke, the ridged band once again "snapped" past the coronal ridge with an erotic mini-startle to the erogenous system, and the foreskin's inner surface once again glided over and stimulated the tender, moist glans as it moved up, as it was designed to do.

I later learned that my circumcised friends sometimes or always used an artificial lubricant during masturbation. I never needed any, as the glans and inner foreskin were naturally moist, and the clear lubrication which was produced soon after having an erection was automatically applied to the glans by foreskin movement.

The glans was extremely sensitive to the touch, and only enjoyed pleasure when it was stimulated by another mucous membrane (such as the inner foreskin or the mouth or the vagina). As an inner organ (covered by the foreskin unless it was retracted), it was much too tender to be rubbed casually.

Orgasms were reached easily (but not prematurely), and they were intense enough to make my knees give way if I was standing.

Everything was different, however, after I was circumcised. Initially, I experienced continuous and disturbing irritation, as the now-exposed glans was very tender. It took about a month for it to become accustomed to constant friction from clothing and sexual activity could be resumed. But the sensations were dulled now.

The glans dried out and became much less sensitive. Even though I still have a frenulum, its nerves have been damaged and it is nowhere nearly as sensitive either.

I now had to masturbate with artificial lubrication (or risk the distinct possibility of an irritated penis). Orgasms often were achieved with extreme difficulty. They were still pleasurable, but they were much, much less intense than prior to circumcision.

I married at age 23, and throughout the next 17 years, my wife and I had a good sex life, but I often had trouble climaxing in intercourse due to a lack of sensation from the glans. I never could climax through fellatio, although this had not been a problem when I was intact. I assumed that my orgasm problems were probably psychological, and supposed that I would simply have to adjust to it (my wife was a virgin when we married, so she assumed that the long time I took to climax was normal, even though it often caused her to become raw during intercourse).

In the late 1980s, I came across references to foreskin restoration, instructions for which I was able to obtain. I was one of the rare and extremely fortunate men who was able to achieve full glans coverage within a year of beginning skin expansion techniques.

The glans is now tender and moist once again. It also has

regained most of its lost sensitivity, although not as much as before circumcision. As a consequence of these changes, I now have no trouble climaxing during either intercourse or fellatio.

My wife enjoys the feeling of the loose, moving shaft skin during intercourse, which gives her a different and "better" (according to her) feeling vaginally. We both enjoy the "glide sensation" of the loose-skinned penis during intercourse, and we like intercourse more than before restoration.

I enjoy masturbating with my restored foreskin (which is almost as good as the original, only lacking the ridged band), and my wife also enjoys playing with my restored foreskin during lovemaking and fellatio. She supports my views that routine infant circumcision is genital mutilation and must be stopped.

Aesthetically, my penis appears quite natural and can pass as intact in locker rooms to all but the most observant. I have even passed as intact during medical examinations, for the circumcision scar is not visible unless the foreskin is retracted. (Knowledgeable physicians, however, may notice the lack of the ridged band at the foreskin opening.)

My wife and I have two sons, born in 1979 and 1983. Although we had to take a stand against the hospital's wishes, we were able to keep both of our sons intact.

Our sons already know why many of their friends are circumcised (which my sons consider horrible), and as they become adults, I will share with them the sexual advantages of the intact penis. Neither they, my father, my brother, nor I ever had any medical problems sometimes associated with keeping the penis intact.

I strongly believe, with billions of persons around the world, that the penis was designed with a foreskin on purpose, and to routinely redesign this organ at birth is a grave mistake and probably a serious crime of child abuse.

****

WE INTERRUPT THIS BOOK
FOR AN IMPORTANT MESSAGE

"Hello. Hello. This is Mother Nature calling all men of America on planet Earth. Your women want you to 'grow' a gently gliding foreskin for your penis. Circumcision is a man-made mistake. A penis with a foreskin is the natural penis for men who diddle on this planet. Now is the time. And this is the place. Natural genitals for Americans will soon become commonplace. Ten-four. 'Tis the key to the mystery door, behind which you'll find the real sexual pleasure you've been searching for. Over and out."

****

Be honest with yourself. If you could just push a button and get your foreskin back, wouldn't you do it? Restoration will take some time and dedication. But in the end, the rewards will be worth it—increased sexual pleasure for the rest of your life. It's always easier to put off until tomorrow what you should be doing today. But in this case, restoration is something you should look into right away, without delay. Procrastination will not get you a new foreskin, but sending for Jim Bigelow's book, *The Joy of Uncircumcising!*, will (see page 215 or Resources at back of book). Also, be sure to visit the website below to see the amazing results restoration can bring.

www.tugahoy.com/Foreskin_Photos.htm

Men seeking support in their restoration efforts may also want to contact NORM at *www.norm-socal.org* or its parent organization *www.norm.org* (also see Resources section).

I wish you the best in your new endeavor.* Remember, the sooner you start, the sooner you'll get results, and the sooner you and your lover will be enjoying the many sexual benefits of the restored penis. (See **Table of Sexual Benefits** after next page.)

---

* DISCLAIMER: Nothing in this book is meant as, or should be taken as, medical advice. If you are interested in foreskin restoration, consult a physician (preferably one who is restoration-knowledgeable, or if not, open to learning about it). Research the subject carefully. Neither the publisher nor the authors can be responsible for the results you achieve through restorative procedures or for any loss or damage allegedly arising from any information or suggestion in this book.

Table of Sexual Benefits

For the Natural, Restored, and

Circumcised Penis

(Next Two Pages)

IMPORTANT

Be sure to check out the Appendixes at back of book.

The secrets they reveal are worth a thousand times
the price of the book.

APPENDIX A:

HOW TO INSURE THAT YOUR PARTNER HAS A VAGINAL ORGASM 99.99% OF THE TIME USING THE MOST COMFORTABLE AND MOST SATISFYING POSITION OF ALL

APPENDIX B:

HOW TO MINIMIZE PREMATURE EJACULATION
AND THE "TAP ME" SECRET
TO PROLONGING INTERCOURSE

APPENDIX C:

A SOLUTION FOR THOSE CIRCUMCISED MEN
WHO TAKE LONGER THAN THEY WANT
TO REACH ORGASM

TABLE OF SEXUAL BENEFITS for <u>N</u>atural, <u>R</u>estored, <u>C</u>ircumcised Penis

	N	R	C
1. Derives pleasure from all erogenous nerves of the foreskin and frenulum.	yes	no	no
2. Experiences a high degree of sensitivity from the nerves of the foreskin's *inner lining*, due to moisturizing and outer foreskin's protective effects.	yes	yes	no
3. Experiences full sensitivity from *temperature-sensing nerves* of the glans because these nerves are reawakened and revitalized by the foreskin's cloaking effects.	yes	yes	no
4. Because the *glans* emerges from a moistened environment and is not abnormally compacted by an overstretched skin, it is relatively pliable; thus its movements create a massaging effect that excites the clitoral tip's pressure-sensitive nerves.	yes	yes	no
5. Because the *glans* is resilient and pliable, the coronal area can flex and stretch, so it doesn't get chafed and sore from intercourse.	yes	yes	no
6. Because the *shaft* is not compacted by a constricting, overstretched shaft skin, the shaft's tissue is pliable, so it experiences more of a massaging effect to its pressure-sensitive nerves.	yes	yes	no
7. Enough shaft skin for a comfortable erection.	yes	yes	may
8. Gliding mechanism of the foreskin reduces friction; sex is more comfortable.	yes	yes	no
9. Foreskin's up-and-down movement alternately stimulates and rests nerves of its inner lining and the coronal area, resulting in high levels of pleasure.	yes	yes	no

10. Foreskin bunches and unbunches to alternately stimulate and rest the pressure-sensitive nerves in the tip of the (male) clitoris.	yes	yes	no
11. Likelier to experience an *effortless* orgasm due to nerve stimulation/rest concept.	yes	yes	may
12. Likelier to experience an *intensified* orgasm due to nerve stimulation/rest concept.	yes	yes	no
13. Experiences the thrill of an erecting penis emerging from its protective foreskin.	yes	yes	no
14. Experiences the pleasure of a relaxed vagina that is more accepting of the penis (vagina is not overly tensed and tightened).	yes	yes	no
15. Enjoys the reward of knowing that his female partner is more truly pleasured by the penis thrusting the way nature intended.	yes	yes	no
16. Enjoys the reward of his female partner's increased frequency of vaginal orgasm.	yes	yes	no
17. Intercourse isn't as physically demanding; less work and less muscle tension are required, so the man can relax and enjoy the subtle pleasures of intercourse.	yes	yes	no
18. Enjoys a mutually shared positive experience with his partner that strengthens their love bond (it does not seem like it was two separate masturbatory-like experiences). More affection during times of non-intercourse may result.	yes	yes	no
19. Likely to have sex more often due to greater interest from his partner, and himself.	yes	yes	no
20. Likelier to have an active sex life in his later years and to have fewer problems in maintaining an erection due to increased arousal capabilities, described above.	yes	yes	no

13

Survey Results of Women Sexually Experienced with Both Circumcised and Uncircumcised Men

This chapter will report the results of a survey of women who have had the comparative experience of intercourse with both circumcised and intact (uncircumcised) men.

THE PURPOSE OF THE SURVEY

The purpose of the survey was to determine the impact circumcision—the surgical alteration of the male genitalia—has on the intercourse experience of the female partner. Specifically, what effect does it have on a woman's ability to:

- achieve vaginal orgasm (both single and multiple)
- maintain adequate vaginal lubrication
- develop vaginal discomfort
- enjoy intercourse

Additionally, the survey sought to find out if women can:

- discern different physical characteristics for both types of intercourse
- discern a difference in various positive and negative thoughts and emotions for both types of intercourse

HOW RESPONDENTS WERE RECRUITED AND SURVEY CONDUCTED

Classified ads were run in various publications (local and national) seeking women who have had experience with both types of men. Respondents were mailed a questionnaire to complete and return anonymously. Surveyed women were aware that their responses and comments could be used in a forthcoming book, though the title of the book was not mentioned.

The survey was conducted intermittently over several years and modified slightly from time to time in that some questions were restructured or reworded to make them more easily understood, but the context of the question was not changed. Women were given a brief introduction to the survey and were presented with line drawings of the two types of penises, both flaccid and erect, including the erection process of the natural penis. The survey questionnaire appears in Appendix F.

Of the 284 surveys sent out, 139 were completed and returned. Of the 139 surveys returned, one considered a man who was undergoing foreskin restoration as having a foreskin. This survey was excluded from analysis. The remaining 138 surveys were analyzed. The thought-provoking results are reported in the pages that follow. Albeit the survey is small, but its findings still tell a big story. Indeed, the survey's results were originally published in a supplement to the *BJU* (British Journal of Urology) *International* in January, 1999, analyzed statistically, and found to have statistical significance. (See Appendix E.)

A PREVIEW OF THE SURVEY'S FINDINGS

The vast majority of women indicated that they overwhelmingly preferred sex with a natural penis. **And they were able to discern specific differences between the two types of intercourse.**

Women were in broad general agreement with the following:

- Natural intercourse is more pleasurable.
- Natural penis thrusts more gently.
- Natural penis's strokes feel more softly-smooth and sensuous.
- Natural man's pubic area is in more constant contact with the woman's clitoral mound (due to the natural penis's propensity for using shorter strokes).

At the same time they concurred:

- Circumcised intercourse is less pleasurable.
- Circumcised penis thrusts rougher and tougher.
- Circumcised penis somehow feels too hard, even discomfortingly harder.
- Circumcised man's pubic area is in much less frequent contact with the woman's clitoral mound (due to the circumcised penis's propensity for using longer strokes).

Of paramount importance, **women overall reported remarkably higher vaginal-orgasmic success rates with intact (uncircumcised) men.** Firstly, they were able to achieve vaginal orgasm with a much higher percentage of intact men vs. circumcised men, coincidentally, exactly double. And secondly, for those men with whom they could achieve it, their rate of success was considerably higher when the man was intact. Thirdly, they achieved multiple orgasms more often with intact men.

Many such astonishing, and disconcerting, revelations turned up when the results of the survey were analyzed. Are these findings destined to change the sex life and sexual attitude of America's men and women forever?

> **"When falling in love and choosing a life partner, it never occurred to me to check the status of his penis first, but this survey has allowed me to see clearly that there are big differences and that I have strong feelings about my sexual experiences with each type."**

A DETAILED ANALYSIS OF THE SURVEY'S RESULTS

Women's responses to the following category of questions brought to light the survey's **MOST IMPORTANT FINDING: Respondents overwhelmingly preferred intercourse with a partner with an anatomically complete penis.**

Question: For YOU, regardless of your vaginal-orgasmic capabilities, which type of intercourse simply **feels better during the overall experience**?

Circumcised	Natural
11 %	89 %

Question: During which type of sex do YOU **feel more relaxed, comfortable, and at ease**?

Circumcised	Natural
13%	87%

Question: You have been shipwrecked and washed ashore onto a descrtcd paradise island in the Pacific. Your rescue ship won't be by to pick you up for five years. On this island is only one other person—a man—a very attractive man, who is interesting to be with and is very likeable. Because you are in paradise, you will probably be having sex fairly often. When you get around to your first lovemaking encounter and you are slowly undoing his belt and pants, would you be wishing that he is

Circumcised	Natural
11 %	89 %

Author's Comment: The above question was designed to eliminate the personality factor and the quandary of some women regarding: Is it the man or the penis?

Question: Of your CIRCUMCISED experiences where the time of ACTUAL intercourse lasted for 8-10 minutes or more, as intercourse progressed,

Did you OFTEN start wishing to just get it over with? Yes No

— OR —

Did you OFTEN really get into it & want it to continue? Yes No

The same question was asked regarding their NATURAL intercourse experiences.

Results: **Circumcised Natural**

Often start wishing to **just get it over with**   70 %   9 %

Often really **get into it & want it to continue**   30 %   91 %

Author's Comment: What a contrast! What a reversal! For circumcised intercourse, 70% of women indicated that they "often start wishing to just get it over with." For natural, inversely, 91 % indicated that they "often really get into it and want it to continue." Isn't the latter the way it should be? Isn't this the basis for "the tie that binds"?

Question: This question will ask you to assess your **overall impression of sexual intercourse with CIRCUMCISED men, rating it as either a positive or negative experience.** You may only indicate ONE number in your response, rating it from a negative (-) 10 to a positive (+) 10.

The same question was asked for NATURAL.

Results:

Circumcised intercourse received an average rating of +2
Natural intercourse received an average rating of +8

Author's Comment: Again, another eye-opener! But even more impressive, provocative, and revealing is the breakdown report for each individual number on the rating scale (Figure 13-1).

Your OVERALL Impression of Intercourse with CIRCUMCISED Men										
Negative Experience	-10	-9	-8	-7	-6	-5	-4	-3	-2	-1
Number of Women	9	4	4	2	5	8	3	4	2	4
							Total Negatives = 45			
Positive Experience	+1	+2	+3	+4	+5	+6	+7	+8	+9	+10
Number of Women	3	6	9	5	13	10	19	17	2	6
							Total +9 thru +10 = 8			
							Total +8 thru +10 = 25			

Your OVERALL Impression of Intercourse with NATURAL Men										
Negative Experience	-10	-9	-8	-7	-6	-5	-4	-3	-2	-1
Number of Women	0	0	0	1	0	1	0	1	1	0
							Total Negatives = 4			
Positive Experience	+1	+2	+3	+4	+5	+6	+7	+8	+9	+10
Number of Women	0	3	3	3	1	4	8	27	20	63
							Total +9 thru +10 = 83			
							Total +8 thru +10 = 110			

Figure 13-1. Breakdown report of overall impression of intercourse with circumcised and natural men.

Women's answers to the next group of questions brought out the survey's **SECOND MOST IMPORTANT FINDING: Respondents overwhelmingly concurred that the mechanics of coitus were different for the two groups of men.**

Question: Do you tend to agree or disagree with the following: The NATURAL man's pubic area stays in closer contact with the woman's clitoral area during intercourse because he tends to use *shorter* strokes in his thrusting movements. He seems to gently "grind" or "jiggle" more, resulting in a pleasant pressuring of the woman's clitoral area which gives her greater pleasure.

Question: Do you tend to agree or disagree with the following: The CIRCUMCISED man's pubic area makes less contact with the woman's clitoral area during intercourse because he tends to use *longer* strokes in his thrusting movements. These longer thrusts result in less physical contact between his pubic mound and the woman's clitoral area.

- **71 % agreed that the natural penis tends to thrust with shorter strokes, resulting in more clitoral contact and greater pleasure.**

- **73 % agreed that the circumcised penis tends to use longer strokes, resulting in less clitoral contact.**

Author's Comment: Nearly 3/4 of the women agreed that the natural and circumcised penis thrust differently.

Question: Do you tend to agree or disagree with the following: In general, intercourse with the CIRCUMCISED man is more rough—they tend to pound or bang away and the penis feels discomfortingly harder during intercourse thrusting.

In contrast, the NATURAL man has gentler and more sensually tender sexual movements, and the penis does *not* feel discomfortingly hard during intercourse thrusting.

Please circle AGREE if you tend to agree with this entire statement, or underline those parts you tend to agree with. Comments:

If you disagree with this entire statement, circle DISAGREE, and explain in what way your experiences differ. Comments:

Author's Comment: Before delving into the results of the above question, first let me state that I eventually came to realize that I made a mistake combining so many concepts into one question. By doing so, it may have made it difficult for some women to agree with the statement *in its entirety*. At the very least, this should have been two separate statements—one for circumcised, one for natural. In the current edition of the survey, this question, for each type, is divided into 12 checkoffs. Although the question could have been constructed better, nevertheless, women were in broad general agreement with it, and the results are as follows:

- **74 % agreed, circumcised sex is rougher**
- **72 % agreed, circumcised men tend to pound or bang away**
- **67 % agreed, circumcised penis feels discomfortingly harder**

- **87 % agreed, natural man thrusts more gently**
- **89 % agreed, natural penis has more sensually tender movements**
- **86 % agreed, natural penis does not feel discomfortingly hard**

Author's Comment: It is interesting to note that more women found it easier to agree with the statements about natural, possibly because these positive experiences stood out in their mind. They were in less general agreement on the statements about circumcised men, possibly because the severity of the tightness of a man's circumcision can vary, and this can impact the intercourse experience.

The survey contained several questions that addressed vaginal-orgasmic capabilities and the results led to:

The THIRD MOST IMPORTANT FINDING: Women overall were less likely to achieve vaginal orgasm with circumcised men. They had considerably more success achieving vaginal orgasm when the man had a natural penis.

Author's Comment: The vast majority of surveyed women were capable of achieving vaginal orgasm, but 15 women were not capable of achieving it with either partner. These 15 women were excluded from analysis for this series of questions. (There may be other reasons why a woman cannot achieve vaginal orgasm besides the type of penis a man has—smoking, alcohol consumption, prescription-drug side effects, low vitamin B12 levels, and low histamine levels, among others, are all possible causes of sexual dysfunction. Also, the man may be at fault if he can't last long enough. And the woman may not be interactive enough to bring about her own orgasm. Position may also be a factor. I touch on these last three topics in Appendix A: How to Have an Orgasm 99.99% of the Time Using the Side-by-Side Position, and Appendix B: How To Minimize Premature Ejaculation.)

The survey defined vaginal orgasm as follows:

A VAGINAL ORGASM* is an orgasm that occurs during intercourse, brought about by your partner's penis and its accompanying pelvic movements and body contact, along with your own pelvic movements, with no simultaneous stimulation of the clitoris by hand. What happens during FOREPLAY is NOT OF CONCERN. But once serious intercourse thrusting begins, a vaginal orgasm is one which you feel was brought about by genital/pelvic movements and body contact/pressure.

Question: With how many CIRCUMCISED men have you been able to achieve a *VAGINAL* orgasm? number of men ___

The same question was asked for NATURAL.

* This definition differs slightly from the one presented in Chapter 3. It is the actual definition used for the survey. Subsequently, it was refined for the book.

The following results were determined by dividing the number of men indicated in the above question by the total number of circumcised, or natural partners.

Women could achieve vaginal orgasm with:

36 % of their CIRCUMCISED partners

72 % of their NATURAL partners

Author's Comment: The percentage for NATURAL was coincidentally exactly double the percentage for CIRCUMCISED. These percentages differ from those in the *BJU* (see Appendix E) because the criteria was changed: women who could not orgasm with either type were excluded for the book's analysis.

Question: With those CIRCUMCISED men *with whom you were able to achieve a vaginal orgasm*, approximately what percent of the time would you say you were able to achieve *vaginal orgasm*? ___ %

The same question was asked for NATURAL.

Among the 123 respondents capable of vaginal orgasm, 12 % reported the same frequency of vaginal-orgasmic success regardless of whether the man was natural or circumcised. However,

76 % reported an increased frequency with NATURAL

10 % reported increased frequency with CIRCUMCISED

Upon closer scrutiny, these results are even more revealing. Forty-seven women (38 %) reported that their vaginal-orgasmic success increased by an **impressive** degree **(by three times or more)** with NATURAL. Conversely, only four women (3 %) reported an impressive increase with CIRCUMCISED. (See Figure 13-2.)

Women Whose Vaginal-Orgasmic Success Increased by 3 Times or More

w/Natural Partners, 47 Women (38%) Increased

% w/ Circ	% w/ Nat	% w/ Circ	% w/ Nat	% w/ Circ	% w/ Nat
0	100	5	99	20	90
0	100	5	95	20	90
0	98	5	90	20	80
0	98	5	70	20	80
0	90	5	50	20	75
0	90	5	50	20	60
0	86	10	100	25	100
0	80	10	99	25	75
0	75	10	98	25	75
0	70	10	80	30	100
0	70	10	80	30	90
0	70	10	75	30	90
0	70	10	75	30	90
0	60	10	60		
0	50	10	50		
0	30	10	30		
2	60				
2	45				

w/Circ, 4 (3%) Increased

% w/ Nat	% w/ Circ
10	60
10	40
15	95
30	98

Figure 13-2. Impressive gains in vaginal-orgasmic success

Note that for these women, more than 2/3 had only a 10% or less success rate with circumcised, and an impressive increase with natural.

In addition, with NATURAL partners, 34 women (28%) indicated **noteworthy** increases in vaginal-orgasmic success. In contrast, for CIRCUMCISED, only 7 women (6%) fell into the noteworthy category. (See Figure 13-3.) ***In all, 66% of women indicated an impressive or noteworthy increase in their vaginal-orgasmic success for natural vs. 9% for circumcised.***

Some women (8%) had limited success with both types of partners and any differences reported were either marginal or nonexistent. Inversely, 18% had excellent rates of vaginal-orgasmic success (80% or above) with both types of partners. Still, even among these highly orgasmic women, 59% reported better success with their natural partners.

When this data was analyzed statistically, women were nearly 5 times likelier to achieve vaginal orgasm with natural partners than with circumcised partners (odds ratio = 4.62, see Appendix E.)

Question: If you are capable of achieving vaginal orgasm during your CIRCUMCISED intercourse experiences, have you generally been able to achieve MULTIPLE vaginal orgasms?

mostly yes___   mostly no___   rarely___   never___

The same question was asked for NATURAL

Results:

Are you able to achieve MULTIPLE vaginal orgasms?				
	Mostly YES	Mostly NO	Rarely	Never
Natural	41%	15%	20%	24%
Circumcised	15%	21%	20%	44%

Women whose Vaginal-Orgamic Success Increase was Noteworthy

w/Natural Partners, 34 Women (28%) Increased

% w/ Circ	% w/ Nat	% w/ Circ	% w/ Nat
0	8	50	100
0	10	50	100
0	10	50	95
0	15	50	75
10	20	50	75
10	25	50	75
20	45	50	70
25	60	50	70
25	60	60	99
25	50	60	85
30	60	70	95
30	50	70	80
40	100	70	75
40	100	75	99
40	60	75	90
40	50		
45	75		
46	78		

w/Circ, 7 (6%) Increased

% w/ Nat	% w/ Circ
0	10
35	85
40	50
50	80
50	75
50	70
80	90

Figure 13-3. Noteworthy gains in vaginal-orgamic success

Author's Comment: It is clear from the results of the above questions that the anatomically complete penis offers a woman a much greater chance of vaginal-orgasmic success. Though the popular press indicates that many women persist in wanting vaginal orgasms, some women indicated that they prefer other types, manual or oral. This is perfectly acceptable, of course, but how much is this influenced by the poor rate of vaginal-orgasmic success they had with their circumcised partners? If these women were conditioned to go for other types of orgasms due to their poor success rates with circumcised partners, this may carry over into subsequent sexual encounters. Of interest is the strong preference women who preferred vaginal orgasms had for natural partners (see Appendix E).

OTHER IMPORTANT SURVEY REVELATIONS

Shorter Duration of Intercourse

Question: Of your CIRCUMCISED intercourse experiences, how many men USUALLY (50-100% of the time) had their orgasm within 2-3 minutes after insertion? ___ number of men

The same question was asked for NATURAL.

Results:

Women indicated that, on average, 42% of their circumcised partners had a problem with premature ejaculation (as defined in the above question). They indicated that for natural 28% had a problem with premature ejaculation.

   Clearly, premature ejaculation is a problem for both types of men, though not as severe for natural as it is for circumcised. My suggestion for eliminating or reducing premature ejaculation is discussed in Appendix B. It's a simple solution, but I found it very effective.

Question: EXCLUDING your CIRCUMCISED intercourse experiences that only lasted 2-3 minutes, how long would you say your average CIRCUMCISED intercourse lasts (intercourse time only, NOT foreplay, etc.). This should be an overall estimated average.

The same question was asked for NATURAL.

Results:

According to these women, the estimated average length of circumcised intercourse is 11 minutes. For natural, 15 minutes. This indicates that natural intercourse lasts about 1/3 longer than circumcised intercourse. (Precious moments filled with pleasure, deepening the love bond—*Author's Comment.*)

Vaginal Lubrication

Question: During those intercourses with CIRCUMCISED men which lasted 5 minutes or longer, as intercourse progressed, did the amount of vaginal lubrication   (circle one)

    lessen   stay about the same   increase

The same question was asked for NATURAL.

Results:

	Lessen	**Stay the Same**	**Increase**
Circumcised	46%	33%	21%
Natural	5%	30%	65%

Author's Comment: If the production of vaginal lubrication is an indication of the excitement of the female partner, then clearly natural intercourse overwhelmingly offers the more rewarding experience.

Vaginal Discomfort

Question: Regarding CIRCUMCISED intercourse, have you experienced vaginal discomfort during sex (or after having sex)? Please circle one.   often   occasionally   rarely   never

The same question was asked for NATURAL.

Results:

	Often	Occasionally	Rarely	Never
Circumcised	31%	45%	17%	7%
Natural	2%	21%	37%	40%

Author's Comment: When the results for "often" and "occasionally" are combined into one group, circumcised is 76%, natural 23% (w/only 2% often). At the other extreme, when the results for "rarely" and "never" are combined, natural is 77%, circumcised is 24%. Evidently, vaginal discomfort is a serious concern with circumcised intercourse. Since freedom from discomfort is a primary factor in the degree of pleasure a woman experiences, natural intercourse clearly offers a woman the better experience.

Negative Thoughts and Emotions Correlated with Intercourse

Question: During or after many CIRCUMCISED intercourses, have you noticed yourself having any of the feelings below? If so, indicate with (S)ometimes or (O)ften

The same question was asked for NATURAL.

Results: See Figure 13-4. Note: Scored as points.

During or after many of my intercourse experiences, I had the following feelings		
OFTEN (scored as 2 points) SOMETIMES (1 point)	Circ	Nat
Irritability	81	11
Unappreciated	97	14
Sexually Violated	66	13
Emotionally Aggravated	69	9
General Out of Sync Feeling	94	9
He Cared Very Little About My Sexual Satisfaction	115	16
Except for My Vagina, He Didn't Seem to Know I Was There	78	8
Bitchy, Argumentative	50	10
Guilty	52	11
We Had Two Separate Experiences (No Feeling of Unison)	114	18
Our Thrusting Rhythms Were Out of Sync	99	18
Felt Like I Was Used as a Masturbating Object	90	22
Incomplete as a Woman	54	7
I'm Glad It's Over	114	17
TOTAL POINTS	820	178
NONE of the above (number of responses)	20	80

Figure 13-4. Negative thoughts and emotions correlated with intercourse

Author's Comment: Note that for natural, 80 women (58%) indicated "NONE of the above." For circumcised, negative thoughts and emotions occurred 4½ times more often.

Question: During intercourse with most CIRCUMCISED men, do any of these thoughts often cross your mind? Please check all those that apply.

The same question was asked for NATURAL.

Results: See Figure 13-5.

During most of my intercourse experiences, the following thoughts often crossed my mind	Circ	Nat
He seems to be distanced from what I'm feeling	53	8
My mind wanders to other things	69	17
He seems to work too hard at it (like it's exercise)	77	5
He seems to concentrate on his sexual needs, not mine	61	8
He seems to work too hard to achieve orgasm	58	12
I seem to be becoming disinterested	56	4
My vagina doesn't seem to be enjoying this	58	12
When he's pumping, I'm afraid he might hurt me	61	6
We seem to be engaging in two separate experiences	41	13
I feel "on alert"	23	9
Frustration	38	5
Discomfort	52	7
A general feeling of discontentment	47	8
TOTALS	693	114
NONE of the above	9	82

Figure 13-5. Negative thoughts correlated with intercourse

Author's Comment: Note that for natural, 82 women (64%) indicated "NONE of the above," while for circumcised only 9 women indicated NONE. Also note, negative thoughts occurred 6 times more often for circumcised.

Positive Thoughts and Emotions Correlated with Intercourse

Question: How would you describe your GENERAL feelings after having sex with most CIRCUMCISED men? Please check all those that apply.

The same question was asked for NATURAL.

Results: See Figure 13-6.

Positive Feelings After Intercourse	Circ	Nat
A feeling of relaxation	45	98
A feeling of being at peace with myself and my partner	27	72
A sense of human warmth and closeness to my partner	43	96
A sense of a mutually satisfying experience	39	93
A sense of completeness and wholeness as a woman	26	80
A wonderful positive-feeling afterglow	37	88
Gee, that was really great	31	74
What a lover!!	15	75
TOTALS	263	676
NONE of the above	56	8

Figure 13-6. Positive thoughts and emotions after intercourse.

Author's Comment: Note that for circumcised, 56 women (41%) indicated NONE of the above, while for natural only 8 women indicated no positive feelings. Also note, positive feelings occurred 2½ times more often for natural.

AGE AND NUMBER OF PARTNERS

Participants ranged in age from 19 to 64. The average age was 37.3 years. The median number of circumcised partners was 8. The median number of intact partners was 2.

QUESTIONS YOU MAY HAVE WONDERED ABOUT WHILE READING THE SURVEY RESULTS

If natural intercourse is so spectacular, why didn't all women prefer it?

From my experience, having noticed such a remarkable difference between the two types of intercourse, I was surprised that the survey wasn't 100% in favor of natural. After carefully looking at the responses and comments of the 14* women who indicated that they prefer circumcised, I offer the following explanation.

First, all people are not equally perceptive. Some are more sensitive, observant, and aware than others. Some are not very perceptive at all. This is simply a characteristic of human nature.

Second, half of these 14 women experienced *only one natural partner* vs. many circumcised partners. If this one intact man happened to have a problem with premature ejaculation, or a foreskin that would not retract over the glans (thus abnormalizing the intercourse experience), or poor personal hygiene, or if the man was in some way a sexual cad, or if the relationship was particularly bad (all of which were indicated in comments), this

---

* The results of the survey were originally published in a supplement to the ***BJU*** (British Journal of Urology) ***International*** (see Appendix E), which reported 20 women. It is reported here as 14 women because the criteria was changed. In the *BJU* article, the criteria was: *one favorable* response (for circumcised) *out of three* questions that asked specifically which type of penis they prefer. For *Sex As Nature Intended It*, the criteria was changed to: *two favorable responses* (for circumcised) *out of three*. Upon re-examining this aspect for the book, it seemed a more accurate assessment of their true opinion—2 out of 3 (a majority) instead of 1 of 3 (not a majority).

would incline these women away from natural in favor of circumcised. It could be inferred that it wasn't so much that they preferred circumcised as it was that they had a disagreeable experience with *one natural partner*. In a sense, it could be said that circumcised won by default rather than by virtue of its merits. These women may have swayed toward natural if they had had a broader base of experience with additional natural partners.

Third, if a woman has a preconceived mindset that the natural penis looks odd, or that it's abnormal, or unclean, etc., this may adversely affect her attitude toward the intercourse experience. She may not be able to relax her prejudices long enough to develop an appreciation for the natural experience. Several women who chose circumcised made prejudicial comments, mostly centered around a concern for cleanliness or a dislike for the look of the natural penis, indicating a tendency to choose the familiar and shun the unfamiliar.

Fourth, some women, who were not able to distinguish much of a difference (their natural experience may have occurred quite some time ago) and were currently engaged in a satisfactory relationship with a circumcised man (usually their husband), may have chosen circumcised because they were pleased overall with the man they were presently with at the time of the survey. Their decision may have been based more on "the man" and the satisfactory relationship rather than on the attributes of the penis.

Other factors may also influence a woman's decision, as discussed in the next section (omitted in this section to avoid repetition).

If all things had been equal—same number of partners; same amount of experience with both types of partners; lack of prejudice because the natural penis is in the minority; lack of preconceived ideas that the circumcised penis is cleaner, etc.; and the fact that most women were currently with a circumcised partner or may have had their sons circumcised, evoking a certain amount of denial and concern—I propose that the natural penis would have approached total approbation.

Although all women did not choose natural, keep in mind that only 14 out of 138 chose circumcised. And of these 14, three women rated circumcised and natural about the same on the negative (-) 10 to a positive (+) 10 ratings question.

The thing that struck me, as I looked over the surveys of women who chose circumcised, was the lack of jubilant accolades. They dutifully checked off choices but rarely applauded the joys of sex in their responses and comments.

In contrast, women who chose natural often spoke glowingly about the sexual charms of the natural penis. Yet, this type of enthusiasm for circumcised was virtually completely lacking when women preferred circumcised. If I were to write this book from a point of view that extolled circumcised, I would have had a pittance of comments to punctuate my points. Essentially, even though these women indicated they favored circumcised, *they "damned it with faint praise."*

Possible reasons why a woman, asked casually, may indicate she doesn't notice a difference between the two penis types.

A male acquaintance, who knew I was writing this book, told me that when he casually asked a few women if they could tell the difference between the natural and circumcised penis during intercourse, they didn't have much to say. I would like to offer an explanation for why this may be so.

First, a woman may actually notice a difference, but may not be inclined to talk about it openly, especially if the person asking the question is a male.

Second, as mentioned, quite a few women commented that they didn't consciously realize the extent of the differences until filling out the specifics of the survey, which prompted them to think about and analyze their past experiences.

Third, a woman may notice differences, but she may not attribute them to the penis. If she has experienced only one intact man (they being so rare in America), she may be inclined to think that "differences are just *his* individual technique."

Whereas, if she were to experience more than one, she may notice a commonality among her natural partners and realize that the differences are due to the type of penis.

Fourth, age (experience) is a definite factor. Some women may have had their natural experience in their earlier years, when they were not as qualitatively discerning, *especially if they were not looking for or expecting a difference.* Age and experience (more exposures to natural intercourse) bring insight into the differences.

Last and most important, a woman may offhandedly reply that she can't feel the physical difference between the two types of penises, per se, during intercourse. And, by and large, this is an accurate statement. Because the vagina is predominantly innervated with *pressure-sensitive nerves* that are not equipped to discern fine-touch stimuli; thus, it cannot definitively delineate differences in the *physical structure* of the two penis types.

However, women of the survey were able to identify several differences between the two *types of intercourse* and the quality of pleasure they experienced. This is because: **It is not the penis's structure that a woman predominantly feels, but rather <u>her vagina's reaction</u> to the penis's structure, movements, and sexing.** The natural penis (with its giveability and foreskin's cushioning) induces the vagina to relax, to soften, to moisten, thereby making it more sensuously receptive to pleasure. The circumcised penis, on the other hand (with its abnormal hardness and scraping action), causes the vagina to tense up, to tighten, to dry out, thus making it comparatively insensitive and less receptive to pleasurable feelings.

The above can vary depending on how tightly the man is circumcised, how vigorously he thrusts, and how long intercourse lasts. If a man is loosely circumcised, is moderately aggressive in his thrusting, or lasts only a few minutes, the vagina's reaction will not be as severely negative. Thus, some women may not notice the degree of negativity that other women notice.

Why is the number of surveyed women so small? Can the results of such a small sampling of women be applied to the general population?

The number of women is small for several reasons. To begin with, only classified ads were used to search for prospects, and even ads run in national publications with large circulations elicited only a few respondents. (Apparently, very few people read classified ads.) Next, women had to qualify by having had sex with both types of men, and since there are so few intact men in America, this narrowed the field. Then, women had to be uninhibited and interested enough to send for the survey. Lastly, after getting the ten-page survey, which might put them off, they had to take their personal time to fill it out and return it. My original goal was 1,000 women, but this would have been beyond my financial capabilities.

However, even though the number of women is small, the results still tell a big story. This was not a close contest. The intact penis was the overwhelming choice, even though it was the underdog, due to its minority status and the derogatory myths that surround the uncircumcised penis.

Although the survey sampled only a small number of women, it did include women of all ages, from all areas of the country. It could be postulated that if the numbers were greater, 1,000 or 10,000, the results might not differ significantly. This is similar to election night results where only a small number of precincts have reported and yet the final results of the election can be predicted within a small margin of error. It is not entirely unreasonable to assume that this sampling of women, although small, represents the opinion of women overall who have experienced both types of intercourse. As mentioned, the results of the survey were originally published in a supplement to the ***BJU*** (British Journal of Urology) ***International*** in January, 1999, analyzed statistically, and found to have statistical significance. (See Appendix E.)

In the final analysis, even if there were no survey of women, previous chapters explaining the sexual functions of the foreskin make it clear that the natural penis, by its very structure, offers an infinitely more rewarding experience for the woman.

Were the survey's results derived from a random sampling of women?

Respondents to my ads in various publications knew I was looking specifically for women experienced with both types of men. Thus, the survey does not represent a random sampling of women from the general population.

When I originally formulated the survey, I knew that I could discern several differences between the two types of penises and the overall intercourse experience, but I wasn't sure other women would notice these differences and be able to express them. Thus, I was interested only in women with the dual experience of both types of men, to see what they had to say on this issue.

A random sampling would have been an exercise in futility, besides being economically infeasible. It didn't make sense to me to run ads soliciting women for a general sexual survey and then have to sift through piles of surveys from women who have not had the comparative experience and are thus not qualified to have an opinion on this matter.

Also, I must add that 64 respondents (slightly over 45%) were solicited through an ad in an anti-circumcision newsletter. However, when their responses were compared with the other respondents, there were no significant differences. Furthermore, at no time were the sexual subjects of this book discussed in the aforementioned newsletter. In addition, I emphasize that virtually all the information contained herein concerning circumcision's effects on adult sexuality is essentially new information and was virtually unknown to even the most avid anti-circumcisionist back in 1993, which is when these particular women took part in the survey (and incidentally, well before the popularity of the internet).

Therefore, respondents could not have collaborated or merely repeat the thoughts they heard from others. The individuality of each respondent's reporting is evidenced by the originality of their quoted comments throughout the book and at the end of this chapter.

CRITICS OF THE SURVEY WILL SAY that a sampling of 138 women isn't large enough to draw any firm conclusions. But just as 100 fatal auto crashes alerted people to the defects in Firestone tires that led to their total recall from the marketplace, these survey findings of 138 voices clearly show consistent patterns that point to abnormalities attendent with circumcised intercourse and may very well lead to the total abandonment of circumcision as a cultural practice.

Critics may say, too, that the way in which women were gathered constitutes a selection bias because some respondents possibly had a special interest in the topic and some may have recognized beforehand that there were differences between the two types. However, this selection bias may be compensated to the degree that each respondent acted as her own control, using her subjective criteria on both types of penises. In other words, it's reasonable to assume that respondents simply reported on their own experiences giving honest evaluations.

Notably, many women commented that they did not give this matter much thought until filling out the survey, and taking the time to contemplate on it. As one woman commented, "I never realized it until I started thinking about it now...but I now realize that I feel natural men are better lovers, generally." And as another commented, "I had to do some thinking on this questionnaire. I was surprised that most of my past sexual encounters that were great were with natural men. I hadn't given it any thought before this." Many women, perhaps most, simply saw the ad, saw that they qualified, and decided to participate because they had never taken part in a sexual survey. In fairness to the importance of this issue, the findings cannot be completely attributed to selection bias.

If I had coldly sampled the general population, many of whom have a preconceived aversion, even repugnancy, to the natural penis due to its minority status and the many derogatory myths that surround it, this in itself would represent a selection bias, heavily weighted in favor of the circumcised penis. For the circumcised penis is considered the norm in this country and is so culturally entrenched, many women may think themselves abnormal if they didn't favor it. Moreover, most women have circumcised husbands or have had their sons circumcised, and thus have a vested interest in seeing that the circumcised penis remains in favor.

Although most women of the survey almost assuredly approached it with an open mind, by sampling a group who were selected to a degree, it may have allowed some women who have an opinion on this important issue to become involved and have a voice. But this is not necessarily a bad thing. In many cases historically, the astute, perspicacious views of the observant few lead the way to the enlightenment of the majority. In the end, it shouldn't really matter how the women were gathered. What matters is: Does the surgically altered circumcised penis affect the sexual pleasure and love bond between a man and woman? And if it does, then why should we continue to defend circumcision just because it represents the status quo?

HAVE ANY OTHER SURVEYS ADDRESSED WOMEN'S PREFERENCES FOR THE CIRCUMCISED VS. UNCIRCUMCISED PENIS?

In 1988, an Iowa survey of 145 women reported in the *Journal of Sex Education and Therapy* concluded that most women prefer circumcised partners for sexual activity. I would like to explain why this study is vastly misleading in its conclusions and does not merit serious consideration.

Most importantly, 83.5% of the participants reported having had sex with only <u>one</u> type of partner (78% only w/circumcised and 5.5% only w/uncircumcised). The 78% experienced with only circumcised are not qualified to make a judgment on which type of penis they prefer for sexual activity because they never had sex with the natural penis. Since the circumcised penis is the cultural norm and thus the only type of experience these women knew, it is a foregone conclusion that they would choose the type with which they were familiar. My comments on the above 5.5% for natural appear after my next point.

Secondly, these women were selected because they had all given birth to sons approximately a month before they were surveyed. Eighty nine percent (89%) had circumcised their sons. Realistically, how could they be expected to choose natural after having just had their sons circumcised?

As stated above, 5.5% had sex only with natural partners. Again, these women are not qualified because they knew only the one type of experience. It could almost be said with certainty that it would never occur to these women that sex could be different with a circumcised penis. Thus, they would think that the only difference between the two types is appearance. In 1988, the circumcised penis was the cultural norm and a woman would likely choose it for this reason alone. Also, as part of the survey, women were shown pictures of the two penis types. A woman might indicate a preference for the circumcised penis because she thought it *looked* sexier—that is, the flaccid circumcised penis, with the glans permanently exposed, closely resembles the *natural* penis in its erect, erotic state. This may lead her to wrongly surmise that it is superior for sexual activity. Some women may only develop an appreciation for the look of the flaccid natural penis after realizing that it offers superior sexual pleasure, compared to circumcised.

The remaining women, 16.5%, had sexual experience with both types of partners. These are the only participants truly qualified to make a judgment on which penis type they prefer for sexual activity. However, for these women, age and degree of experience are at question. We can safely assume that most of these women were young, since they had recently given birth. As stated several times, age (experience) is a definite factor in a woman's abililty to discern the sexual differences between the two types of penises. These might not jump out at them at a young age, and even if they did notice differences, they would most likely attribute them to *the man's technique* and not the penis type. Also, the study did not indicate the degree of experience these women had with natural partners. Since these were young women, they might have based their judgments on one-night stands or short-term relationships. These kinds of sexual encounters may not provide enough experience for a young woman to realize that the natural penis is sexually superior.

FINAL COMMENTS

This survey has shortcomings that may garner it more than its fair share of criticism, especially since its iconoclastic findings strike home personally to so many people. My experience has taught me that there is a great deal of hardheadedness and emotionalism associated with the circumcision issue, particularly since many parents have circumcised their sons. And circumcised men, themselves, may have difficulty facing up to the idea that they could be deficient or inferior in their sexuality.

But despite its small sampling of women and other shortcomings, its message is clear. Circumcision is not only an extreme tragedy for the male victim, but also has adverse effects on the sexual pleasure of the female partner. And this may ultimately prove to have a detrimental effect on the love bond, affecting the very core of our society—the family unit. To deny this concept and defend circumcision is, in a word, nonsensical. We must confront this issue, acknowledge it, change our attitudes, embrace its truths, and get on with our lives, knowing that tomorrow's child will enter the world in a better way, and that humanity, and the world, will be a better place because of it. And for those men of today, who have been the victims of this absurd and tragic practice, we must now give our wholehearted support in their endeavors to restore.

BE SURE TO READ WOMEN'S COMMENTS
ON THE PAGES THAT FOLLOW

WOMEN'S COMMENTS

The quotes that follow were compiled from survey comments. The seriousness of their worth and the heartfelt sentiment they express are epitomized in the words of the following respondent:

> "I'm so glad you're working on this topic. Women who have had sexual experience with both types have an important message to send to the men of America—spoken from the deepest tissues of our bodies."

WOMEN'S COMMENTS REGARDING NATURAL

> "With natural, all the rainbow of sensations is there."

> "I have never been anything but ecstatic when having intercourse with my natural husband, nor have I ever refused him entry, since I looked forward to it as much as he."

> "My sexual experiences with three natural men were extraordinary in the gentleness, sensuality, and mutuality of the experience."

> "A natural man is more sensitive, affectionate, wanting to please, maybe because they know the true feeling of sensitivity and stimulation."

> "Natural is incredibly more erotic and attuned to me. Penis felt softer, velvety, lovely."

"Couldn't get enough of him!" (Draws a Smile Face)

"Ongoing phases of unfolding, deepening passion and fulfillment."

"My husband is the only natural man I have ever had intercourse with, and he has almost always been able to help me experience a vaginal orgasm, whereas with circumcised men, it happened rarely."

"It was better, he seemed more excited and his response to my touch made me feel like I was really a great lover."

"More comfortable, more moisture, less of the rubbing that leaves you sore."

"One reason I prefer the natural penis is because it greatly enhances my enjoyment of giving oral sex. I have two sons who I have chosen to leave natural."

"Another very distinctive difference in my experience with circumcised versus natural partners was that the natural men were more *embracing* during intercourse. They held me close and rubbed against me more overall. Whereas, in contrast, circumcised men just want to prop themselves up on hands and knees and stroke themselves, so there's not as much overall body contact."

"I like the way natural men thrust."

"Natural men have a more laid-back approach. They don't seem to feel as rushed or pressured to achieve orgasm. They seem to enjoy the act more than the resulting orgasm."

"I feel totally satisfied with my natural partner's penis. Natural is more relaxing! I love to make love to a natural penis!"

"I felt as if I wanted the natural penis inside me all the time. It felt so wonderful."

"Wow, Wow, Wow!"

"The man I lost my virginity to was the son of Greek immigrants. I do remember that when stroking him, it just seemed to flow easily, naturally exciting him. I didn't need any lubricant. However, you can't stroke my circumcised husband's penis dry. It is uncomfortable to say the least."

"I've experienced very *deeply satisfying* intercourse only with natural men."

"My last natural intercourse was more than 20 years ago but I remember it very well. I have two sons by my circumcised husband. My decision to leave them natural was greatly influenced by the sweet and gentle natural man I knew in Kentucky in 1977."

"The uncircumcised man is a much better sexual partner, leaving emotional issues aside."

"I believe natural sex is better sex."

"Natural feels very different; my first circumcised penis felt like a dildo."

"I do notice that there is almost constant contact with my clitoris and he does jiggle quite a lot."

"My first lover was natural, and when I later went with my second lover who was circumcised, I found I liked thinking about my natural lover's penis more, but I did love him more." [*Author's Comment:* Did she love the natural man more because sex with him was better? Did she love the circumcised man less because the sex was not as good?]

"Natural intercourse is a much more pleasant experience—soft. I felt that I contributed to our mutual pleasure."

"I've always felt there was quite a difference in the two types of penises and I strongly favor natural men. It's a real tragedy that any male should undergo circumcision. The foreskin is there for a reason."

"Natural intercourse felt more right somehow. More appropriate and normal."

"The first few times with my husband, who is natural, I was surprised that I didn't have the pain afterwards that I did with my circumcised ex-boyfriend, especially since my husband's penis was larger."

"Intercourse with the natural man gives me a lot more pleasure and is much more satisfying. I would rate it higher than 10 if I could."

"There does not seem to be a feeling of mutual satisfaction with circumcised men in my experience. I feel natural men are better lovers.

"There is much more tenderness, it's much more a joint experience rather than one-sided."

"Gentler and less abrasive, the man seems more male and I, in turn, more female."

"I'm very surprised because I thought the gentleness had to do with the individual himself... but maybe not."

"There is definitely more clitoral area stimulation with natural."

"I hear a lot of women saying they think a natural penis is ugly and wouldn't want to have sex with one, but they've never tried it. I felt that way too before I had sex with a natural man."

"It felt great, like nothing I had ever felt before. I was easily brought to a vaginal orgasm."

"Pelvic thrusting and body contact is more tender."

"The whole experience is better. It's more intimate."

"Softer, deeper, less friction, more sensuous."

"Even when it goes on for a long time, I never feel bruised or abraded."

"I much prefer sex with an uncircumcised man. It is much more pleasurable. There's something very nice about it that's hard to explain."

"With natural, fellatio is much easier. On circumcised men, I always felt like I was choking and gagging because my mouth, throat, and hands had to do all the work. With the natural penis, the extra skin does the work."

"I have chosen a partner that is circumcised. I wish he weren't. My fantasies are usually about natural penises. I love the look of a natural penis and I do believe that just seeing it adds to the pleasure felt during intercourse. Natural penises are much more fun to have oral sex with."

"My natural partner kept more constant contact and pressure on my whole genital area during intercourse, so I never felt like he was 'banging away' but that he was with me and pleasuring me."

"My natural lover seems more aware of where my body is in relation to his; we become one in motion, not two using each other for our own separate ends, as with circumcised."

"I wish it could last all night long. Once a natural penis is in your vagina, you wish it could stay forever."

WOMEN'S COMMENTS REGARDING CIRCUMCISED

"I cried a lot in the dark—both during and after circumcised intercourse."

"I had a feeling of sadness, lack of satisfaction, emptiness, and frustration after intercourse with my circumcised husband. I never remember feeling like a whole woman during my marriage."

"It takes a lot of *work* to achieve vaginal orgasm with a circumcised partner."

"I have experienced a situation where a circumcised man has difficulty entering me as a result of my vaginal muscles tightening up."

"I've often said to myself, after one of these circumcised encounters: 'I'd have been better off masturbating.' Certainly once a woman has had good sex with a natural man, a circumcised man is like a cripple in comparison."

"When the man is too forceful with his thrusting, I lose all sense of feeling. I no longer desire to reach an orgasm."

"After a while, I began to realize I liked the natural penis better. When I was a little younger and more socially active, the first thing I wanted to know about a man wasn't 'What's your sign?'—it was, 'Are you circumcised?'"

"The glans of the circumcised male feels rough, and the shaft is very hard, unnatural. It is not the same as with a natural penis."

"Most of the time after the initial romantic stage was past, I felt like a blow-up doll could have done the job."

"Sometimes it's too much work for too little reward. When it's over, I think to myself, 'Thank God he finally came!'"

"Circumcised penis is hard and unforgiving—less elasticity."

"I never made the connection between this feeling of hostility and circumcised sex until now. I can't believe the BIG difference with a natural man."

"With circumcised, the pain was sometimes excruciating."

"I sincerely hope *something* can be done to eliminate the practice of circumcision. I have suspected for many years that it is a primary factor in the problems between the sexes—everything from the divorce rate to domestic violence."

"Afterwards, it was just as if we were strangers that didn't even connect. I often wondered why I was even putting myself through all the trouble of this unenjoyable sex!"

"Sometimes it seemed that I was simply a receptacle for him to use instead of a partner and lover."

"When you have to apply lubrication and provide your own stimulation and you're sore afterward the whole thing seems like an exercise in futility. Often, I've sensed the man wasn't *really* satisfied either—and this mutual dissatisfaction contributes to problems elsewhere in a relationship."

" I have gone as far as to get into arguments directly after intercourse, upon which I'd end up kicking the guy out for being a lousy lover! I'd often find myself wondering, 'Is that all there is?' "

"I dried out and suffered from post-intercourse irritation and soreness."

"During intercourse, the thrusts hurt my insides; after, the pain way up in my vagina lasts about a day."

"I admit to feeling aggravated toward the circumcised man. Mostly because of our poor relationship or my not being able to reach orgasm. It seemed like he should do something about it but he would or could not."

"Circumcised men feel like a dry stick inside you—and the way they pound away trying to get off leaves the woman's pubic mound and cervix bruised. Either that, or they get off so quick they leave you wondering what happened."

"I desire to get it over with—it gets very uncomfortable. I've gently told my husband this. I try to have enough foreplay so that he is close to orgasm when we start insertion."

"Vaginal tissues get rubbed raw with a circumcised penis. I always thought sex was painful until I had intercourse with an uncircumcised man. With the natural penis, I didn't experience abrasion."

"Yes, with circumcised, have difficulty being entered—vagina tightens up. Many times this experience was as if the vagina was rejecting the circumcised man. I have not had this feeling with a natural man."

"Circumcised thrusting seems to be hard and fast, therefore eliminating any pleasure I might feel in my clitoris."

"The prolonged, long thrusts were too exhausting and not very pleasurable. I generally feel frustrated, that I am a failure as a woman. Sometimes it leaves me feeling irritable, but I don't express this to my partner."

"With circumcised men, my vaginal muscles tighten up. With natural men, my vaginal opening is much more relaxed and accepting of the penis. I always seem so relaxed with my natural man. Never with the circumcised."

"I often think and feel that he is not paying attention to me or in sync with my breathing or thrusts."

"Long thrusts for extended periods of time cause great discomfort."

"They seem to need a lot more violent thrusting to achieve orgasm."

"An absence of moisture and rubbing that leaves you sore are a real problem with circumcised penises."

"I've always had to use a lubricant with a circumcised partner—and the ones who aren't 'minutemen' tend to take so long that I feel blistered afterward."

"It has often crossed my mind that circumcised men should be issued one of those blow-up dolls—and stay away from living creatures with feelings!"

"These longer thrusts can sometimes make the cervix sore both during and after intercourse."

"I feel very strongly that I experienced a lot of pain with my circumcised partner. The circumcised penis hurts. But with my natural partner, I have no pain, only pleasure."

"A lot of circumcised men seem to be so desensitized they have to really work to achieve orgasm—and being partner to one of these types is a real punishment! You dry out and start feeling sore and it just isn't any fun at all. But with my natural experiences, it was just the reverse; it feels good to begin with, I produce copious amounts of lubrication, and the longer the encounter lasts, the more the pleasure escalates."

"Feelings of sadness at my partner's apparent numbness and disconnection."

"Unfortunately, men of my generation, born here in the U.S., all seem to be circumcised. I wonder what deep-rooted psychological problems circumcision has caused them."

"We women with circumcised partners are living our whole lives without the holy experience of true sexual communion, and it is a loss of monumental proportions. It hurts our souls, our spirits. I know I am deeply wounded by it, and I sense that most women also are. Tragic."

"In my experiences with circumcised men, they just don't have the desire, passion, and erotic behavior."

14

How Americans Came to be Routinely Circumcised

Who were the first people to practice circumcision? When did it begin? And why was it begun? No one really knows. The answers are lost in antiquity. Theories abound, but no one can say with certainty when, where, or why male circumcision began.

It is not known whether the practice began with one group and then spread to others or if it developed independently among a number of different groups. But the fact that various circumcision styles are practiced by different groups suggests that the practice had more than one origin.

Artifacts 6,000 years old show that the practice was well established in Egypt long before it was adopted by the ancient Jews. This is confirmed by the *Encyclopedia Judaica*, which states, "It seems that Abraham did not start the practice of circumcision" (1).

Regardless of where it started, male circumcision is currently practiced by various peoples and countries of the world, primarily by the Muslims (historically, more often called Moslems) and Jews worldwide, some African countries, and the United States. And to a much lesser extent, Australia and Canada (where rates have been gradually declining and are presently estimated to be about 10 and 20 percent, respectively). Approximately 20% of the world's males are circumcised.

Although Jews can trace the origin of their ritual to passages in the Old Testament, Moslems, on the other hand, practice it primarily as a cultural ritual, with religious overtones. Although circumcision has come down through Moslem culture to symbolize religious purity, the word "circumcision" does not appear anywhere in the Koran (the Moslem equivalent of the Christian Bible) (2). Still, male circumcision is a ritual strictly adhered to by the Moslems. In Moslem culture, circumcision is usually performed sometime between adolescence and marriage. It is often part of a village ceremony in which young men are initiated into manhood, their circumcisions also serving as a symbol of a "true believer" in Islam.

Religion is not a major factor in the circumcision rates of the United States, Canada, and Australia, which practice it primarily for its presumed medical benefits or simply because the father was circumcised and the parents feel the son should match.

THE BRITISH EMPIRE ADOPTS CIRCUMCISION AND EXPORTS IT TO NORTH AMERICA

Everyone familiar with the story of Robin Hood knows how King Richard's crusade to the Holy Land created grave problems for the people he left behind in England. But what people don't know is that the Crusades set in motion the forces that would eventually lead to the circumcision of millions of males in England, Canada, Australia, and the United States.

In the 12th century, King Richard, along with other European rulers, organized an army that invaded the Middle East in hopes of freeing the Christian Holy Lands from Moslem occupation. The more culturally advanced Moslems looked upon these intruding Europeans, who raided and plundered their land, as barbarians, and called them "uncircumcised dogs." For in the eyes of the Moslems, the Christian uncircumcised penis was an affront to Allah and Islamism (3). Captured Europeans were routinely circumcised by force, and many a knight in shining armor returned to Mother England without his foreskin (4).

Over the next several hundred years, as England expanded its economic and colonial ambitions into other Moslem countries, Arabs, Turks, Afghans, and Indian Moghuls all had a turn at cutting off British foreskins. For example, 300 English workers at the Old London Company offices in Cossimbazar, India were stripped and publicly circumcised by the Moghul troops who captured the British outpost (5). On a different occasion, a Scottish officer and many of his subordinates were forcefully circumcised during an elaborate ceremony in which their foreskins were burned as an offering to Allah (6).

According to historian Allen Edwardes, after great battles, "the slashed prepuces [foreskins] of the Unbelievers, [were] heaped in mounds....in accordance with the rigid martial code of the Moghul Empire, the warrior rose in rank according to the number of foreskins he brought in from the field" (7).

As the British Empire continued to send soldiers, adventurers, and government clerks into Moslem lands, an increasing number of men returned home circumcised. Some, however, did not return because they bled to death. To prevent the tragic consequences of a poorly performed impromptu circumcision, some English companies began, as early as the mid-1600s, to have their representatives circumcised before sending them off to foreign lands. It was a lot safer to have it done at home than to risk the knives and swords of the overzealous Moslems. Thus began the first circumcisions of Englishmen by fellow Englishmen.

By the early 19th century, the circumcised penis had become fashionable among British aristocracy, who wore it proudly as a badge of honor—proof of having served the Motherland in foreign service. Gradually, this mark of distinction gained a prestigious recognition among the privileged upper class, and young squires of elite all-boy schools began to get circumcised to match their parents or peers.

Except for the upper classes, however, the majority of English males remained uncircumcised. But upon the publication (1891) of a paper by the president of the Royal College of Surgeons entitled, "On Circumcision as Preventive of Masturbation," an anti-masturbation frenzy swept through Britain and even working-class boys began to be routinely circumcised (8). This anti-masturbation mania soon invaded America.

Why would the foreskin be blamed as a cause of masturbation? Because, during urination, or when retracting it for cleaning purposes, a male has to handle the penis and pay attention to it. This extra handling and attention was blamed for an increased incidence of masturbation, and in the 1800s, the medical community was beginning to associate masturbation with a wide variety of purported ills. Reports like the following began to commonly appear in medical literature ascribing many harmful effects to masturbation:

> One of the two men who indulged in excessive masturbation became insane; the other dried out his brain so prodigiously that it could be heard rattling in his skull.... The effects of masturbation range from impotence to epilepsy, and include 'consumption, blindness, imbecility, insanity, rheumatism, gonorrhea, priapism (painful continuous erection due to disease), tumors, constipation, hemorrhoids, female homosexuality, and finally lead to death' (9).

When anti-masturbation mania took possession of the medical psyche, the scientific practice of medicine was in its rudimentary stages of development. The causes, contagions, and cures for nearly all diseases were unknown. One of the prevailing British theories of illness was that "All disease could be reduced to one basic causal model, either the diminution or increase of nervous energy" (10). This theory was picked up by a famous American physician, Dr. Benjamin Rush, who espoused that if nervous energy were the basis of all disease, then orgasm was a target to control. In 1812, Dr. Rush wrote that overindulgence in sex or masturbation resulted in:

> ...seminal weakness, impotence, dysury, tabes dorsalis, pulmonary consumptions, dyspepsia, dimness of sight, vertigo, epilepsy, hypochondriasis, loss of memory, malangia, fatuity and death (11).

The above ideas seem recklessly crude and completely overblown compared to our present-day knowledge, but at the time, the purported destructive effects of masturbation were a serious issue. Dr. Rush's statements were picked up and persisted, in one form or another, well into the 20th Century. Among the leading champions of this theory interrelating sexuality and disease was Dr. Sylvester Graham, the developer of graham crackers, who wrote a book on the evils of excessive sexuality in which he added dozens of diseases to Dr. Rush's list, including disturbances of the stomach, heart, lungs, skin, and also of the brain, into which masturbation induced insanity, he claimed (12). Graham's book went through 10 editions from 1834-1848.

In 1855, an editorial in the New Orleans Medical Journal stated:

> Neither the plague, nor war, nor small pox, nor a crowd of similar evils have resulted more disastrously for humanity, than the habit of masturbation: it is the destroying element of civilized society (13).

Another opponent of masturbation was John Kellogg, whose breakfast cereals are still well known. In 1882, he wrote that masturbation was a sin against nature, causing "urethral irritation, inflammation of the urethra, enlarged prostate, bladder and kidney infection, priapism, piles and prolapse of the rectum, atrophy of the testes, variocele, nocturnal emissions and general exhaustion" (14). Kellogg also noted that a masturbator could be detected by 38 suspicious signs, including: changes in disposition, sleeplessness, bashfulness, round shoulders, lack of breast development (in females), use of tobacco, acne, biting of the fingernails, and the use of obscene words (15). Masturbation and its telltale signs understandably evoked fear among parents, who did not want their children to suffer the horrible physical and emotional consequences of this evil.

Another opponent, Dr. P. C. Remondino, published a detailed book, in 1891, taking the evils of the male sex organ one step further, blaming the foreskin itself for various undesirable traits and illnesses. In his medical opinion:

> The prepuce [foreskin] seems to exercise a malign influence in the most distant and apparently unconnected manner; where like some of the evil genii or spirits in the Arabian tales, it can reach from afar the object of its malignity, striking him down unawares in the most unaccountable manner; making him a victim to all manner of ills, sufferings and tribulations; unfitting him for marriage or the cares of business; making him miserable and an object of continual scolding in childhood, through its worriments and nocturnal enuresis, later on beginning to affect him with all kinds of physical distortions and ailments, nocturnal pollutions, and other conditions calculated to weaken him physically, mentally, and morally, to land him, perchance, in the jail, or even in a lunatic asylum. Man's whole life is subject to the capricious dispensations and whims of this Job's-comforts-dispensing enemy of man (16).

In 1903, Mary R. Melendy wrote *The Ideal Women—For Maidens, Wives And Mothers*, which stated:

> It (self-abuse) [masturbation] lays the foundation for consumption, paralysis and heart disease. It weakens the memory, makes a boy careless, negligent and listless. It even makes many lose their minds: others, when grown, commit

suicide. How often mothers see their little boys handling themselves, and let it pass, because they think the boy will outgrow the habit, and do not realize the strong hold it has upon them! I say to you, who love your boys—'Watch!' Don't think it does no harm to your boy because he does not suffer now, for the effects of this vice come on so slowly that the victim is often very near death before you realize that he has done himself harm. It is worthy of note that many eminent physicians now advocate the custom of circumcision, claiming that the removal of a little of the foreskin induces cleanliness, thus preventing the irritation and excitement which come from the gathering of the whitish matter under the foreskin at the beginning of the glans. This irritation being removed, the boy is less apt to tamper with his sexual organs. The argument seems a good one, especially when we call to mind the high physical state of those people who have practiced the custom. Happy is the mother who can feel she has done her duty, in this direction, while her boy is still a child (17).

With typical writings like the above, the early 20th century found the American medical establishment in general agreement that masturbation and hypersexuality had devastating and damaging effects on one's physical and emotional well-being.

The evil foreskin, and its supposed propensity toward masturbation, had to be eliminated, according to the belief of the time. This dangerous activity had to be brought under control —for one's own good! Thus, routine circumcision began its infiltration into American society and subsequently escalated throughout most of the 20th century.

Any custom that infiltrates a society may continue on after the original reasons for its inception have been forgotten. In America, circumcision continued to be practiced long after the medical profession and the general public had abandoned, even forgotten, its original purpose, which was to thwart the supposed evil effects of masturbation. Once circumcision became accepted, a variety of straw medical benefits were attributed to its practice during the 1900s, thereby perpetuating its further acceptance and continuance.

Although circumcision never gained universal acceptance in the United States, it persisted and gradually picked up momentum, for two reasons. Firstly, hospital births became increasingly common, and the medical profession in these situations began doing routine circumcisions "for the child's own good." Secondly, World Wars I and II brought with them an epidemic of venereal disease. Taking the advice of their British counterparts, who associated VD with the foreskin, American military doctors presumed that soldiers without foreskins were less likely to contract venereal disease. Thus began the "unofficial" campaign of the United States Armed Forces to circumcise the troops "for health and cleanliness" reasons. This policy of "short-arm" inspections followed by circumcisions became routine throughout the military and did not abate until the human rights of GI's were finally given some recognition during the Vietnam Conflict. Even so, many American soldiers who still had foreskins were routinely circumcised if they picked up any "problems" from the "girls" in town. By 1970, the circumcision rate had risen to an estimated 80%, mainly because of the greater number of hospital births. This, combined with the military's policy of circumcising for "health and hygiene" reasons, left the great majority of American men without foreskins. The rate continued to rise until 1980, when circumcision was at its peak, estimated at 85%.

CIRCUMCISION RATE

How many men in America are circumcised? This question cannot be easily answered. Exact circumcision rates are impossible to determine because hospitals apparently considered circumcision so routine and so trivial they usually did not enter such a "routine" procedure in the records. In addition, if a child was circumcised later in the doctor's office, this very likely went unreported. However, even though there is a lack of precise national data, the conservatively estimated rates of infant male circumcision in the United States show a steady increase from 1870-1980, after which it began to decline (see Figure 14-1) and is presently (1998) estimated at 60% (20). This decline was primarily brought about by the publication of books like *Birth Without Violence*, by Dr. Frederick Leboyer (1976), which had an impact on the psyche of hospital maternity wards and on the greater number of women returning to home births.

This, then, is where the beginning of the Foreskin Restoration Revolution now finds us, with the majority of the American male

Estimated U.S. Circumcision Rates (Percent)

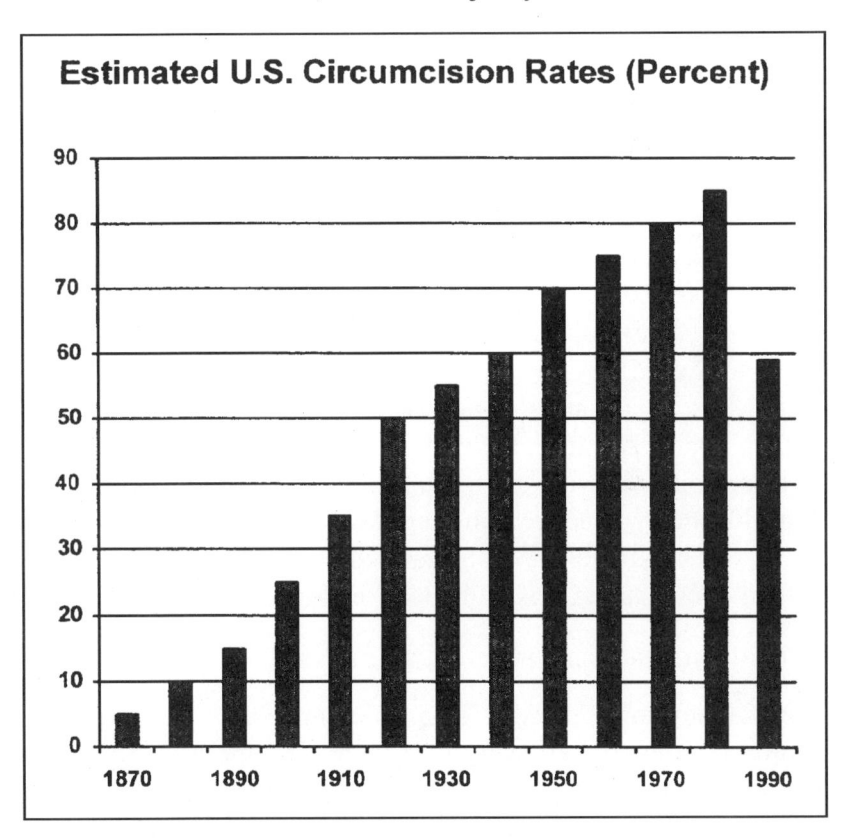

Figure 14-1. Estimated percentage of males circumcised from 1870-1980, according to Wallerstein (18). Estimate for 1990, source NOCIRC (19).

population circumcised. Nevertheless, I believe this is about to be reversed, and that America is on the eve of becoming a non-circumcising country. Soon, the circumcision rate of infant males in America will drop to near zero percent, and countless men will be restoring their foreskins. As you will recall, England was at one time obsessed with circumcision, and yet in the late 1940s, as a result of information released favoring non-circumcision, England's rate plummeted, almost "overnight," to less than 1 percent. The changeover in America will undoubtedly be just as sudden and complete.

15

35 Reasons Why You Should Not Circumcise Your Son

Circumcision may be only a 15-minute operation, ***but it affects a male for the next 72 years of his expected life.*** Doesn't it seem prudent that you should forego circumcising your son and wait for the controversy on this issue to settle, and then let your son decide if he wants to be circumcised? After all, it's *his* penis.

1. The idea that the child should "match" the father is one of the most common reasons parents give for having their son circumcised. But in light of the information in preceding chapters, we now realize that the father should not have been circumcised in the first place, so it makes no sense to circumcise the child just because the father is circumcised. No man who understands how circumcision affects his sexual functioning would have consented to his own infant circumcision.

    The father will have to be magnanimous and accept the fact that his son's penis will be different from his. But after all, isn't one of the purposes of parenthood to make a better life for our children than we had for ourselves? Besides, if the father restores his foreskin, the two of them will actually match very well.

2. Perhaps you already have a son who is circumcised, and you may therefore be considering that subsequent sons should be circumcised too, so they will not be "different" from one another. It is unfortunate that your previous son was circumcised, but each child is an individual. Your decision should be based on what you now know.

3. Some parents have their son circumcised so he will look like "the other kids" in the locker room, but keep in mind that since 1980, the U.S. circumcision rate has dropped about 25 percent (1). America's attitude about circumcision is changing, and in the years ahead, more and more kids in the locker room will be sporting natural penises.

4. Nature had her reasons for giving your little boy a foreskin. Doesn't it seem prudent to trust Mother Nature's judgment on this matter?

5. Approximately 80% of the world's men have natural penises. Circumcision is not the standard in the world; it is the exception.

6. Circumcision is a human rights issue. To retain the genitals one was born with is a birthright. It is the child's body, not the parents'. Why should parents be allowed to authorize amputation of a perfectly healthy piece of the child's flesh, one that provides vital protective and sexual functions? Removing part of the child's penis censors him from perceiving, experiencing, sharing, and enjoying his existence.

7. Circumcision is unwarranted surgery and has been thought so for some time. As early as 1978, the Executive Board of the American College of Obstetricians and Gynecologists (ACOG) issued a statement of policy headed: STATEMENT ON NEONATAL CIRCUMCISION. The opening pronouncement reads:

The American College of Obstetricians and Gynecologists (OB/GYN) supports the position of the AAP [American Academy of Pediatrics] ad hoc Task Force on Circumcision (1975) that 'there is no absolute medical indication for routine circumcision of the newborn' (2).

Unlike the AAP, which published its 1975 position in *Pediatrics*, its official journal, thereby achieving wide dissemination, ACOG sent the STATEMENT ON NEONATAL CIRCUMCISION to its own members via the *ACOG Newsletter*. The "STATEMENT" was not published in the *ACOG Journal* and is not listed in *Index Medicus* (3).

Unfortunately, many members of the medical community were not then, and are not now, aware of the above proclaimed (and subsequent) official positions on circumcision, so they continue to recommend it. Therefore, it is your responsibility to tell your doctor that you do not want your son circumcised. By reading this book, you have acquired information that your doctor may not be aware of. Assertively tell your doctor that you do not want your son circumcised. Take care to see that your wishes are followed through. In some hospitals circumcision is so routine it may be done even though you've indicated otherwise. Beware!

8. As the facts of this issue unfold, more and more childbirth educators are advising against routine circumcision.

9. The Delegates of Family Practice and the College of Pediatric Urologists are in general agreement that infant circumcision is contraindicated and provides no valid medical or hygienic benefits (4).

10. Prince Charles of England is circumcised, as it has long been the custom of British royalty to do so. Princess Di insisted that her sons *not* be circumcised. Attitudes are changing. More people are deciding against circumcision.

11. The natural penis is capable of providing greater sexual pleasure than the circumcised penis, for both the man and his female partner. There are immeasurable differences between natural and circumcised sex, and although the psychological and sociological repercussions are just beginning to be discussed, I am confident that we will find that the two types of sex have different effects on the emotions and love bond of the participants.

12. Premature ejaculation is more common among circumcised males according to the results of the survey.

13. The penis head (glans) is designed by nature to be an *internal* organ, like the tongue. Removing the protective foreskin makes the glans an *external* organ.

14. Circumcision may leave psychological scars, the extent of which are only now beginning to be recognized. Below are excerpts from three letters received at the office of UNCIRC (5).

> "I have been angry about the subject of infant circumcision for some time. It started when I realized that it was one of the factors in my taking so long to climax with my sexual partner. How could a country that calls itself civilized do such a horrible thing to its little boys? My thought is that parents have no right to consent to unnecessary surgical procedures on their children anyway." S.R., Ohio

> "Throughout my entire life, I've always felt frustrated, never sexually fulfilled, always feeling as if something were missing...now I know...I was robbed of the most sensitive part of my penis on day one." B.Y., Arkansas

"This subject is unfortunately for me a lifetime nightmare. It all started the day I was born, March 7, 1951, at Tampa General Hospital in Tampa, Florida—a time when routine genital mutilations were performed. Ever since I can remember, I always knew something was wrong with my penis. I guess it was 1959 or 1960 when I realized what was wrong. My best friend's oldest brother was intact, and it was the first time I ever saw a complete penis. I knew then what was wrong with mine. I remember feeling this sick sense of loss, and continue to until this day in 1990, and will probably go to my grave with it." M.H., Oregon

15. Circumcising your son may cause you grievous guilt feelings later, after you realize that you should have kept him intact. Since the circumcision rate is dropping and in all probability will continue to drop, by the time your child reaches adulthood, the natural penis will be the accepted norm.

16. If you have your child circumcised, he will very likely mourn your decision when he is older. Circumcision can make a child feel distressed, when he's an adult, about the hostile feelings he has toward his parents because they had him circumcised.

17. The natural penis is more visually appealing. All of the famous sculptures in Europe depict intact men. Some American parents may consider circumcising because they think the natural penis looks funny or odd. But this is because they are not used to looking at a natural penis; they have been conditioned to think of the circumcised penis as the "normal" look. In the future, when the natural penis is the norm, people will think that the circumcised penis looks mutilated. Many survey respondents found the natural penis more visually appealing. Here are a few of their comments:

> "To me, looking at the bared circumcised glans routinely in a non-sexual setting is a complete turn-off."

> "I like to look at the natural penis much better than to see a circumcised penis. A natural penis looks more beautiful and desirable."

> "The visual effect of seeing an impending erection just starting to peek out of its foreskin is just so much sexier."

> "I like to look at the natural penis, and it tends to turn me on more than circumcised ones."

> "I have come to prefer the natural penis because it is visually and emotionally more appealing to me."

18. The natural penis does not need any special care during infancy. Its foreskin should never be forcibly retracted during bathing or routine visits to the doctor. Simply wash the exterior of the penis in the same way you normally wash any other part of the body. In the words of the American Academy of Pediatrics:

> Care of the uncircumcised boy is quite easy. 'Leave it alone' is good advice. External washing and rinsing on a daily basis is all that is required. Do not retract the foreskin in an infant, as it is almost always attached to the glans. Forcing the foreskin back may harm the penis, causing pain, bleeding, and possibly adhesions. The natural separation of the foreskin from the glans may take many years [usually by age 5, but occasionally into the late teens]. After puberty, the adult male learns to retract the foreskin and cleanse under it on a daily basis (6).

19. Leaving the foreskin intact will *not* cause your child to masturbate excessively. An adolescent or adult male will usually masturbate whether he is circumcised or not. In fact, more and more authorities are acknowledging that masturbation is a natural part of development.

20. The foreskin glides up and down the shaft during masturbation. When the foreskin is missing, the man's hand frictionizes the shaft and usually requires an artificial lubricant. When the foreskin is present, artificial lubrication is unnecessary.

21. The foreskin is necessary in order to give the erect penis the extra skin it needs for a comfortable erection. In contrast, the tight, taut skin of the erect circumcised penis can be uncomfortable, even to the point of pain.

22. By removing the penis's only moving part, it makes foreplay less fun for his sexual partner. One survey respondent stated this best when she said:

    The natural penis offers variety—skin forward, skin back, etc.—like the excitement of a convertible car.

23. A common misconception is that if you don't have your son circumcised in infancy, he will have to have it done later in life. This is simply not true. American doctors, who have little experience with adult (or boyhood) foreskin problems (which rarely occur), such as infection, are quick to recommend circumcision as the only solution. However, if a child were to develop an ear infection instead, the doctor's approach would be to first try conservative treatments like warm compresses, increased fluid intake, dietary changes, supplementary vitamins, antibiotics, and if necessary, an incision to drain the area—but not amputation. In Europe, this is the type of treatment physicians administer for a rarely occurring infection of the foreskin, rather than

amputation, because they have a greater appreciation for the importance of the foreskin. This is discussed in more detail in Chapter 17.

24. Circumcising an infant to prevent cancer of the penis in later life runs contrary to sound reasoning. Cancer of the penis is extremely rare and does not usually occur until old age. Why should a man be denied the pleasures of a fully functioning penis for his entire lifetime when only about one male in 100,000 ever contracts the disease, and then, only in his old age? Keep in mind, these statistics indicate there is a 99,999 chance in 100,000 that he will *not* get cancer of the penis. Furthermore, there is no guarantee that circumcision will absolutely prevent penile cancer, as both circumcised and uncircumcised men can contract it. This topic is discussed in Chapter 18.

25. Routinely circumcising baby boys to prevent venereal disease in adulthood also runs contrary to sound reasoning. Venereal disease is rampant in this country, even though the vast majority of males are circumcised. Clearly, circumcision does not prevent VD. Chapter 18 contains a more detailed discussion.

26. Routinely circumcising males as a preventative for infant urinary-tract infection (UTI) is the latest medical excuse advocated to justify circumcision (discussed in detail in Chapter 18). UTI's are rare and can be effectively treated with antibiotics. Furthermore, the rate of infant UTI among females is significantly higher than that for males, yet no one is advocating routine female circumcision.

27. Some proponents of routine circumcision erroneously believe that it helps prevent cervical cancer in women. Those who have seriously studied the facts found no correlation between cancer of the cervix and the presence of a foreskin on a woman's sexual partner. Chapter 18 discusses this more thoroughly.

28. Circumcision hurts. Infants feel pain, and this unwarranted surgery, done without anesthesia, is traumatic for the newborn child. Most babies scream frantically during their circumcisions. Some stop breathing and lapse into a semi-conscious state. The degree of psychological effects of this pain, inflicted so early in life, may be more profound than most Americans realize (7). See Chapter 17 for more details.

29. Circumcision can result in serious medical complications, and there are definite surgical risks involved. Hemorrhage, infection, scarring, fistula, meatal ulceration, excessive penile skin loss, accidental injury or amputation of the glans or part or all of the penis, as well as other complications, are not uncommon. Circumcisions have occasionally resulted in death. Much of the acceptance by parents of infant circumcision is based on the false belief that circumcision is insignificant, trivial, inconsequential, painless, and free of risks. Nothing could be further from the truth.

   Actually, it could be said that the complication rate for circumcision is 100%, since each little boy's future sexuality is compromised as a consequence. This entire topic is discussed more thoroughly in Chapter 17.

30. Many insurance companies will no longer pay for circumcision. Why put out the extra money when circumcision is not medically necessary?

31. The foreskin protects the glans from abrasive clothing.

32. The foreskin provides for a nice little jacket during cold weather. Having a foreskin over the penis head is like having fur-lined gloves for your hands.

33. The foreskin will not restrict the penis from growing to its normal length, as some people believe. Keeping him natural insures a fuller look.

34. If you have your son circumcised and public opinion swings in the anti-circumcision direction, he will undoubtedly want to become surgically or non-surgically restored when he matures because of the popularly proclaimed advantages of the foreskin. Why not let him keep all the equipment nature gave him so he will not have to go through the hassle and expense of restoring? (Besides, even though he can restore, restoration does not restore the penis to its true, original condition.)

35. According to my husband, who is restored, and according to Bud Berkeley, an intact man and founder of the Uncut Society of America, the sensation of an erecting penis expanding inside its foreskin and then bursting forth and having the foreskin slide down the shaft is so incredibly great, no man should miss out on it. Berkeley describes it this way in his book, *Foreskin: A Closer Look:*

> During erection...the uncut man receives his most exquisite experience as the skin stretches out its nerves to accommodate the engorged penis. The best sensation comes as the skin slides down over the shaft (8).... [H]ow could anyone deprive a man of such an experience? All the medical, religious, and fashion excuses for circumcision suddenly become insignificant upon discovering the ultimate male experience of s-t-r-e-t-c-h (9).

16

Valid Reasons for Circumcising Your Son

1.
2.
3.
4.
5.
6.
7.
8.
9.
10.
11.
12.
13.
14.

15.
16.
17.
18.
19.
20.
21.
22.
23.
24.
25.
26.
27.
28. **There Is No Reason To Circumcise A Child**
29. **Valid Enough**
30. **To Justify**
31. **Compromising His Adult Sexuality**
32. **And Future Marital Happiness**
33.
34.
35.

17

Common Myths That Popularized Circumcision

As Americans, we tend to think of ourselves as pacesetters, as leaders for the rest of the world to follow. We think that if other countries aren't doing things our way, they soon will. But as far as circumcision is concerned, "We are the laughing stock of the other industrialized nations...[because] we are the only nation on earth to circumcise the majority of...[our] infant males for nonreligious reasons" (1). The other English-speaking countries (England, Canada, and Australia) that adopted the practice at the same time we did have either discontinued it almost entirely or its incidence has been rapidly declining. England's neonatal circumcision rate is now at about one-half of one percent. The rates for Australia and Canada are about 10 and 20 percent, respectively.

CLEANLINESS IS NOT A VALID REASON FOR CIRCUMCISION

The myth that the natural penis is difficult to care for and keep clean is one of the most common reasons given for circumcision. In numerous conversations with friends and relatives, the one comment I heard repeatedly was, "Isn't it supposed to be cleaner?" While the bared, dry, circumcised penis head does seem easier to keep clean, the fact remains that keeping the glans and foreskin of the natural penis clean requires minimal effort, no more than it takes for a woman to keep her genitals clean.

In infancy, the foreskin does not usually retract. The advice of the American Academy of Pediatrics is simply to wash the outside of the penis as you would any other part of the body. Do not try to forcibly retract the foreskin because it can hurt the child and damage the penis. Retractability will take place in time (anytime from infancy or childhood to the late teens), whereupon the child can be taught to retract his foreskin and clean beneath it, just as little girls are taught proper hygiene for keeping their genitals clean.

In childhood, adolescence, and adulthood, keeping the penis clean requires no more effort than we pay to other parts of our body, such as shampooing our hair or washing our ears. Surely, a male's most prized possession—his penis—is worth this minimal effort. Retracting the foreskin and washing behind it once a day, or perhaps just before having sex, should not present a problem for most men. A few males may neglect their hygiene, but this is not a justification for removing the foreskins of millions and millions of infants.

Although the secretions of the female genitalia emit an odor, sometimes quite strong, we don't cut away parts of a woman's genitalia to make her cleaner and odor free. Let me stress that some genital odor for both male and female is normal and natural, and many people even consider it an aphrodisiac. Certainly, many men perform oral sex on women and admit they find a woman's genital odor erotically stimulating.

However, if your mate objects to the odor of your genitals, there is a simple remedy: Take vegetable oil (like Wesson oil) and apply it around the inside of the foreskin and glans, or for the woman, around the clitoris and vulval lips. Leave the oil on for about a minute, then blot it off with a tissue. The oil will absorb the odor and transfer it onto the tissue. Then rinse with an unsoaped washcloth. This method is better than washing with soap because it will not leave a soapy residue on the genitals if you decide to engage in oral sex.*

* During showers, when you do wash with soap, be aware that some soaps can dry out and irritate the genitalia. I recommend Dove soap (classic version, not the unscented) because it is gentle and moisturizing as well.

The vegetable oil technique really works. If you are a person who is easily offended by your partner's odor, I highly recommend this procedure.

WHAT IS SMEGMA, AND IS IT A PROBLEM?

The inner lining of the foreskin is mucous membrane, which secretes a clear, lanolin-like lubricant, that facilitates the foreskin's movements and prevents it from adhering to the glans. (Likewise present within the female vulva area.) This substance does not presently have a medical name and is usually referred to by doctors simply as "subpreputial wetness," or erroneously as smegma. I propose that this transparent, lanolin-like, lubricating secretion be called *lanofore*. Smegma, in contrast, is an opaque, whitish substance that is *sometimes* present under the foreskin and can emit an odor if hygiene is neglected.

Critics of the natural penis often point to smegma as evidence that the natural penis is unclean, and they use this as a justification for circumcision. But in light of the points below, does this make sense?

First, keep in mind that smegma is easily removed by occasionally wiping or washing the penis.

Second, *women's genitals also produce smegma*, yet no one makes any big fuss about this, and rightly so.

Third, let me stress that smegma develops a potentially offensive odor *only when penile hygiene is grossly neglected*, just as it would if a woman grossly neglected her genital hygiene.

Fourth, ironically, with all the concern about smegma, I propose that it is actually an *unnatural excretion*—a by-product of the incomplete digestion of dairy products—this is why it may develop a cheesy odor when allowed to accumulate, if hygiene is neglected. The explanation below elaborates.

In their mega-million-selling book, *Fit For Life*, authors Harvey and Marilyn Diamond make a strong case for why milk and dairy products are an unnatural food for human beings (2).

According to the Diamonds, and others (like Robert Cohen, author of *Milk: The Deadly Poison*), who have thoroughly researched this topic, the human digestive system cannot properly process the dairy products of cows. It is becoming widely known that many people have great difficulty digesting dairy products, and several dairy-product digestive aids are currently on the market. Also milk substitutes, like soy milk, are now a basic constituent of many infant formulas, due to the fact that infants exhibit digestive disturbances from cows' milk.

The Diamonds point out that in the wilds of nature, no other animal continues to drink milk after it has been weaned from its mother. *Moreover, milk, as it exists in nature, is not subjected to extensive processing—like pasteurization, homogenization, irradiation, and preservatives, etc.—that modern commercial dairy products receive, which further adds to their indigestibility by destroying vital enzymes.*

I propose that in the absence of dairy products, smegma would virtually not exist. In this regard, a prospective examination of over 4,500 uncircumcised males was done in Japan, where dairy products are not part of the typical everyday diet. Only 0.5 % (5 in a 1,000) had smegma (3).

My husband notices that he develops smegma only after he has ingested dairy products, which he rarely eats. Fortunately, when he does occasionally have smegma, it is easily eliminated with the vegetable oil method described earlier or by washing the penis with Dove soap and water.

It is common for dairy-product residues, trapped in skin crevices, to develop a cheesy smell. You can easily test this on yourself. Go for a couple of days without washing behind your ears and then run your finger in the crevice behind your ear a few times. If you have eaten dairy products, you will notice that your finger may present a residue and will smell a bit cheesy. This is an indication that your body is using the pores of the skin to excrete dairy product residues. The same thing can happen under the foreskin. The body uses the pores of this thin, mucous membrane to expel the residues of incompletely digested dairy products—in fact, there is a medical term, *smegmalith*, which *Dorland's Medical Dictionary* defines as "a calcareous [calcium rich] concentration of smegma." The fact that this substance is calcium-rich suggests that smegma may have its origins in dairy products.

It should be stressed that some sloughing off of dead skin cells (desquamation) is normal and natural and takes place on both the circumcised and uncircumcised penis. But I propose that dairy products may somehow exacerbate this process and cause excessive desquamation.

Each individual must decide for himself the merits of eating or not eating dairy products. I merely wish to make the point that the intact penis does not naturally have an offensive, cheesy odor as its critics (who have a vested interest in having the circumcised penis remain in favor) claim. Nor is the intact penis automatically accompanied by smegma. And it certainly does not make sense to cut away an important component of a man's sexuality to correct an odor problem that may be caused by dairy products—postulated to be an unnatural substance for humans to eat—and can be eliminated by giving them up, *or by practicing simple hygiene.* It is well known that dietary habits are changing. Who knows, in 10 or 20 years, dairy products may no longer be an important constituent of the American diet, just as it is not an important component in the diet of billions of people around the world. Who knows, at some point in the future, we may all be drinking soy milk instead.

Smegma is a terrible sounding word, and since it is used almost exclusively to identify the opaque, potentially odorous substance sometimes present under the foreskin, I suggest it be used specifically to describe that substance. On the other hand, *lanofore* is a pleasant sounding word, and I propose that it be used to designate the natural, clear, lanolin-like, lubricating secretion of the foreskin, which does not have an objectionable odor.

In short, the solution to the smegma problem, if indeed it is perceived as a problem, is a simple cleansing of the genitals on a daily basis—not amputation of the foreskin.

NEWBORNS DO FEEL PAIN

There is a common myth that newborn infants do not feel pain. Or, more recently, that they do feel pain during circumcision, but it is minor, of short duration, and is not remembered.

The mistaken idea that the newborn does not feel pain has been commonly believed for quite some time. *The Mothers' Medical Encyclopedia* (1972) stated, "Circumcision of a newborn boy is not painful for the child" (4).

Dr. E. T. Wilkes said that circumcision is "not very painful" (5). Dr. F. W. Rutherford stated that "circumcision is only momentarily painful" (6). Moreover, Dr. Charles Schlosberg declared that "the infant feels as much pain momentarily as he would while receiving an injection" (7).

Another common misconception is that the cries of the child are due more to the restraints used during the operation than the actual operation itself. Dr. Seymour Isenberg and Dr. L. M. Elting express this belief this way:

> As for anesthesia, none is needed. Although the baby may scream and kick during the procedure, this seems to be more of a reaction to being bundled to the circumcision board than actual pain...Since a good portion of the baby's nervous system is not yet formed, especially that part that localizes pain, circumcision done at this age the first few days after birth is probably the best time (8).

The fact is: ***Infants do feel pain, and there is now a great deal of research evidence to substantiate this*** (9).

A newborn baby is as sensitive to pain as anyone else is, yet, babies are routinely circumcised **without anesthesia**. Perhaps this would be a little like having a root canal without Novacain. Probably worse, much worse. Make no mistake about it, circumcision causes your baby excruciating pain and agony.

Babies cry and scream frantically while they are being circumcised. Some stop breathing and lapse into a semi-coma.

Others go into a state of immobilized shock, in which they can't even cry. (I would like to interject this important point. In television presentations of the circumcision topic, a video of an actual circumcision is sometimes presented in which the baby is shown distressed and crying. But there is actually more distress than meets the eye, because underneath the surgical cloth that covers the child, the infant's arms and legs are strapped down. If he were not strapped down and covered, the infant's distress would be considerably more visible; he would be thrashing his arms and legs about quite violently. Because his head is the only part of the body that can move, his crying and the thrashing of his head are all we see. These television videos do not present an accurate depiction of the infant's suffering.)

Dr. Howard J. Stang, et al. (1988) describes the infant's pain as follows:

> There is no doubt that circumcisions are painful for the baby. Indeed, circumcision has become a model for the analysis of pain and stress responses in the newborn. Not only does the unanesthetized newborn cry vigorously, tremble, and, in some cases, become mildly cyanotic because of prolonged crying, but other stress-related physiological reactions have also been demonstrated, including dramatic changes in heart and respiratory rates and in transcutaneous oxygen and plasma cortisol levels (10).

In an interview with Rosemary Romberg, author of *Circumcision: The Painful Dilemma*, Dr. Howard Marchbanks stated:

> In medical school I was taught that the baby's nervous system is not developed sufficiently to be aware of the pain of circumcision. But my experience in doing it and observing the baby's reactions tell me otherwise.... Anyone who has a foregone conclusion that it was not painful for the baby and therefore one should not hesitate to do it only has to listen to the baby while it is being done (11).

In March, 1999, the American Academy of Pediatrics released a new report entitled, "Circumcision Policy Statement," wherein it acknowledges, *for the first time*, that "newborns who are circumcised without analgesia experience pain and stress" and recommends using analgesia to reduce circumcision pain. But the report does not explain that *analgesia doesn't eliminate pain, it only relieves it somewhat*. Analgesia is not equivalent to anesthesia. Infants cannot be anesthesised due to the risks involved. Despite the policy statement of the AAP, many American infants undoubtedly continue to be circumcised without analgesia because it takes time for this type of information to permeate down to the everyday practitioner. An additional factor that could potentially impair this information getting to the right people is that it was published in the journal, *Pediatrics*, and many circumcisions are performed by interns, obstetricians, and others, not pediatricians.

CIRCUMCISION IS A VIOLATION OF AN INFANT'S HUMAN RIGHTS

Every year, about 1,200,000 million American baby boys are strapped down and stripped of their foreskins *without their consent,* which, of course, they cannot give. But that's the point. Would an infant consent to his own circumcision if he had a choice? As a nation, we've come a long way in our awareness of human rights. But we still have a long way to go. An infant's right to the genitals he was born with is only now beginning to be recognized. Genital mutilation—circumcision—call it what you will—is a violation of an infant's rights as a human being. For the infant will soon grow to be a man, and as a man, isn't he entitled to the basic human right of the genitals he was born with?

Many articles written about infant circumcision make the assumption that it is the right of the parents to make the decision. Some parents and/or doctors think that it is their duty to make the circumcision choice for the child. However, in the last analysis, the infant's genitals belong to him, and no one should have the right to cut off a healthy part of the child's body.

The male penis is the only organ of the human body over which parents are given such authority. There is no other healthy structure of the human body that can be amputated at the parent's request. Why should parents be allowed to choose whether the child—the child who will soon grow to be a man—will get to live out his life with a complete, natural penis or go through life with an incomplete, circumcised penis?

During his circumcision, the infant may struggle and scream with all his might, but unfortunately, no one who is listening believes he has any "voice" in the matter. If the infant were not preverbal, perhaps it would be a different story, for surely he would tell the circumciser in no uncertain terms what to do with his knives, scissors, and clamps.

ADULT CIRCUMCISIONS ARE RARELY NEEDED

There is a general myth that sooner or later the foreskin is likely to develop medical problems and it is therefore better to have the child circumcised in infancy to avoid having to have it done as an adult. But getting a circumcision performed later in life and *needing* to get a circumcision done are two different matters. Adult foreskin problems rarely develop, but if they do, there are other solutions besides circumcision.

When Edward Wallerstein, author of *Circumcision: An American Health Fallacy*, questioned the health departments in non-circumcising countries like Norway, Denmark, and Finland, he found that very few adults ever require a circumcision. He reports:

> In Oslo, Norway, over a 26-year period in which 20,000 male babies were cared for, 3 circumcisions were performed —a frequency rate of 0.02%. In Denmark, 1,968 children up to the age of 17 were examined over a period of several years. In this group, 3 circumcisions were performed—a frequency rate of 0.15%. In this study, in retrospect, the physician believed all three operations might

have been avoided. Both of the above studies related to the infrequency of circumcision in infancy and puberty; they did not deal with the issue in adulthood.

Health officials of each Scandinavian country were queried about adult circumcision.... None of the health officials could provide precise data, because the numbers were so small that they were not worth compiling. Each official stressed that foreskin problems were presented but said they were largely treated medically—surgical solutions were extremely rare (12).

In America, doctors are quick to recommend circumcision as the only remedy for conditions that are treated and cured by other means in non-circumcising countries. American doctors simply have not had the diversity of experience their counterparts in non-circumcising countries have had because in America there are so few foreskins. Consequently, when a problem arises— even something simple like a minor local infection—they generally recommend circumcision without considering simpler, alternative solutions, like prescribing an antibiotic or soaking the penis in a warm bath of Epsom salts.

PHIMOSIS DOES NOT REQUIRE CIRCUMCISION

Below is a story received at the offices of NOCIRC, a clearinghouse for information about circumcision.

> My parents not only resisted medical advice for circumcision but also let my foreskin loosen at its own slow rate. I was about 12 before my urethral meatus was visible and 16 before I saw the corona of my glans. Even with this slow loosening of the foreskin, I never experienced irritation or inflammation. Before becoming sexually active, I spent a few minutes per day over a period of months gradually stretching the foreskin by hand until it would easily retract. This approach was simple, painless, and effective (13).

Since the early 1970s, several articles have been published in the medical literature outlining a variety of surgical techniques that doctors can use to expand a phimosed* opening, thereby eliminating the need to circumcise (14). This new attitude is commendable, but in most cases, perhaps all, surgery may not be needed at all, as discussed below.

Surgical intervention for phimosis may soon be superceded by a promising new *non-surgical* treatment developed in China, which uses a balloon catheter to stretch the foreskin opening. This technique was judged successful if within two weeks there was free retraction of the foreskin over the coronal sulcus (coronal ridge). The success rate in 512 boys was almost 99%; only three patients required a second or third dilation (15). The procedure is simple and safe, and is well tolerated by the patient. Balloon catheters are commonly used in medicine today, most notably to dilate coronary blood vessels.

Another approach used in France gently stretches the foreskin with graduated speculums (16).

In addition, there are prescription steroidal and non-steroidal topical ointments (like betamethasone valerate 0.05%) now available that can effectually render a tight foreskin opening elastic and expandable, thereby resulting in retractability. Also, in some cases, a tight foreskin can be corrected simply by periodically stretching the foreskin manually while in a warm bath.

Visit *www.cirp.org/library/treatment/phimosis* for more information about correcting phimosis non-surgically.

Fortunately, phimosis and paraphimosis (defined in the next section) are extremely rare. The Finnish National Board of Health provided Wallerstein with case records for 1970 for both phimosis and paraphimosis. A total of 409 cases were reported for males 15 years of age or older, which represents only 2/100ths of 1% (0.023%) of the total male population in that age group. *This means 99.997% did not develop a problem.* Moreover, according to Finnish authorities, only a fraction of the reported cases required surgery—a number too small to reliably estimate (17).

* Phimosis is a rare condition sometimes present in adulthood, in which the foreskin is too tight and will not retract over the glans.

The causes of phimosis have not yet been determined, but it seems logical that this condition may be a consequence of insufficient levels of nutrients that promote skin elasticity (like vitamins C, B6, E, and the mineral zinc). (Consult the plethora of literature that is available in health food stores and your local library, bookstore, and/or visit a professional versed in nutritional therapy.)

THE FORESKIN USUALLY DOES NOT RETRACT IN INFANCY AND EARLY CHILDHOOD, AND SOME MALES MAY NOT DEVELOP FULL RETRACTABILITY UNTIL THEIR LATE TEENS

The myth that the foreskin should retract at birth has been, and continues to be, widely believed by the medical community, when in fact, about 96% of male babies have non-retractable foreskins at birth that gradually become retractable during childhood (18). At birth, the penis is not yet fully developed, as is the case with all parts of the body. *Foreskin retractability is a gradual process.* Partial retractability is often achieved by the age of five. However, *full retractibility may not occur until some time later, occasionally as late as puberty, or the late teens.* This normal developmental stage should not be misdiagnosed as phimosis. (A detailed discussion of phimosis can be found at *www.infocirc.org/top.htm*)

Because doctors see so few intact penises in this country, many are not aware that the foreskin is usually tight during infancy and early childhood. Many doctors will advise parents to forcibly retract the foreskin for cleaning purposes, but this is painful, damaging, and unnecessary. The penis as a whole should simply be washed like any other part of the body until such time as the foreskin does retract. By this time, the child is usually able to take care of his own penis and can be taught how to do so.

If an infant is not circumcised at birth, various circumstances may lead to an *unnecessary* circumcision later in childhood. Because doctors are generally unaware that the foreskin is non-retractable in infancy, several things may happen, all of which may result in the child getting circumcised. First, during routine office visits, the doctor may notice that the foreskin is non-retractable and try to force it back. This is painful for the child and bleeding may occur. The doctor may then misdiagnose the condition as phimosis and advise the parents to have the child circumcised.

Second, if the mother follows the doctor's advice to retract the foreskin to clean the glans, she may find it psychologically uncomfortable. She may feel it's too much like "playing with the child." Besides, it may hurt the baby and cause crying and bleeding. As a result, in many cases, the parent(s) may decide to get the child circumcised after all.

And third, if the mother does continue to forcibly retract the foreskin, causing bleeding and little tears between the glans and the foreskin, it can result in a condition called *acquired phimosis,* where the little tears continually heal over, causing scarring and adhesions. This condition can result in a non-retractable foreskin, in which case circumcision will generally be prescribed, all because the foreskin should not have been forcibly retracted in the first place.

There is one more condition caused by improper care of the natural penis that requires discussing. This condition is called *paraphimosis*. Paraphimosis can be brought about when the foreskin is forcibly retracted and then gets stuck behind the glans. Circumcision is usually advised for this condition, but such does not have to be the case. It is my understanding that another solution is possible—applying ice to the penis head. Ice causes the penis head to contract, thereby allowing the foreskin to slide back to its original position. Or one can simply clamp down on the glans with the thumb and index finger to reduce its size and then ease the foreskin back in place over the glans.

Until recently, very little information was available to health care professionals concerning the proper care of the uncircumcised penis. Consequently, they assumed that proper care required forcible retraction of the foreskin in order to clean underneath it. Due to lack of information, American doctors, most of whom are circumcised themselves, were left on their own regarding advice to new mothers on the care of the natural penis.

The medical community is making progress, however, and the American Academy of Pediatrics now has a pamphlet entitled, "Newborns: Care of the Uncircumcised Penis." Yet it is important to note that the first edition of this pamphlet was not published until 1986 (19). Many doctors and nurses who have not yet read this pamphlet may continue to advise mothers incorrectly.

The following is taken from the above-mentioned American Academy of Pediatrics pamphlet, presented previously but reported here because of its relevancy to this section:

> Care of the uncircumcised...[penis] is quite easy. 'Leave it alone' is good advice. External washing and rinsing on a daily basis is all that is required. Do not retract the foreskin in an infant, as it is almost always attached to the glans. Forcing the foreskin back may harm the penis, causing pain, bleeding and possibly adhesions. The natural separation of the foreskin from the glans may take many years. After puberty, the adult male learns to retract the foreskin and cleanse under it on a daily basis (20).

THE FORESKIN IS AN INTEGRAL PART OF THE PENIS ITSELF. CIRCUMCISION DOES CAUSE HARM AND DOES NOT ALLOW THE PENIS TO FUNCTION NORMALLY

Most Americans believe that circumcision does not impair the functioning of the penis. But as discussed throughout the book, this is an erroneous belief. Of course the circumcised penis can still be used for urination and procreation, but we are just beginning to understand that circumcision damages normal sexual functioning, on sensory and mechanical levels, and does not allow the penis head proper protection.

The above has been adequately dealt with in previous chapters. There is, however, one harm of circumcision I would like to elaborate on and re-emphasize. This concerns the "tight" circumcisions many men have received as a result of having had too much skin removed.

Many circumcised men who contact organizations like NOCIRC and NORM complain of tight, taut shaft skin, and even painful erections. Over and over men complain, "I was cut too tight," "I have no slack skin on the shaft of my penis," and "I was cut so tight my penis bends up (or down or to one side)" (21).

Some men are cut so tight that it causes hair from the penis base to be pulled up onto the penis shaft during erection. These hairs would normally remain at the base of the natural penis, but when the foreskin is missing, the lower penis shaft skin is pulled forward to accommodate the erection. One electrolysist I spoke with said that he is seeing more and more men for removal of these hairs, which are frequently pulled forward as far as midway onto the penis shaft during erection. Some of these men confided that their female sexual partners found these wiry hairs uncomfortable during intercourse and caused them vaginal irritation.

CIRCUMCISION'S RISKS AND COMPLICATIONS

Doctors commonly tell parents that infant circumcision is a simple operation with few risks. The procedure may be easy to perform, but like any other surgical procedure, it has its risks and complications. A few of these are hemorrhage, infection, a badly executed circumcision resulting in a mutilated appearance, excessive skin loss, scarring, fistula, fibrosis, ulceration, accidental injury or amputation of the glans, and even death. Medical literature clearly reflects such complications and tragedies (22). Wallerstein notes:

> The most common circumcision complication is hemorrhage.

According to Dr. John Denton (1978) the 'rate reported at times as being up to 2%' (23). In some cases, hemorrhage was so severe that heroic measures had to be taken, including blood transfusion (24).

Below is a portion of a presentation made to a subcommittee of the California Medical Association on March 4, 1989. The presentation was made by Dr. James L. Snyder (25):

In 1986, I presented to the Virginia Urologic Society two infants who had been circumcised with disastrous results. One had suffered a degloving injury with the loss of all the skin of the penile shaft and required further surgery. The second infant suffered gangrene and necrosis of the entire glans and penis due to electrocautery. I was called as a consultant to see both of these infants within hours of the injuries and can tell you that both of these children will be lifetime genital cripples.

Since my two personal experiences witnessing tragic infant circumcision, I have gathered data which I bring here before you on other tragic results of infant circumcision.

In 1982, an Iowa infant bled to death after circumcision.

In 1983, another Virginia child suffered a degloving with his circumcision, requiring skin grafting.

In 1984, a Louisiana child's penis was destroyed by a circumcision and sex-change surgery was advised.

In 1985, two children in an Atlanta hospital suffered destruction of their penis at circumcision. One underwent sex-change surgery.

In 1986, an Alaska child's infected circumcision led to convulsions and massive brain and kidney damage.

Numerous children are circumcised so severely that their sexual functioning is devastated, and recently the medical literature and the lay press have reported on significant numbers of adult men who were so displeased with their circumcisions they have sought and submitted to plastic surgical reconstruction of their penis.

Electrocautery devices have caused severe damage in several incidences since the 1970s. In one case, reported by Dr. S. John Money and Patricia Tucker, the entire penis sloughed off. In this case, the child underwent sex-change surgery and was raised as a girl (26). (In Jan/Feb, 2000, this story was featured on *Dateline NBC, The Oprah Winfrey Show*, and *20/20*). In August 1985, as noted in Dr. Snyder's report, two babies in Atlanta were burned so severely by an electrocautery device that one boy also required a sex-change operation and is also being raised as a "girl." The other boy, whose parents refused a sex-change operation, will, according to a 1991 news report, "never be able to function sexually as a normal male" (27).

HEALING MISHAPS

Sometimes the circumcision incision (scar) bonds to places on the corona of the denuded infant glans during the healing process. This is known as a "skin bridge." Skin bridges usually occur unevenly so that they do not involve the entire scar around the penis. These "bridges" form tunnels between the scar and the glans, where dirt and debris can get trapped, causing irritation.

Acquired phimosis is another healing mishap. Sometimes enough of the foreskin is left so that the remaining skin collapses back over the raw glans and attaches to it. These bonds form true adhesions and require medical attention. Rosemary Romberg, author of *Circumcision: The Painful Dilemma,* cites a mother's account of a doctor freeing her 20-month-old son's post-circumcision adhesions:

> My sister accompanied us and the doctor instructed my sister and me to each pin down one of Colin's arms and legs. He then—using no anesthesia—tore the foreskin from all around the glans. It was minutes of horror!! Perhaps it was worse than his original circumcision, for now he could recognize exactly what was happening. Here were three adults, two of

them close love-figures, restraining him and putting him through this agony!! He screamed, 'Mamma, Daddy, Lola...I'm sorry, I'm sorry...Mamma...' over and over again. My poor baby, sorry for what!!?? I was the one to be sorry.... After the doctor was done with Colin, he had us put ointment on the wound until it healed. This took two adults just to pin him down again to get the ointment on. For weeks after this ordeal, Colin wouldn't allow anyone near his penis (28).

MEATAL STENOSIS

This is one of the most common circumcision complications. Normally, the foreskin cloaks and protects the glans and urinary opening. But circumcision removes this inherent protection and exposes the bared glans to abrasive diapers, urine, and feces. Diaper rash and abrasion on the glans and urinary opening can bring about ulceration, scarring, and meatitis, which may lead to meatal stenosis. Meatal stenosis is a stricturing or closing of the urinary opening due to ulceration and scarring. When meatal stenosis occurs, the infant must have an operation called a "meatotomy" to reopen the urinary channel (29).

INFANT DEATH

Death is something no one recovers from. It is a life gone forever. Nevermore to return. Deaths due to circumcision are truly tragic for the parents and family of the infant involved. Dr. Hank Streitfeld states that, "In America, with millions of elective circumcisions performed annually, about five little boys will die each year as a result of infection or bleeding" (30).

18

Medical Myths
Perpetuate Circumcision in America

If the American penis is circumcised, it is because the twentieth century has been 'the 100-year reign' of routine infant circumcision in this country. During this century, only a handful of doctors and parents have questioned or opposed the practice. With such near-universal acceptance, many beliefs about the penis and infant circumcision have come to be accepted without question. Many of these beliefs have become, in fact, national myths. That is, they are simply believed to be true and are often repeated without any demand that they be reconsidered and demonstrated to be true.

Myths only survive in a culture when at least some authority figures give them credence and benefit from them. Circumcision myths survive in America in part because a very large segment of the medical community in this country continue to repeat them...(1).

MYTH: The foreskin is a mistake of nature—a superfluous and unnecessary skin that extends beyond the actual penis.

Dr. S.I. Millen stated the myth as follows:

> The human male is cursed with a super abundance of foreskin over the penis. Circumcision...remedies the fault by removing the excess of foreskin (2).

Dr. Sherman Silber had this to say about the foreskin:

> The foreskin is essentially just an extension of the outer penile skin that is redundant and extends well beyond the actual tip of the penis. It is this extra skin that is removed during circumcision (3).

A. A. Lewis, together with Dr. Eli Bauman and Dr. Fred Klein, had this to say:

> The foreskin has no sexual significance for the healthily formed male. It neither impedes nor increases his coital pleasure. With erection, the foreskin naturally rolls back to uncover the head of the penis and, from then on, plays absolutely no part in any sexual activity. The head usually has extreme erogenous sensitivity, but the foreskin has none. It is as useful as one's appendix and, like the appendix, can sometimes be troublesome enough to need surgery (4).

With statements like these coming from the medical community, America has not been a very safe place for foreskins.

FACT: The foreskin is not extra, purposeless skin.

It is unfortunate that doctors have been routinely removing foreskins for nearly a century without understanding or questioning what they have been removing. Incredibly, the medical community has been debating circumcision's risks and potential benefits for decades, yet virtually no one addressed the question: Does the foreskin have a purpose, and if so, what is it? (In defense of the medical community, let me reiterate that until somewhat recently, sexual topics and the study of sexuality have been taboo. In a country where the vast majority of the adult male population, including doctors, are circumcised, no one was looking for the sexual purposes of the foreskin.) But now we know, the foreskin is alive with sensory nerves and serves several functions during intercourse. It is a living, vital part of the complete penis. To cut it away is to leave a lifetime scar on the body and mind of the victim, who must then go through his life denied his full sexual existence.

THE CANCER MYTHS

There are three cancers that have been alleged to be linked with the natural penis: cancer of the penis and/or prostate in men, and cancer of the cervix in women.

Cervical Cancer

In the early 1960s, Dr. S. I. McMillen published a book entitled *None of These Diseases*, in which he reported on several studies linking increased rates of cervical cancer in women whose sex partners had uncircumcised penises. He took the position that Old Testament "ordinances" are God-given protection against such diseases. Dr. McMillan noted that 13,000 women had died of cervical cancer during a representative year and then went on to say, "[T]he large majority of deaths could have been prevented by following an instruction that God gave to Abraham [to circumcise]" (5).

In 1981, Dr. Sherman Silber took this attitude:

> A...benefit of circumcision is that wives of circumcised men are less commonly afflicted with cancer of the cervix (the opening of the women's womb). There is controversy currently among doctors on whether it is circumcision that protects against cancer of the cervix, or whether it is some other aspect of hygiene in circumcised men that is responsible. Regardless of the reason, these women are much less likely to suffer the most frequent cancer of the female organs (6).

In response, Jim Bigelow, Ph.D., author of *The Joy of Uncircumcising!*, states:

> It is interesting to note in Dr. Silber's statement above that he questions whether it is circumcision *in men* or some other aspect of hygiene *in men* which governs the female's susceptibility to cancer. Nowhere during this period was the cause associated with the woman's behavior relative to cervi-

cal cancer. The debate lasted for several years, but finally even the most dedicated proponents of infant circumcision had to acknowledge that factors other than the circumcision status of the male sex partner accounted for cervical cancer (7).

By 1984, Dr. S. I. McMillen, in the second edition of *None of These Diseases*, had modified his indictment of the foreskin as it related to cancer of the cervix:

> In the first edition of this book, I cited the evidence that cancer of the uterine cervix...was primarily a disease of sexual partners of uncircumcised males. In the intervening years, however, cervical cancer has been more firmly related to multiple sex partners.... A recent study found evidence of venereal warts virus in 73 of 80 women who had cervical cancer. Thus it seems that cervical cancer is, for the most part, a result of venereal disease...(8).

Edward Wallerstein, in his comprehensive book, *Circumcision: An American Health Fallacy*, goes into considerable detail about the various invalidities of several studies linking cervical cancer with uncircumcised sex partners. To report on this in detail is beyond the scope of this book. However, one aspect of his research is highly important in the cervical cancer debate, for when he compared the new case data for the United States with the non-circumcising countries of Sweden and Norway, the results showed that the United States had a *higher* rate, not the lower rate you might expect, if circumcision status of a sexual partner were the sole determining factor. In 1972, the rate per 100,000 for the United States was 32.0; for Sweden (1968) 25.0; and for Norway (1967) 20.2 (9).

After all his years of research, Wallerstein concludes, "Correlations exist between cervical cancer and poor state of health, poor nutrition, poor hygiene, poverty, early onset of sexual activity, promiscuity, number and spacing of children, etc., but not circumcision" (10).

The capper for this inaccurate claim is that in the American Academy of Pediatrics' recent exhaustive review of the scientific data on male circumcision (discussed at the end of this chapter), the cervical cancer myth was not even dignified with a historical mention, let alone asserted.

(Cited references, fore and aft, may appear dated, but keep in mind that they represent the time frame when these issues were being discussed—from which the myths to this day survive.)

Last Minute Insert: While this 2nd edition was at the press, the cervical cancer issue was resurrected when a study published in the *New England Journal of Medicine* (April 11, 2002) reported that women married to uncircumcised men were slightly more at risk in contracting it. Subsequent public discussion pointed to various flaws in the study's methodology and interpretation of its statistics, calling into question its validity. However, even if its findings were valid, circumcision should not be advocated as a preventative because CIRCUMCISION IS A GREATER HARM since it severely damages the sexuality of both the man and his female partner throughout their life, every time they make love. And what about the vast millions of women who will never contract cervical cancer: Should they, and their male partners, be made to suffer the lifetime of sexual deprivation (routine circumcision would bring), and the havoc it wreaks on relationship happiness? Also, periodic pap smears detect cervical cancer in its early stages, which is treatable. In addition, leading scientists anticipate a cure for cancer before the end of the decade.

Penile Cancer

Cancer of the penis is often used in the arguments of circumcision proponents even though it is one of the rarest cancers to strike males. Dr. George Denniston homes in on the crux of the penile cancer issue with the following statement:

> Cancer of the penis is very rare—one case in 100,000—usually in older men. Even if circumcision could prevent it, 100,000 foreskin amputations would be necessary to prevent one [case of] cancer of the penis. One hundred thousand infants would be mutilated, and several infants would die to prevent that one case of cancer. Who could scientifically advocate foreskin amputation for this reason? (11).

If circumcision were a factor in reducing penile cancer, we would expect to see significantly less of it in circumcising nations as compared to non-circumcising nations. This does not appear to be the case. For example, when Wallerstein researched this topic, he found that the penile cancer rate of the U.S. (a circumcising country) and the rates of Finland, Norway, and Denmark (all non-circumcising countries), were approximately the same, about one new case annually per 100,000 population (12).

On its web resource The Penile Cancer Resource Center (13), the American Cancer Society states:

> This practice [circumcision] has been suggested as conferring some protection against cancer of the penis by contributing to improved hygiene. However, the penile cancer risk is low in some uncircumcised populations, and the practice of circumcision is strongly associated with socio-ethnic factors which in turn are associated with lessened risk [that is, these other factors, and not circumcision, account for the lower risk]. The consensus among studies that have taken these other factors into account is that circumcision is not of value in preventing cancer of the penis.

Even if the foreskin were a risk factor in penile cancer, which it does not appear to be, why should a man be denied a lifetime of sexual pleasure when there is only one chance in 100,000 that he will ever contract the disease—and then, only in his old age? Considering the foreskin's many functions, circumcising to prevent the possibility of cancer of the penis makes about as much sense as routinely removing women's breasts to prevent breast cancer.

Prostatic Cancer

In 1972, in *Today's Health*, Dr. Marvin Eiger stated, "The uncircumcised man is more than twice as likely to develop this [prostatic] form of cancer" (14).

Dr. Eiger's conclusion was based on a study by Dr. A. Apt that compared incidences of prostatic cancer in Sweden (non-circumcising) and Israel (circumcising) (15).

Importantly, Dr. Apt did not take age into consideration. It is well established that prostatic cancer is most often found in men over the age of 55-60. Dr. E. N. Preston re-analyzed Dr. Apt's data taking into account the proportion of the population in both Sweden and Israel aged 60 and over. He found that Sweden had 7.2 times as many men in this older age group as did Israel.

Based on this increased number of men, Sweden would be expected to have 7.2 times as many incidences of prostatic cancer as Israel. The data, however, showed a difference of only 4.7 times that of Israel's. Dr. Preston asked, "Would this mean that non-circumcision protects against prostatic cancer?" (16).

In summarizing his discussion on prostatic cancer, Wallerstein states:

> [W]e see that the overwhelming epidemiological data demonstrate that the cause of prostatic cancer remains a mystery. Its etiology has nothing to do with circumcision, yet the myth persists in current medical literature (17).

And finally, in a definitive statement, E. Grossman and N. A. Posner assert:

> No one today seriously promotes circumcision as a prophylactic against cancer of any form. No significant correlation between cancer and circumcision has ever been proved (18).

In summary, the American Academy of Pediatrics has never aggrandized this one-time myth, which is no longer parroted by even the most uninformed.

VENEREAL DISEASES

MYTH: Uncircumcised males are more likely to contract venereal disease than circumcised males.

Many statements by members of the medical community have perpetuated this myth. Dr. Vincent Vermooten bluntly states, "Circumcised men are less prone to venereal infection" (19). Dr. Marvin Eiger stated in 1972: "Certain types of venereal disease are rarer among the circumcised possibly because their penises are less subject to slight breaks in the skin that might admit disease germs" (20).

In 1973, Dr. Abraham Ravich published a book entitled, *Preventing V.D. and Cancer by Circumcision* (21). And in 1974, Dr. David Reuben published, *How to Get More Out of Sex*, in which he writes, "...military doctors discovered that circumcised men were less susceptible to Venereal Disease...(No one knows exactly why—maybe the foreskin...gives germs a place to hide)" (22).

Although the above statements are from somewhat older literature, it is exactly this type of reporting that gave rise to the myth that circumcision could somehow protect against the ravages of VD.

More recently, Dr. Aaron Fink wrote, "...estimates of relative risk suggest that uncircumcised men are twice as likely as circumcised men to develop genital herpes or gonorrhea and five times as likely to develop yeast infection or syphilis" (23).

FACT: According to Bigelow, who investigated this subject extensively, "No study has ever substantiated the claim that circumcision prevents or significantly reduces the risk of venereal disease" (24).

There have been studies that found a higher percentage of cases of a particular venercal disease in uncircumcised males, but in each case, other factors emerged to explain the reason behind these findings (25).

For example, two famous studies, one in 1854-55 in London and the other in 1882-83 in New York, each found that, of all religious groups, Jews had the lowest incidence of venereal disease. Since male Jews are circumcised in infancy, the researchers concluded that circumcision helped prevent VD. However, Orthodox Jewish religious practices, Jewish social life, as well as the social isolation of Jews, were not factored in (26).

To put it in plain language, the Jews in these studies didn't sleep around; if you don't sleep around, you won't contract VD. This, not circumcision, was the primary factor in their low incidence of venereal disease.

As Wallerstein points out:

> If circumcision were the remedy, because of the high circumcision rate in the United States, all venereal diseases, including Herpes II, should have largely disappeared. They have not (27).

The Center for Disease Control, located in Atlanta, has been maintaining figures and estimates for sexually transmitted diseases since 1941. Each year more than 12,000,000 new cases are reported to The Center (28).

There are basically two kinds of sexually transmitted diseases (STDs)—viruses and bacteria. There are more than 40 million people in the United States with STD viruses—1 million documented cases of HIV, 30 million cases of genital herpes, and 12-24 million cases of genital warts (29).

STDs caused by bacteria include syphilis and gonorrhea. There is presently an epidemic of these bacterially related STDs. Syphilis has been increasing annually since 1986. More than 50,000 infectious-stage cases were reported in 1990. This is the largest number of cases reported in the past 40 years (30).

Gonorrhea is the most frequently reported bacterially related STD. Approximately 700,000 new cases were reported in 1990. The Center for Disease Control estimates, however, that the actual cases were double (1.4 million) because many cases are not reported (31).

In light of the above and considering that the vast majority of sexually active American men are circumcised, we can clearly see that circumcision does not offer a magical form of protection against sexually transmitted diseases.

AIDS

The following chart (Figure 18-1) demonstrates that circumcision clearly does not ensure protection against the HIV virus leading to AIDS.

Did you know?

The United States has the sixth highest AIDS rate in the world. It is preceded by Zimbabwe, Congo, Malawi, Kenya, and Chad. All are circumcised nations. How protective can circumcision be?

AIDS Cases per 100,000 (1994)
Source: World Health Organization

Circumcising Nations:	
Zimbabwe	96.7
Congo	58.4
Malawi	49.2
Kenya	24.8
Chad	20.2
United States	**16.0**

Non-Circumcising Nations:	
Japan	0.2
Finland	0.9
Norway	1.5
Sweden	2.0
Germany	2.2

Figure 18-1: Comparative AIDS Cases

On the contrary, circumcision may possibly help to spread AIDS. In a letter to the New England Journal of Medicine, Dr. John Swadey writes, "...common speculation tends to link American circumcision practice to AIDS." Dr. Swadey says that his examination of circumcised American males "discloses a very significant incidence of persistent suture holes, micro-sinuses, skin tabs and bridges, irregular scarring" around the circumcision scar which are subject to tearing from abrasion (32). During circumcised intercourse the taut penis shaft skin is continually frictionized against the vagina, possibly resulting in minute abrasions to both the vaginal entrance and the penis shaft skin. Consequently, microscopic amounts of blood may be exchanged and the HIV virus passed. Some respondents to the Awakenings Survey done by NOHARMM (33) confirmed Dr. Swadey's observations when they stated that their circumcision "scars still bleed to this day" and that "...[my circumcised penis] sometimes bleeds from being cut so tight." In addition, some respondents to my survey indicated that bleeding and/or abrasion during intercourse was sometimes a problem.

> "My husband was cut too close—the skin on his penile shaft occasionally 'splits' much like a paper cut, causing him much discomfort."

> "My ex-boyfriend, who was circumcised, seemed desperate to achieve orgasm and would thrust quite violently, occasionally making me bleed. He always felt bad about it, but it would happen again."

The AIDS rate in America (and those of other circumcising countries) shown in the AIDS chart demonstrates the inanity of promoting circumcision as a means of stemming the tide of HIV. The United States has the highest rate of HIV among first world nations, by a large margin. The United States also has the highest circumcision rate among first world nations, again by a wide margin. Clearly, circumcision has not been effective in preventing AIDS in the United States. The best protection against AIDS is to always wear a condom when with a partner whose sexual history is in question.

URINARY TRACT INFECTIONS

MYTH: Circumcision is effective in preventing and/or treating urinary tract infections.

Beginning in 1985, Dr. Thomas Wiswell, et al. published studies reporting a statistical correlation between infant circumcision and a reduced rate of urinary tract infections (UTI).

His findings indicate that from 1 to 4% of uncircumcised infants boys could develop UTI before their first birthday, which may require a short hospitalization (34).

FACT: Any body part may, in fact, become infected, but foreskin amputation as a preventive treatment for UTI is a drastic overreaction for a problem that is readily treatable by other means, such as antibiotics. Dr. Wiswell's research findings and conclusions have been challenged on a worldwide basis.

The amount of research and rebuttals set off as a result of the Wiswell studies are too numerous to fully report here, but a few of the more striking issues should be explained.

First, nearly half of the infants involved in Dr. Wiswell's research were baby girls, and their UTI rate of 0.57% was nearly twice the 0.31% UTI rate of the infant males (combined circumcised & uncircumcised) (35). The recommended treatment for baby girls is antibiotics. But for prevention in baby boys, Wiswell recommends circumcision. Isn't circumcision a rash measure considering that the treatment for girls is antibiotics?

Other studies that followed Wiswell's questioned the validity of his findings. Dr. Martin Altschul presented the results of his UTI study at the First International Symposium on Circumcision (1989). He reported that he:

> ...found not a single confirmed case of UTI in a normal male infant. All of the confirmed cases occurred in infants who had clear-cut urinary birth defects (36).

Dr. Altschul also examined the records of all infants under one year of age with UTI admitted to Northwest Region Kaiser Foundation Hospitals from 1979 to 1985. Out of approximately 25,000 infants (boys and girls), he found only 19 UTI cases, 14 female and 5 male. Three of the males were uncircumcised, which computes to a rate of 0.12% (or 3 out of the approximately 2,500 males in the group who were uncircumcised). Dr. Altschul concludes that such a rate "is not high enough to justify routine circumcision" (37).

Another physician, Dr. Leonard Marino, states:

> It has been my custom for the last 15 years to do a routine urinalysis at 2 months of age. Rarely is any abnormality found. In 15 years, I have admitted only 3 infants to a hospital with illness of the urinary tract: two girls with hydron-ephrosis and a circumcised male with UTI.
>
> ...My experience reinforces the practice of discouraging routine circumcision, a cause of more morbidity than benefit (38).

Why would there be such a difference in findings and conclusions between Wiswell and his contemporaries? Dr. Altschul speculates that the differences between his findings and Dr. Wiswell's may be due to "differences in foreskin care" (39). Parents in the Wiswell study were instructed "to gently retract the foreskin to allow the easily exposed portion of the glans to be cleaned." As previously discussed, authorities in the know, including the AAP, recommend that the infant penis be left alone until it can be retracted naturally by the boy himself. Forcible retraction may actually open the way for infectious organisms.

A second possible explanation comes from information provided by doctors from five different Swedish hospitals, which suggests that increased incidence of UTI among uncircumcised males may be related to the hospital birthing environment, not the foreskin (40). It has been noted that "Kaiser hospitals (from which Altschul got his figures) commonly offer rooming in. Military hospitals (source of Wiswell's studies) frequently do not" (41). New medical research indicates that when an infant is allowed to room in with its mother, staying in close physical contact, it picks up natural antibodies from the mother, which help the infant to resist infectious germs (42). In addition, The American Academy of Pediatrics and the Canadian Paediatric Society have both recently pointed out that breastfeeding has a protective effect against urinary tract infection in infants (43)(44).

Finally, there is a question as to the relative seriousness of UTI. Dr. George Denniston puts this entire issue into perspective:

> The largest number of infections that could be prevented by foreskin amputations, according to the author Dr. Thomas Wiswell, is 20,000 per year in the United States. So we should do 1,500,000 foreskin amputations [annually] to prevent infections, *now treatable with antibiotics*, in less than 2% of the infants? (45). (Emphasis added)

It seems self-evident that circumcising to prevent potential medical problems for a minute few is not a valid reason to routinely remove the foreskins of millions and millions of infants.

While there has been an ongoing controversy for decades in the medical literature concerning circumcision's possible health benefits—the stark, hard fact remains that these articles consistently failed to discuss the possibility that the foreskin could have a purpose and should not be casually cast into the trash can of medical waste. This remissness on the part of the American medical community seems unbelievable, but it must now be acknowledged, and somehow lived down.

Why have doctors been so slow to open their eyes to this issue? First, there is the economic consideration—doctors collectively make hundreds of millions of dollars annually from this surgery. Second, there are deep personal psychological connections to the custom—imagine how embarrassing and humiliating and ego-threatening the foreskin/circumcision controversy must be for a male doctor who 1) is himself circumcised, 2) had his sons circumcised, and 3) has circumcised other males (and, in the case of a female doctor, the latter two, plus her husband is probably circumcised). Circumcision simply perpetuated itself—doctors were psychologically blinded to the idea that circumcision could have harmful sexual repercussions.

Yet, for every troubling issue that cries out for resolution, there is a day of reckoning. And the contents of this book portend that that day has arrived. The medical community can no longer escape the inescapable truth—the foreskin is an intrinsic element in male sexuality and it is every male's birthright to retain the genitals he was endowed with by nature. To this end, an organization has formed called Doctors Opposing Circumcision (D.O.C.), which has members in all 50 states and all the Canadian provinces, as well as many other foreign countries. Doctors and nurses can get more information by visiting these websites

> www.DoctorsOpposingCircumcision.org
> www.cirp.org/nrc

This chapter was written in the mid-1990s as a brief overview touching on the major topics discussed in the medical literature. Since that time additional articles have been published both for and against circumcision. These I did not attempt to include because in 1996 the American Academy of Pediatrics (AAP) formed a Task Force to review the medical literature on circumcision from the last 40 years. After an intensive two-year study, they released their findings on March 1, 1999, and published a new "Circumcision Policy Statement" in the journal, *Pediatrics*, excerpts of which follow (46)(47). Their position is summarized in their opening statement:

> Existing scientific evidence demonstrates potential medical benefits of newborn male circumcision; however, these data are not sufficient to recommend routine neonatal [infant] circumcision.

The statement cites hygiene and protection from urinary tract infections, penile cancer, and sexually transmitted diseases as the "potential health benefits" not compelling enough to warrant recommending routine newborn circumcision. The reports that:

- "there is little evidence to affirm the association between circumcision status and optimal penile hygiene."
- "the absolute risk of developing a UTI in an uncircumcised male infant is low (at most, ~1%)."
- "behavioral factors appear to be far more important risk factors in the acquisition of HIV infection than circumcision status."

- "Penile cancer is a rare disease" and "the risk of penile cancer ... is low."

The statement acknowledges that the "true incidence of complications after newborn circumcision is unknown," then adds that complications include bleeding, wound separation, infection, skin bridges, meatitis, meatal stenosis, urethral fistula, inclusion cysts, scalded skin syndrome, sepsis, meningitis, partial amputation of glans, penile necrosis, and others.

The new AAP statement acknowledges that "newborns who are circumcised without analgesia experience pain and physiologic stress" and recommends using analgesia to reduce circumcision pain, but it does not explain that there is no analgesia that eliminates the pain.

The statement* advises that, "Parents and physicians each have an ethical duty to the child to attempt to secure the child's best interest and well-being," but fails to mention that legal experts and medical ethicists in the U.S., Canada, and Europe have questioned the legality of routine circumcision and have determined that it constitutes a violation of human rights.

However, by rejecting potential "medical benefits" as justification for routine infant circumcision, the American Academy of Pediatrics has struck a major blow against the practice of circumcision, and the already declining circumcision rate in the U.S. should therefore drop dramatically.

In August, 2000, the AMA (American Medical Association), the largest medical association in America, joined the AAP in renouncing the reputed medical benefits of circumcision in a statement entitled, "Neonatal Circumcision," saying that routine circumcision is "non-therapeutic"—not medically necessary. For details visit website: *http://www.ama-assn.org/ama/pub/article/2036-2511.html*

* Readers interested in reviewing the AAP policy statement, with supplementary comments for non-medical persons, should visit:

www.cirp.org/library/statements/aap1999/

19

Will the Jewish People Disavow Circumcision?

> This is my covenant which ye shall keep, between me and you and thy seed after thee; every man child among you shall be circumcised.
>
> And ye shall circumcise the flesh of your foreskin; and it shall be a token of the covenant betwixt me and you.
>
> Genesis 17:10-11

It is impossible to write a book of this nature without addressing the issue of Jewish circumcision, for it is widely known that Jewish infant boys are circumcised for religious reasons.

The Jews did not "invent" circumcision, however. Circumcision was in practice in Egypt and other parts of Northern Africa long before the Jews began to practice it in adherence to the above Abrahamic covenant about 4,000 years ago. What effect will the information in this book have on Jewish ritual circumcision? Could a ritual practiced for so long be changed? These are the questions this chapter will address.

All Jews are not automatically in agreement with circumcision just because they are Jewish. Though not well known, some Jewish parents do not circumcise their sons, and there are many Jewish people currently involved in the anti-circumcision movement. As far back as the mid-1800s, some Jews, through the Jewish Reform Movement, sought to abolish circumcision. But their attempts were unsuccessful. Thus, circumcision remained as a religious tenet.

If you are a present-day Jew, you should ask yourself if the Abrahamic covenant in Genesis has any real meaning to you in today's modern world. Do you really believe that God spoke to Abraham and told him to cut off part of the penis of all male Jews?

The majority of today's Jews probably do not have the Abrahamic covenant in mind when they choose to have their child circumcised. They choose it for the same reasons as non-Jews—because they have heard that it supposedly has medical benefits, etc.—or merely to conform with the religion of their parents, a religion in which they themselves, however, are not truly active. Many Jews who elect the circumcision ritual are simply following the tradition among their people, with little or no awareness of the religious meaning ascribed to the ceremony (1).

Some Jews believe that circumcision had its beginnings as a health measure. Edward Wallerstein, himself a Jew and author of *Circumcision: An American Health Fallacy*, maintains that this is not true. He asserts that for the Jews, circumcision began solely as a religious ritual, and Jewish religious leaders throughout history have abhorred the idea that circumcision is done for health benefits (2). In the words of Wallerstein:

> In summary, there are no substantive data in Jewish circumcision history or practice to support the thesis that circumcision is a health measure or that health benefits are in any way derived from it. Historically, the methods employed in performing the surgery were anything but sanitary or scientific. To this day [1980], little or no control is exercised over its practitioners, who can and do cause harm, even death.
>
> Religious Jews vehemently deny any health benefits and insist that circumcision is purely a religious rite. Nonreligious Jews who accept circumcision for its supposed health benefits derive support for that theory from the wide acceptance of routine circumcision by non-Jews. Thus, a brief overview of Jewish circumcision sheds no light as to its health origins and no proof of its purported hygienic benefits in its past or current practice (3).

The Jewish ritual of circumcision is done solely for religious reasons. Changing the ritual must come through the religion itself. If you are a Jew who has come to a greater understanding of circumcision by the information in this book, you now realize that a way must be found to reconcile the disparity between circumcision's harmful effects and God's covenant as "communicated" through Abraham. For this issue affects the lives of children who are soon to be born and generations yet to come. If you believe this ancient ritual should be re-evaluated, express your feelings to your rabbi and to others within your religion. To anyone informed on this issue, the importance of an intact foreskin takes on new significance. I assert that non-circumcision is an idea whose time has come for all races and creeds.

Unknown to most Jews, the ritual of circumcision has already undergone several changes throughout its history, according to Wallerstein (4). In the earliest days, the Jews practiced a circumcision style called Milah, in which only the very tip of the foreskin was cut away. This early form of circumcision was nothing like the fully-bared-glans style of today's circumcision.

When the ancient Jewish circumcisers cut off only the protruding tip of the infant foreskin, a great deal of the natural foreskin remained intact to cover a substantial portion of the glans (when flaccid). However, because the *ridged band* was destroyed during the Milah procedure, the foreskin could not function entirely the way nature intended, although it did leave the penis shaft some extra skin to expand into during erection and provided somewhat of a gliding mechanism during intercourse.

DAVID'S FORESKIN

Many people have wondered, and explanations have been debated, as to why David, in Michelangelo's famous statue of him, has a foreskin. Surely, a man with Michelangelo's knowledge of the male anatomy and Biblical history would have known not to put a foreskin on a Jewish youth. Did he consider the circumcised penis unaesthetic? Was he simply too embarrassed to chisel the intimate details of a bared glans? Were all his models natural (uncircumcised), so he therefore sculpted what he was familiar with? These are some of the speculations that have been raised regarding the statue of David "mystery," which was chiseled in stone.

The carving of David was not a hasty affair. Michelangelo labored over it for years. Why, then, would he sculpt a Jewish youth with a foreskin? Recently, a very convincing theory has been put forward by Wallerstein. He states:

> Michelangelo probably knew exactly what he was doing. First, it is necessary to examine the precise method of circumcision in 1000 B.C. [around the time of David's birth]. Originally, the procedure called for removing only the very tip of the foreskin. Known in Hebrew as Milah....
>
> The glans of David's penis is almost completely covered by the foreskin. This factor probably prompted physicians to claim that Michelangelo sculpted the penis as uncircumcised. ...In addition, the sculpting of this statue was not a hasty affair. Michelangelo labored on it for four years. We can assume that with his astute knowledge of anatomy, he was as meticulous in penile details as in all others.
>
> It is therefore probable that Michelangelo correctly portrayed David as circumcised, based upon the surgical procedure of that period—that is, with only the very tip of the foreskin removed (5).

In any event, Milah was in use for almost 2,000 years and was not changed until the Hellenistic period (circa 300 B.C.-1 A.D.). At that time, the Greeks were trying to convert the Jews to paganism. Some Jews, in order to "restore" their foreskins, resorted to blistering the tip of the remainder of the foreskin in order to enlarge it, thereby appearing more uncircumcised. So many Jews adopted this practice that the rabbis of that period decided to alter the circumcision procedure in order to make it impossible for a circumcised Jew to try to appear uncircumcised. This was accomplished by a procedure known as Periah, in which the entire foreskin was cut off, including the inner lining and frenulum, torn by specially sharpened fingernails of the Jewish ritual circumciser (mohel).

The next change in the ritual, although not universally adopted, began in the Talmudic period (circa 500-635 A.D.). At this time an additional element was added—Messisa (sometimes spelled Mezziza or Metzitzah, its phonetic pronunciation). Messisa consisted of moistening the lips with wine and then taking the bleeding penis into the mouth to suck the blood. This was done several times, and a special receptacle was provided to receive the blood that was spit out.

These two parts of the ritual—Periah and Messisa—remained in general use until about 100 years ago. The above procedures became, for the majority of the Jewish community, radically changed in the last quarter of the 19th century by the introduction of advances in aseptic surgery. The total foreskin was still removed, but the use of fingernails was often replaced by a knife or scissors (although Orthodox Jews continue to use fingernails as an instrument for tearing the tissue of the inner foreskin and the frenulum). Sucking blood directly from the penis was also discontinued, or at least replaced with a glass tube to avoid direct mouth-penis contact. This practice has also, for the majority of Jews, been discontinued.

In addition to the above changes, the first half of the 20th century brought an increase in the number of hospital births. Many Reform Jews began using doctors instead of mohels to perform the surgery. Over the years, even Conservative Jews adopted this practice. Orthodox Jews, however, have never allowed doctors to replace mohels.

As noted above, the Jewish religious ritual of circumcision has undergone several changes throughout its history. In light of the new information we now have about the deleterious consequences that can result from cutting off the foreskin, it is hoped that Judaism will re-evaluate this ancient practice and make one final change—abolish it. This, I believe, may be accomplished through Judaism's own Talmudic Laws, which are presented below.

TALMUDIC LAWS AS A MEANS TO DISAVOW CIRCUMCISION

During the Talmudic period of Jewish history, making vows was, in general, considered a sign of bad upbringing because if a vow could not be fulfilled it could cast reproach upon the honor of one's family. Mainstream rabbinical tradition was opposed to the making of vows and discouraged people from making them (6).

> "If you forbear to vow, it shall be no sin in this." (Deuteronomy 23:23)

> "Do not form the habit of making vows." (Babylonian Talmud—Nedarim 20.a)

But since some people did make vows, the rabbinical authorities were confronted with the dilemma of how to resolve a situation in which one made a sacred vow but, for various reasons, could not fulfill it.

During the Talmudic legislation period, many sages maintained that Jewish law should have a way of annulling a vow. They argued that a person might regret making a certain vow, and there should be some remedy for its retraction. They succeeded in establishing a methodology for annulling a vow which was implemented into standard Jewish law and is still operative today (7).

Here is how a vow is undone by one who wishes to have it annulled: (8) The person who has made the vow which cannot be fulfilled appears before a sage or a quorum of three knowledgeable men, who ask the person: "If you had known the consequences of making this vow, would you have done it?"

If the person replies, "I would not have taken the vow," the sage or the quorum of three pronounces him absolved of his oath.

Another remedy for the failure to fulfill a vow can be found in the "Kol Nidre" ("All Vows") recited at the beginning of the Jewish holiday Yom Kippur, the Day of Atonement. This holiday is a 24-hour fast for transgressions and oaths that could not (or cannot) be fulfilled, which one regrets having sworn to:

> All vows, bonds, promises, obligations, and oaths wherewith we have vowed, sworn, and found ourselves from this Day of Atonement unto the next Day of Atonement. They shall be absolved, released, annulled, made void, and of no effect; they shall not be binding nor shall they have any power. Our vows shall not be vows; our bonds shall not be bonds (9).

Rabbis are also familiar with a lesser known ceremony which focuses more closely on individual vows. In the Jewish religion, it is referred to as Hatarat Nedarim, the Annulment of Vows. The traditional time for this ceremony is just prior to Rosh Hashanah, the New Year. During this ceremony, three or more individuals band together and take turns representing a quasi-ecclesiastical court. Each individual, in turn, recites a formula whereby he renounces all oaths and promises. Reference in this formula is made to vows and various promises forgotten, and vows of which one is still aware (10).

Finally, the Formula for Annulment of Vows is as follows: (11)

The three "judges" sit while the petitioner seeking annulment stands before them and states:

> Listen please, my master, expert judges: every vow or oath or prohibition, or restriction that I adopted by use of the term *konam* or the term *cherem*, that I vowed or swore while I was awake or in a dream, or that I swore by means of God's Holy Names that it is forbidden to erase, or by means of the name Hashem, Blessed is He; or any form of Naziritism that I accepted upon myself, even the Naziritism of Samson; or any prohibition, even a prohibition to derive enjoyment that I imposed upon myself or upon others by means of any

expression of prohibition, whether by specifying the term *prohibition* or by use of the term *konam* or *cherem* [konam means any vow of abstinence, cherem is any ban]; or any commitment even to perform a *mitzvah* that I accepted upon myself, whether the acceptance was in terms of a vow, a voluntary gift, an oath, Naziritism, or by means of any other sort of expression, or whether it was made final through a handshake; any form of vow, or any custom that constitutes a good deed to which I have accustomed myself....

Therefore I request annulment for them all. I regret all the aforementioned whether they were matters relating to money, or whether they are matters relating to the body or whether they were matters relating to the soul. Regarding them all, I regret the terminology of vow, oath, Naziritism, prohibition, cherem, konam (i), and acceptances of the heart.

The judges then repeat three times:

May everything be permitted you, may everything be forgiven you, may everything be allowed you. There does not exist any vow, oath, Naziritism, cherem, prohibition, konam, ostracism, excommunication, or curse. But there does exist pardon, forgiveness, and atonement. And just as the early court permits them, so may they be permitted in the Heavenly Court.

Finally, the ceremony is concluded with the petitioner declaring for the final time that he "cancels from this time onward all vows and all oaths."

CIRCUMCISION CONTRADICTS JEWISH MORAL PRINCIPLE

Another important consideration is that Judaism teaches that enjoyment of life is an authentic goal of life. Furthermore, rabbinical teaching maintains that "in the world to come" we will be judged for the failure to enjoy life's legitimate pleasures (12). Since circumcision drastically interferes with one of life's fundamental joys—a man's and his female partner's ability to both give and receive pleasure during intercourse—with detrimental effects on their love relationship—another quintessential joy, it seems prudent that Judaism re-evaluate religious circumcision for this reason alone.

Let me close this chapter with a statement from *Circumcision: The Hidden Trauma*, by Ronald Goldman, Ph.D., himself a Jew:

> I hope that the review of American circumcision practice is independent of religious considerations. In particular, I encourage those individuals and groups who may take a position on the issue to do so regardless of how their position may be received by Jews. Though concern for the feelings of Jews is appropriate, Jewish discomfort with this issue is inevitable....
>
> [T]he Jewish community has a considerable role to play in the national circumcision dialogue. That role, I believe, is to act and speak responsibly. I am concerned that a small but vocal minority of Jews may use reckless charges of anti-Semitism to respond to arguments against circumcision. Thoughtful questioning of circumcision is not anti-Semitic because Jews are also questioning the practice. Furthermore, it is possible to question the actions of a person or group without being categorically opposed to the person or group. In fact, questioning an action that causes harm is more likely to be motivated by concern rather than ill will. I believe that most Jews will not stereotype those opposed to circumcision and impugn their motivation.
>
> Jews have long-held repressed feelings about circumcision. The growing debate will certainly stir them. In my view, the proper response for Jews is to support each other as we air these feelings within the Jewish community (13).

20

A Call to Reason

This chapter is dedicated posthumously to Edward Wallerstein, inventor of cable TV and author of *Circumcision: An American Health Fallacy* (Springer Publishing, 1980). Edward was a man who looked forward into time. When he first called out into the bewilderment of circumcision's unanswered questions, very few ears were tuned to his call. But that was then—and this is now—where we stand on the edge of a solemn vow.

A Call to Reason

For Now, Forevermore, and a Season

Yes, it's a call to reason
For now
Forevermore
And a season
For all the time that's yet to come
Until there be not one more sun

Look hard and deep now
Into the eyes of time
Which must never again deceive us,
For the time has come
To take a vow—to slash no more
The secret parts between another's legs
While that infant screams and sobbingly begs,
Crying out in agonizing pain,
"Please, mister circumciser, please,
Please do not bloody and slice me
And leave your lifetime scar,

Please—put those clamps
And sharp scissors away,
Please, mister circumciser, please,
Ohmygod—please put that razor-sharp scalpel away"

Yes, if we could hear the "words"
In the cries of his pre-verbal days
(While strapped down spread-eagled on a Circumstraint tray)
That's precisely what we'd hear
That helpless little infant say,
If he could speak at all
Between his gasping-for-breath sobs and his ear-piercing screams

But that was then,
And this is now,
Where we stand on the edge
Of a solemn vow
And the time that has now come to say
—BURY the circumciser's knives TODAY!
So deep within the burial ground
That they shall never again be found
—BANISH these circumcision weapons of pain
Upon whose screaming-steel blades remain
All the blood-stained memories
Of each and every victim
Who has ever cried out in vain

With our newly opened eyes,
Surely now we are appalled and despise
The damage we've so savagely done,
But still, what's done is done
And cannot be undone,
It is only the road to the future
That we can hope to shape and change

And so, with our eyes focused determinedly
On the future,
See now each and every little boy
Who shall ever come into this life,
Who shall now be left intact and unsliced
From the silent skin
Which shall bring him such joy,
With its pleasure-receptor nerves
He was born to enjoy

Yes, there is a time
And there is a place
For vows whose time has come,
And surely this
Is now the time,
And surely this
Is now the place,
To leave the circumcisions of the "past"
Far, far behind
In the inner recesses of our mind,
Forgotten,
But never to be forgotten

Some may say, "go slow"
(Coming up somewhere from behind)
"Let the sands of time settle this issue
—this issue is going to take time"
But I say NO!
This is no time for slowed-down faint-hearted reactions
—For action is the word of the day
NOW is the time,
And THIS is the place,
Natural genitals for the whole human race

They cannot wait
These infants of the United States
Stripped down and strapped
To Circumstraint trays
Where passion is torn so savagely
From their flesh of youthful innocence
—And they cannot wait
These children of foreign lands
Who see ahead only the sand in the hourglass
And the fateful, dreadful day
When ritual will claim them as victim
As the swipe of the razor sweeps past
"NO! NO!—a thousand times NO!"
Is what the children say
"Tomorrow will not be soon enough"
Is what the infants say

Yes, yesterday's child
Is but one day old
And that little face
Will soon be tear-streaked
And older than its little look at time
If we do not think of that infant child
As a child of yours and mine...

We must begin TODAY,
For today is the first day
Of the rest of their lives,
And so we must not be delayed,
We are standing at this crossroads
And it's time to tear the page
From the history
Of the circumcision age,
Let tomorrow's generations
Look back at this time and see

That we acted with firm determination
To make unmutilated genitalia
A universal reality

Yes, it's a call to reason
For now
Forevermore
And a season,
Calling out to one and all,
There is no time like the present
To read the writing on destiny's wall

Circumcision
Has had its day in our history
But the time has now come for its fall,
It's all but over now for circumcision
Says the writing on destiny's wall,
Yes, you had your bloody day in our history
But the time has now come
For
Your
Fall

       ...The End

But this ending is only the beginning
Of everything that will ever come to pass,
Where tulips shall spring forth from damnation
In the hearts and minds of a new generation
This generation...
This time...
This place...
This human race...

Afterword

by George C. Denniston, M.D.

This book has the potential to make the world, and especially the United States, a happier place to live, by opening our eyes to the importance of the foreskin as an inherent element of sexual pleasure. Its comprehensive explanations show how some humans, in sanctioning circumcision, have acted to deprive other humans of their full sexual functioning and experience.

While the author has put forth some advanced, controversial ideas that are sure to invite scientific scrutiny, she demonstrates that she knows far more about the true value and functioning of the foreskin than most American doctors. Sadly, many of these doctors have bought into the illogic of cutting away healthy, natural tissue without ascertaining its worth. In their defense, it must be admitted that the bizarre paradigm of circumcision has been fraught with numerous myths that have pervaded our culture and confused even the brightest of minds.

Doctors Opposing Circumcision (D.O.C.) was founded to help end routine neonatal circumcision in America, and its members, in 50 states and on 6 continents, are working to bring out the facts concerning this tragic practice.

All non-religious circumcisions in the U.S. are performed by doctors. Yet, paradoxically, routine circumcision violates not only the Golden Rule, but also the first tenet of medical practice: *First, Do No Harm.* In fact, circumcision violates *all seven* Principles of the A.M.A. Code of Ethics.

Doctors' licenses do not authorize them to cut people unless they are performing surgery. And circumcision is not surgery, *by definition*. Surgical procedures have been defined as: repair of wounds, extirpation of diseased organs or tissue, reconstructive surgery, and physiologic surgery (i.e., sympathectomy). Routine circumcision does not fall into any of these categories. Therefore, ethically, doctors performing this operation are outside their authorized domain.

American men, circumcised in infancy, are now documenting the harm that has been done to them by doctors who operated on them without their consent. The bizarre practice of parents telling the doctor to operate and remove healthy tissue occurs nowhere else in medicine. According to modern medical ethics, parents do not have the right to consent to a procedure that is not in their son's best interests. The removal of a normal, important part of the male sexual organ is not in their son's best interests.

America has the highest rate of AIDS in the industrialized world, and also circumcises the majority of its males. There may be a connection. We do not yet know. Before a doctor performs a circumcision, he should first have the answer to this question: *Might this baby have an **increased** risk of AIDS as a result of circumcision?*

The time is approaching when doctors will be unwilling to perform this painful, contraindicated procedure. Already, an ever-growing number of physicians are opposed to routine neonatal circumcision. These doctors recognize that no one has the right to forcibly remove normal sexual body parts from another individual. They recognize that doctors should play no role in inflicting this painful, unnecessary procedure on newborns or children.

In order for a doctor to stop circumcising babies, he or she must take a courageous step. The doctor must recognize that what has been done in the past was not in the best interest of the infant, and he must say, "I will not circumcise any more babies."

Many doctors have already taken that sometimes personally challenging step, and we honor them. Those who lack the courage to change continue to circumcise.

We have the greatest admiration for men who, having been cut themselves, have moved past their denial and refused to permit the circumcision of their sons. Countless millions of American parents have said NO! to circumcision, increasingly more as time has progressed. Every parent and grandparent now has the opportunity to learn what circumcision does to the penis and its long-term potential consequences. With this knowledge, the tragedy of circumcision will not be passed on to their descendants—saving them much grief and enriching their lives. To this end of greater understanding, this book serves a valuable purpose. And if the revolutionary ideas it asserts hold up and make their mark, we will undoubtedly see an end to circumcision in America, and hopefully, someday soon, the world.

George C. Denniston, M.D.
President, D.O.C. (Doctors Opposing Circumcision)
www.DoctorsOpposingCircumcision.org
September, 2000

Appendix A

How to Have a Vaginal Orgasm 99.99% of the Time Using the Side-by-Side (Face-to-Face) Position

> "I use the side-by-side (face-to-face) position. Neither partner is totally dominant and both probably attain their maximum pleasure. I think that because the woman is able to move quite freely, she is able to control the pressure on her clitoral area and help herself to achieve orgasm."
>
> "The side-by-side position definitely helped our sexual relationship. I would maybe orgasm 40% of the time with other positions, but the side-by-side position guarantees me orgasm 100% of the time!"
>
> — Comments from survey respondents

My husband and I strongly recommend this position. We believe the side-by-side position is the most satisfying for both partners. It will very likely become your favorite position. It allows freedom for either partner to set the pace of the thrusting rhythm, and enables deepest penetration. Also, it is extremely comfortable, makes sex almost effortless, and leaves the hands free to fondle and caress one another. And the big plus is, it virtually guarantees that the woman will achieve orgasm.

The simplest way to achieve this position is to first get into the man-on-top position, wherein both partners are face-to-face, with the woman on her back (commonly known as the missionary position).

Once in the missionary position, the woman, keeping the man's body between her legs and the penis within the vagina, carefully rolls him onto his side. Both partners will then be on their sides, face-to-face. I recommend rolling the man to the left, but I am not sure if this varies for left- and right-handed people (I am right-handed).

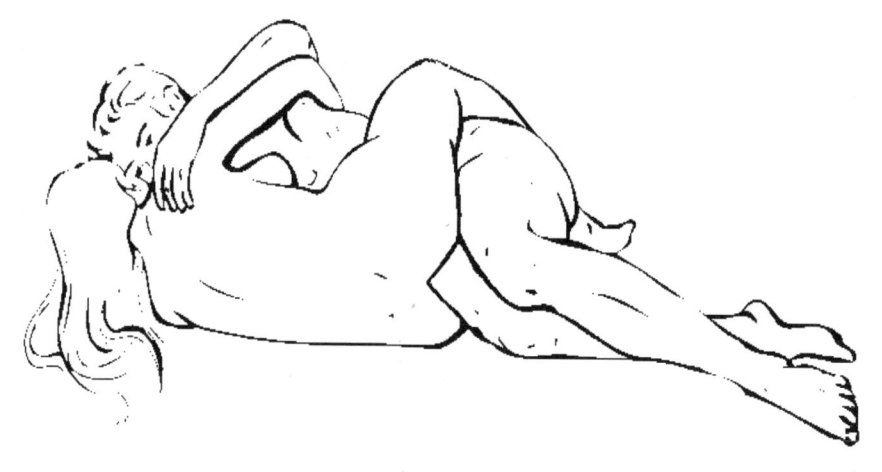

The first few times, you try this you will have to be a bit careful, because the penis may slip out of the vagina. But within a few tries, you should become good at it.

In the roll-to-the-left position (described above), when properly positioned, the woman's left thigh will be under the man's side, at about waist level (and the knee-to-thigh area of her left leg will be positioned under the man's waist to chest area).

Once in this position, the woman's right hand is free to do whatever, especially to pull the man's buttocks in tightly to her as her passion increases, or to twiddle her partner's nipples intermittently. (She can also free her left hand, and by crossing it over her right, can twiddle both of her partner's nipples simultaneously, thereby exciting him and helping to assure that he maintains his erection.)

Instead of keeping his legs straight, the man may find it more comfortable to draw his knee(s) up closer to his partner's buttocks, almost as if he is making a seat for her.

During prolonged intercourse, either partner can temporarily stop their thrusting to reduce sexual tension, thereby maintaining prolongation. **(See the "Tap Me" Secret to Prolonging Intercourse in Appendix B.)**

Most importantly, in this position, the woman's clitoris is pressed up against the man's body and she can maintain even closer contact by pulling the man's buttocks in toward her.

Although it is probably somewhat of an individual matter, I recommend that when the woman is ready to go for her orgasm, she should "grind" away for a while and then totally relax the pressure against her clitoris by loosening up and temporarily remaining inactive for 10-15 seconds. During the woman's momentary inactivity, if the man uses a very short, rapid, vibrating-type stroke, he will send the woman to Cloud Nine. (*More precisely, while the woman is momentarily resting and remaining motionless, with the penis deep within the vagina, the man should press his pubic area tightly against the woman's clitoral area and then jiggle rapidly. This will give the woman mini-orgasms. These jiggling movements do not involve any actual thrusting of the penis. It's more of a vibrating action against the woman's clitoris.*) You simply must try this technique. You'll be praising it forever.

The woman's sex organs need this respite from thrusting to rejuvenate, and varying the tempo through this relaxed type of movement is important for achieving multiple orgasms. It not only helps to relax things in between orgasms, but it may also be helpful in building up to the first orgasm as well.

The woman must take responsibility for her own orgasm and should abandon any inhibitions she may have about thrusting wildly, **with pressure,** *against her partner's body. Go for it like there's no tomorrow.*

And don't be timid about relaxing for a moment or two after orgasm and going for another. You'll be surprised at your capacity in this gratifying position and will very likely find that you will often be able to achieve multiple orgasms. And the man benefits, too, because it lengthens the time of his copulatory pleasure.

In the side-by-side position, both bodies are relatively close to one another, which adds to the feeling of intimacy. However, when the woman is seeking orgasm and still has trouble achieving it, she should position herself so that *his body is at 12 o'clock* and *hers is at 9 o'clock*. This position applies even greater stimulatory pressure to the clitoris, which some women may need. (In the 9 and 12 o'clock position, both partners are still lying on their sides, face-to-face.)

If your partner is circumcised—until he restores—you may find it necessary for him to remain motionless, that is, *he should not thrust his penis when you are actively working toward your orgasm,* for two reasons: 1) his thrusting is likely to pull his body away from yours, taking pressure off your clitoral mound, 2) the movement of his coronal ridge "hook" may work to lessen your excitement and may inhibit your ability to achieve orgasm.

For maximum comfort, from time to time, it may be necessary for the woman to roll her partner somewhat back into the missionary position in order to reposition her left leg back into place, approximately at his waistline.

It is also nice to roll back into the missionary position periodically to let the man take up most of the work, and for a momentary change of pace. But when you want to bring yourself to orgasm (again?), roll him back on his side to bring about more direct clitoral stimulation against his body.

You're really missing out if you don't give this position a try. We sometimes get set in our ways, but if you are having trouble achieving vaginal orgasm every time, or multiple vaginal orgasms, I strongly suggest this position. Once you start using it, I think you will use it all the time.

One further note: Although it's not an essential piece of equipment, we think that sex (and sleep) is always better on a waterbed. We prefer the original, full-flotation type mattress.

Land and Sky Quality Sleep (which I have no financial affiliation with) sells a superior basic mattress for a very reasonable price, along with everything else you need to get set up. Visit *www.landandsky.com*. Be sure to not overfill your mattress. You should be able to sink into it somewhat. If the mattress feels too firm, and you're rolling around on top, it's too full. Also, I recommend a zip-around mattress enclosure to temper motion somewhat. For a mattress pad, use a European featherbed or a down-filled comforter. For maximum comfort, I recommend all-cotton sheets and natural fiber blankets. Also, wear all-natural sleeping clothes. Poly/cotton blends and synthetic fibers will cause you to toss and turn all night and during prolonged intercourse, can give you sheet burns.

You won't believe the vast superiority natural fibers will make in your sexual and sleeping comfort.

Important: This Appendix focused on the woman's pleasure. Tips on maximizing the man's copulatory pleasure should be reviewed at pages 227-230.

Appendix B

How to Minimize Premature Ejaculation and the "Tap Me" Secret to Prolonging Intercourse

In my own personal experience with a man who was prone to premature ejaculation, we found the following solution.

He would enter me very slowly. After he was fully inserted, we would both remain motionless for about a half-minute to a minute. This allowed him time to get used to being in me. (I think some men—or their partners—begin overly active thrusting too early, and this can quickly lead to a loss of control over the ejaculatory reflex.) Then, while fully inserted, he would wiggle in a side-to-side motion for another moment or two. We both found this very arousing, but not overly stimulating for him, because there is no wildly active thrusting.

After he could tolerate this amount of stimulation, he would proceed to use very short thrusting strokes, while simultaneously pressed up tightly against my clitoral mound. Within another minute or two, he would have complete control over his ejaculatory reflex and could continue to perform actively for as long as we wanted, often for a half-hour or more.

However, if we were at some point thrusting vigorously and he felt I was bringing him too close to ejaculation, he would lightly *tap me on the shoulder*, and I would immediately stop my pelvic movements. After about 15 seconds, we could then proceed to thrust again as actively as we wished. However, if at any time he felt I was stimulating him to orgasm prematurely, he would "tap me" again. We'd again rest for about 15 seconds, more or less, until he felt he had his ejaculatory reflex under control.

I found this technique to be wonderful because he didn't have to disrupt our erotic state with an unwelcomed verbal command like, "Stop for a minute." The non-verbal approach is far superior, in my opinion. It sends the message in a gentle way and does not disrupt the ecstasy of the moment. Also, as a side benefit, the few seconds of rest recharged our sexual organs, so our pleasure was enhanced when we resumed.

As time went on, he increasingly gained greater control over his ejaculatory reflex, and it was rare that he had to tap me at all. Through this method, he developed complete control over his orgasmic response.

The idea in using this technique is for the man to maintain his sexual excitement at a level that provides great pleasure *without striving headlong towards orgasm.* This involves thrusting with short strokes and wiggling and jiggling a lot. My husband says that he finds it much more pleasurable to prolong the sex act at sub-orgasmic plateaus for an extended period of time rather than approaching it with the intent of achieving orgasm relatively quickly. And I agree.

Male readers should keep in mind that helping your female partner to achieve multiple orgasms will, in itself, keep the act alive longer. Experimenting with the sexual position described in Appendix A should help her to accomplish this.

The "tap me" technique and the technique in Appendix A will have their greatest benefit after restoration. Sadly, women of the survey indicated that they do not enjoy prolonged intercourse with the circumcised penis.

Appendix C

A Solution for Those Circumcised Men Who Take Longer Than They Want to Reach Orgasm

(And a Sexual Improvement in General)

This is only an interim solution, for after a man restores, he will find it much easier to come to orgasm (but not prematurely). Yet even after restoration, he may still find this technique desirable on occasion, or even routinely, for it may heighten his orgasm significantly.

Some circumcised men complain that they have to work too hard to achieve orgasm. Some have to pump away for a considerable time—they want to orgasm but find it difficult or impossible. This is not only frustrating for the man, but prolonged aggressive thrusting can also be discomforting for his female partner. Here is a suggestion which should prove helpful.

When the man is ready to go for his orgasm, the couple should assume the missionary position, wherein the woman is on the bottom with her legs open and the man is on top with his legs together. The woman should then close her legs—sliding them together to a point that is comfortable for the man. The man should in turn open his legs so that his legs are straddling her legs, i.e., ***his legs will be spread apart over her legs, which are now almost, or completely, closed together***. In this position, greater pressure is applied to the penis. This added pressure may be enough to allow the man to come to orgasm virtually at will. Additionally, if the woman twiddles her partner's nipples, this will also help to bring the man to orgasm.

And finally, if prolonged thrusting has caused nerves to become over-stimulated, taking the penis out of the vagina for a moment should revitalize their sensitivity.

Appendix D

Supplementary Evidence Concerning the Male Clitoris

The concept of a male clitoris is sure to be surprising to many readers. Therefore, as an elucidative aid, this appendix is devoted to Josephine Lowndes Sevely's explanations on the topic from her book, *Eve's Secrets* (excerpted from pages 16-22). Keep in mind that her book, subtitled, *A New Theory of Female Sexuality*, was concerned almost exclusively with female sexual anatomy. Her discovery of the male clitoris came about as a result of her seven-year Harvard-approved investigation into the similarities of the female and male genitalia. Sevely's text begins below:

The Lowndes Crowns Theory

[Italian anatomist Gabriel] Fallopio [1523-1562] is credited with the first fully detailed description of the clitoris. He was the first to dissect its deeper internal structure—a part of the female anatomy unknown to scientists before him. In the process of making this important discovery, however, he made the error of assuming, and providing a basis for others to assume, that the clitoris was a miniature penis. The curious historical fact is that this belief came about not through valid scientific research, but as a result of an ingrained male perspective that viewed the female as inferior [the penis being so big, and the female clitoris so small] and an unquestioning acceptance of incorrect translations.

Even more curious is the fact that the erroneous nature of the penis/clitoris idea could have gone undetected for so many centuries. As I propose to show, an argument can be made on the basis of a reevaluation of existing anatomical facts to convincingly demonstrate that the old inadequate notion should be replaced by a new, much more plausible concept.

The new theory advanced here proposes that the clitoral tip and the penile glans are *not* counterparts of each other; the true counterparts are the female tip and the tip of a male structure *inside* the penis. The male structure is the part that fills with blood and brings about erection, a capsule-like part called the corpora cavernosa, meaning literally "cavernous bodies." It can now be stated with some certainty that the true counterpart of the female clitoris is not the penis but rather this internal part of the penis that can only be called—and that I now identify as—the male clitoris. The tips of the male and female clitorises are the Lowndes crowns, named by the author who identified the correct homology, in the tradition of anatomical parts being named by the person who makes the discovery.

Many people may be surprised to learn that the female clitoris has deeper structures under the skin. These deeper structures are the organ's two leglike parts that run along the lower part of the pubic bones at either side of the lower vagina between the inner thighs. Simple names exist for all the parts of the clitoris: they are the crown (the tip); the corpus (the body); and the crura (the legs). The crown is the part most familiar to us; indeed, along with its covering fold, it is usually thought of as the clitoris, as if it represented all of it. If the covering fold is drawn back, the crown is easily visible—a highly sensitive tip of flesh about the size of a small pea.

The corpus (or body), on the other hand, is not visible, but it can be felt with the fingertips just under the surface of the skin. It is usually about a quarter of an inch in diameter and somewhere less than an inch in length.

The crura (or legs), since they are internal structures, are not visible either; nor can they be easily felt. The two crura taper; in thickness, each one is somewhat less than the width of a little finger....The shape in nature that most closely resembles it is the seed of a maple tree.

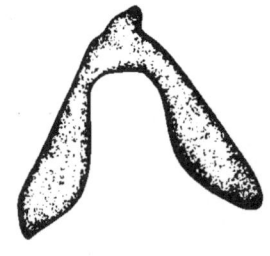

The idea of a male clitoris is startling to most people. Understandably, the visible parts of the male sexual organs are much more familiar than those inside the penis. For instance, just about everyone knows about the shaft of the penis, the foreskin, the glans, and the urethral opening through which both sexual fluids and urine are passed; but perhaps less well known is the body of tissue that surrounds the male urethra, called the spongiosum. And although everyone knows that the penis gets erect because it fills with blood, up to now very few have known about the part into which the blood flows, which is the male clitoris.

The following illustrations of life-size [reduced for this publication] schematic models of the male and female clitoris make it clear that the male and female organs are very much alike; like the female, the male clitoris contains two crura, a corpus, and a crown (see Figure below).

The two organs are also fairly close in size. A careful measure of the [specimens'] overall length shows five inches for the male and four inches for the female, making a 5:4 ratio. Since on the average men weigh approximately 160 pounds and women 128, one would expect such a difference to be reflected in the sizes of the parts that make up these weights, and the 5:4 ratio is exactly in line. On reflection, therefore, the traditional premise that the sexual parts of men and women are vastly different in size must be reconsidered.

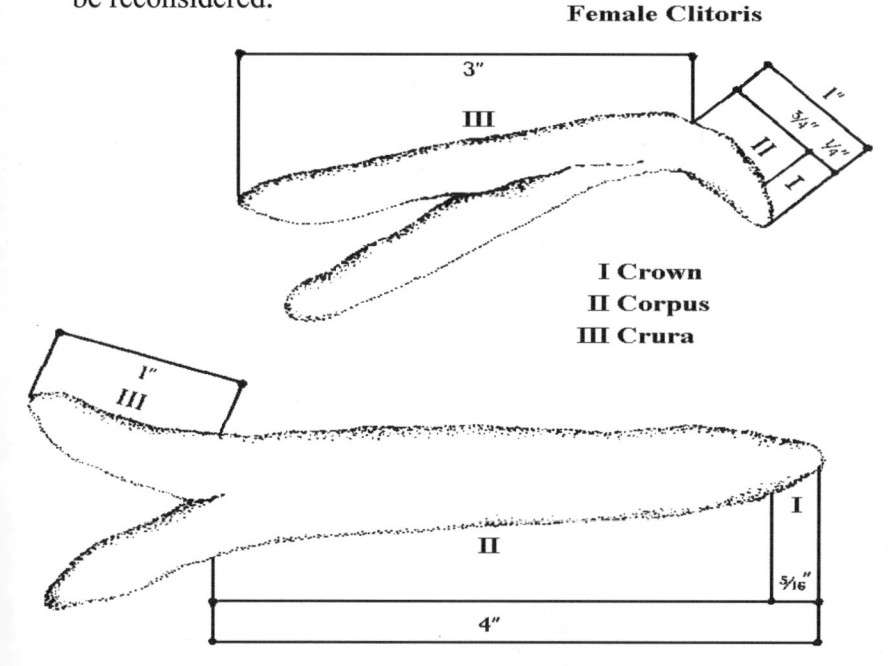

Female Clitoris

I Crown
II Corpus
III Crura

Male Clitoris

370 *Supplementary Evidence Concerning the Male Clitoris*

The female clitoris has a *short* body that splits in two to form the long, separated legs, while the male clitoris has a *long* body that splits into two to form only very short, separated legs. But this difference is one of organization, not of substance. The female and male clitorises are composed of basically the same erectile substance.

...If the tip of the female clitoris is not the counterpart of the penile glans, is there another female part that *is?* There is indeed, and the part can be easily located and observed. If the inner folds (the labia minora) are spread apart, the opening of the urethra [urethral meatus] becomes clearly visible...The [urethral] meatus is surrounded by a relatively prominent area shaped like an acorn.... [This] area... has heretofore been left unnamed. This acorn-shaped prominence is the woman's glans.

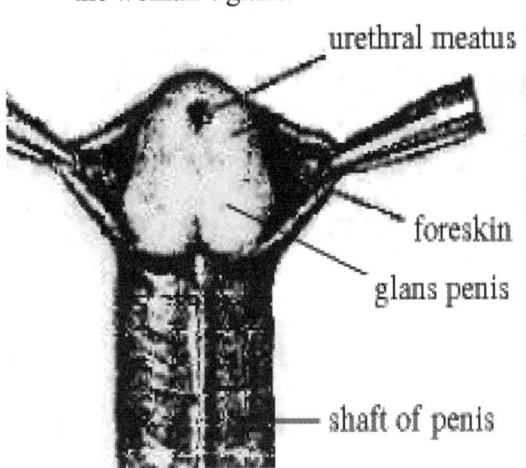

(These two figures were not in *Eve's Secrets'* presentation.)

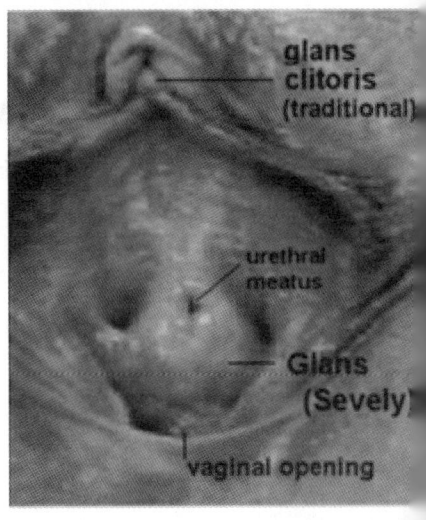

Close-up photo of female vulva showing location of true female glans per Sevely

[*Author's Comment:* The above drawing of the penis and close-up photo of the female genitalia illustrate that the male and female glans have a similar appearance and that both are perforated by, and surround, the urethral meatus. Since the urethral meatus of both genitalia are obvious homologues, it seems logical that the tissue housing them are also homologous. If the female glans (pictured above) is the true homologue to the male glans, then the female clitoris is not the homologue to the male glans, as traditionally believed. Thus, Sevely's Lowndes crown theory deserves serious consideration and in all probability will be later affirmed as true.]

Appendix E

Reprint* from *BJU* (British Journal of Urology) *International*, January, 1999, Volume 83, Supplement 1, pages 79-84

The effect of male circumcision on the sexual enjoyment of the female partner
by K. O'Hara and J. O'Hara

Introduction

Male circumcision, the most commonly performed surgery in the USA, removes 33-50% of the penile skin, as well as nearly all of the penile fine-touch neuroreceptors [1]. To date no study has investigated whether this dramatic alteration in the male genitalia affects the sexual pleasure experienced by the female partner or whether women can physically discern the difference between a penis with or without a foreskin. The impact that male circumcision has on the overall sexual experience for either partner is unknown.

Just as female circumcision was advocated in some Muslim and African countries to control women's sexuality, so too was male circumcision introduced into English-speaking countries in the late 1800s as a method of treating and preventing masturbation [2]. While there has been debate over whether circumcision affects the sexual sensations of the penis, there have been few relevant studies. Four men circumcised in adulthood reported decreased sensitivity [3]. Writing under a pseudonym, a physician circumcised as an adult argued that the loss of sensitivity he experienced was favourable, as it gave him more control over his orgasms [4]. Another man, circumcised as an adult, lamented that the decrease in sensation could be equated with seeing in monochrome rather than colour.

Laumann *et al.* [5] found that circumcised men had different sexual practices from genitally unaltered men. Circumcised men were more likely to masturbate,

---

* Contains a few changes as noted.

to engage in heterosexual anal and oral sex, and to engage in homosexual anal sex. In the male rat, removal of the penile sheath markedly interferes with normal penile reflexes and copulation. When circumcised rats were paired with sexually experienced females, they had more difficulty obtaining an erection, more difficulty inserting the penis into the vagina, and required more mounts to inseminate than did unaltered males [6]. Preputial secretions in mice and rats are a strong attractant for female mice and rats [7-11], and may provoke the onset of oestrus in mature females [12].

There may be a histological explanation for these findings. The tip of the foreskin, and some or all of the frenulum, are routinely removed as part of circumcision. This tissue contains a high concentration of the nerve endings that sense fine touch [1]. After circumcision, the surface of the glans thickens like a callus. The glans is innervated by free nerve endings that can only sense deep pressure and pain [13].* Over 30 years ago, Masters and Johnson, using undocumented methodology, tested the sensitivity of the glans in men with and without foreskins and found no difference [14]. The absence of fine-touch receptors in the glans could explain their findings, as Masters and Johnson may have been measuring the wrong variable. Without knowing what was measured or how, these results constitute little more than anecdotal evidence. A study from Iowa in the late 1980s [15] found that young mothers (who had recently given birth to sons) preferred intercourse with a circumcised man; however, the importance of this study is compromised, as only 16.5% of the women surveyed had sexual experience with both circumcised and intact men. The study results may reflect the tendency of people to choose the familiar and shun the unfamiliar. In a survey conducted on the Internet, circumcised men were significantly more likely to use additional artificial lubricants during sexual activity (odds ratio, OR=5.64, 95% CI=3.65-8.71) [16].

The 12th century physician and rabbi Moses Maimonides advocated male circumcision for its ability to curb a man's sexual appetite [17]. Further, he implied that it could also affect a woman's sexuality, indicating that once a woman had taken a lover who was not circumcised, it was very hard for her to give him up. The impact of male circumcision on the sexual pleasure experienced by both males and females is largely unstudied. While the brain is

* Since the article, subsequent investigation has caused me to consider the information in this sentence inaccurate. See my discussions in Chapters 4 and 8B.

often cited as the primary 'sexual' organ, what impact does surgical alteration of the male genitalia have for both partners? Based on anecdotal reports, a survey was developed to determine the effect of male circumcision on a woman's ability to achieve vaginal orgasm (both single and multiple), to maintain adequate vaginal secretions, to develop vaginal discomfort, to enjoy coitus and to develop an intimate relationship with her partner. This review presents the findings of a survey of women who have had sexual partners both with and without foreskins, and reports their experiences.

Methods

Women having sexual experience with both circumcised and anatomically complete partners were recruited through classified advertisements in magazines and an announcement in an anti-circumcision newsletter. Respondents to the advertisements were mailed a survey to complete and return, the comments then compiled and the responses analyzed statistically. The survey is continuing and this article reports the preliminary results.

Of the 284 surveys, 139 were completed and returned; no attempts were made to characterize the demographic details of those who did not respond. The women completing the surveys were aware that their responses and comments could later be published anonymously in a forthcoming book. The survey included over 40 questions; the results were analyzed for age, number of lifetime partners, preputial status of the most recent partner, preference for vaginal orgasms (as defined below) and their preference for a circumcised or intact penis. Multiple choice answers were assigned numeric values, i.e., 'increased', 'stayed about the same' and 'lessened' of 1, 0, and -1, respectively. Likewise, questions with answers of 'mostly yes', 'mostly no', 'rarely' and 'never' were assigned values of 3, 2, 1 and 0.

The survey defined 'vaginal orgasm' as 'an orgasm that occurs during intercourse, brought about by your partner's penis and pelvic movements and body contact, along with your own body's pelvic movements, with no simultaneous stimulation of the clitoris by the hands'. Premature ejaculation was defined as the man 'usually (50-100% of the time) has his orgasm within 2-3 minutes after insertion'. The survey included three sets of responses for the respondents to rate their sexual experiences with their circumcised and unaltered male partners; the questions and possible responses are listed in Appendix 1. Comparisons between responses are expressed as the OR and 95% CI.

Results

Of the 139 surveys returned, one considered a man who was undergoing foreskin restoration as having a foreskin; this survey was excluded from analysis. Not all questions were answered by all respondents. Contradictory answers to questions showed that not all respondents understood the questions; these responses and unanswered questions were excluded from the analysis. The demographic profile of the respondents is shown in Table 1.

Table 1 The demographics of the respondents

Variable	Mean/median/number
Mean (SD) age (years)	37.3 (9.2)
Number of partners:	
Mean (SD)	14.7 (11.2)
Median	10
Preferred vaginal orgasm	71
Preferred position for attaining vaginal orgasm:	
woman on top	54
man on top	57
side to side	12
rear entry	4
no preference	9

Comparisons of experiences with circumcised or intact partners are shown in Tables 2 and 3. With their circumcised partners, women were more likely not to have a vaginal orgasm (4.62, 3.69-5.80). Conversely, women were more likely to have a vaginal orgasm with an unaltered partner. Their circumcised partners were more likely to have premature ejaculation (1.82, 1.45-2.27). Women were also more likely to state that they had vaginal discomfort with a circumcised partner either often (19.89, 5.98-66.22) or occasionally (7.00, 3.83-12.79) as opposed to rarely or never. More women reported that they never achieved vaginal orgasm with their circumcised partners (2.25, 1.13-4.50) than with their unaltered partners. Also, they were more likely to report never having had a multiple orgasm with their circumcised partners (2.22,

1.36-3.63). They were also more likely to report that vaginal secretions lessened as coitus progressed with their circumcised partners (16.75, 6.88-40.77).

During prolonged intercourse with their circumcised partners, women were less likely to 'really get into it' and more likely to 'want to get it over with' (23.32, 11.24-48.39). On the other hand, with their unaltered partners, the reverse was true; they were less likely to 'want to get it over with' and considerably more likely to 'really get into it.'

When the women were divided into those older or younger than 40 years, the older women were more likely to rate the frequency of orgasm as higher, with an unaltered partner ($Z=2.04$, $P=0.02$). Women 29 years and younger were more likely to prefer orally induced orgasms (2.61, 1.14-5.97), while women over 40 years preferred vaginally induced orgasms more than those aged ⩽ 29 years (3.00, 1.16-7.32). The older women also had more lifetime unaltered partners ($Z = 2.95$, $P = 0.002$). This may reflect the decreased availability of unaltered men of similar age for the younger women.

When the women were divided into those with more or fewer than 10 lifetime partners, those with >10 were more likely to have orgasms with their circumcised partners than those with fewer partners, but still less frequent orgasms than they had with their unaltered partners. Women who preferred a circumcised partner overall were more likely to have had ⩾ 10 partners (3.52, 0.92-13.50).

When women who preferred vaginal orgasm were compared with those preferring orally or manually induced orgasm, the former rated unaltered men higher ($Z=2.12$, $P=0.016$), had more positive postcoital feelings (Set 3; $Z=2.68$, $P=0.003$) with their unaltered partners, and rated these men higher overall ($Z=2.12$, $P=0.016$). These women were more likely to prefer being on top during coitus to achieve vaginal orgasm (2.46, 1.21-4.98). They were also more likely to have an unaltered man as their most recent partner (1.74, 0.87-3.47).

The women who preferred circumcised partners (as elicited in one of three questions, n=20*) were more likely to have had their first orgasm with a circumcised partner (3.10, 1.09-8.79) (when they often had not yet experienced

* In the survey chapter (Chapter 13) of *Sex As Nature Intended It*, this figure was reported as 14 women. This is because the criteria was changed for the book. Notice that the above says "as elicited in one of three questions." In re-examining this aspect for the book, the criteria was changed to *two out of the three questions*. This seemed a more accurate assessment of a woman's true preference—2 out of 3 (a majority) instead of 1 of 3 (not a majority).

an unaltered partner), and more likely to enjoy prolonged intercourse with a circumcised partner (8.38, 2.88-24.35) than those who preferred unaltered partners. Although these women preferred circumcised partners, they still found unaltered partners to evoke more vaginal fluid production, a lower vaginal discomfort rating and fewer complaints (Sets 1 and 2, Table 3) during intercourse than their circumcised partners. In women who preferred circumcised men, there was no difference in their comparison of circumcised and unaltered men other than overall rating and a higher rate of premature ejaculation in their unaltered partners (4.63, 2.36-9.07). These women had fewer unaltered partners (2.47 vs 3.78, $Z= -1.68$, $P=0.045$), which suggests that their limited exposure to unaltered men may have been a consequence of 'premature ejaculation'. The inability to detect a difference in orgasm frequency, coital duration, coital complaints or satisfaction, and 'yet to formulate a preference', suggests that factors of conformity may be influential.

When women were grouped based on the preputial status of their most recent partner, women with unaltered partners had a higher rate of orgasm with them, at a mean (SEM) of 70 (31)% vs 56 (40)% ($Z= 2.28$, $P=0.01$). They were more likely to rate circumcised partners lower ($Z= 2.61$, $P=0.0047$) and unaltered partners higher ($Z=2.83$, $P=0.002$). When only women whose most recent partner was circumcised were considered, the results were consistent with the results from the entire study population.

Discussion

These results show clearly that women preferred vaginal intercourse with an anatomically complete penis over that with a circumcised penis; there may be many reasons for this. When the anatomically complete penis thrusts in the vagina, it does not slide, but rather glides on its own 'bedding' of movable skin, in much the same way that a turtle's neck glides in and out on the folded layers of skin surrounding it. The underlying corpus cavernosa and corpus spongiosum slide within the penile skin, while the skin juxtaposed against the vaginal wall moves very little. This sheath-within-a-sheath alignment allows penile movement, and vaginal and penile stimulation, with minimal friction or loss of secretions. When the penile shaft is withdrawn slightly from the vagina, the foreskin bunches up behind the corona in a manner that allows the tip of the foreskin, which contains the highest density of finetouch neuroreceptors in the penis [1], to contact the corona of the glans, which has the highest concentration of fine-touch neuroreceptors on the glans [18]. This intense stimulation discourages the penile shaft from further withdrawal, explaining the short-thrusting style that women noted in their unaltered partners. This juxtaposition of sensitive neuroreceptors is also seen in the clitoris and clitoral hood of the Rhesus monkey [19] and in the human clitoris [18].

As stated, circumcision removes 33-50% of the penile skin. With this skin missing, there is less tissue for the swollen corpus cavernosa and corpus spongiosum to slide against. Instead, the skin of the circumcised penis rubs against the vaginal wall, increasing friction, abrasion and the need for artificial lubrication. Because of the tight penile skin, the corona of the glans, which is configured as a oneway valve, pulls the vaginal secretions out of the vagina when the shaft is withdrawn. Unlike the anatomically complete penis, there is no sensory input to limit withdrawal. Because the vast majority of the fine-touch receptors are missing from the circumcised penis, their role as ejaculatory triggers is also absent. The loss of these receptors creates an imbalance between the deep pressure sensed in the glans, corpus cavernosa and corpus spongiosum and the missing fine-touch [20]. To compensate for this imbalance, to achieve orgasm, the circumcised man must stimulate the glans, corpus cavernosa and corpus spongiosum by thrusting deeply in and out of the vagina. As a result, coitus with a circumcised partner reduces the amount of vaginal secretions in the vagina, and decreases continual stimulation of the mons pubis and clitoris.

Respondents overwhelmingly concurred that the mechanics of coitus were different for the two groups of men. Of the women, 73% reported that circumcised men tended to thrust harder,* using elongated strokes, while unaltered men by comparison tended to thrust more gently, to have shorter thrusts (while deep within the vagina),** and tended to be in contact with the mons pubis and clitoris more, according to 71 % of the respondents.

The responses in Sets 1, 2 and 3 (Table 3) are more a measure of intimacy than physical differences in thrusting patterns. While some of the respondents commented that they thought the differences were in the men, not the type of penis, the consistency with which women felt more intimate with their unaltered partners is striking. Some respondents reported that the foreskin improved their sexual satisfaction, which improved the quality of the relationship. In addition to the observations of Maimonides in the 12th century, one survey

* Notice of Correction: The words "and deeper" were deleted.
**Notice of Correction: The words "(while deep within the vagina)" were added.

found that marital longevity was increased when the male had a foreskin [21]. Why the presence of a foreskin enhances intimacy needs further exploration.

When this information is compared with that collected by Laumann *et al.* [22] during the same period, the women in the present survey had more lifetime partners (a median of 2 and 10, respectively). When the women with one partner in the former study were excluded (because having sexual experience with both a circumcised and unaltered partner necessitates at least two partners), the women in the present survey were more likely to have had >4 partners (7.26, 4.46-11.83), > 10 partners (5.83, 4.02-8.48), and > 20 partners (4.16, 2.48-6.98). The high number of lifetime partners is a consequence of the inclusion criteria for the present study. If a woman were to randomly find partners among American sexually active males, 70-90% of whom are circumcised, 3-7 partners would be needed for a woman to have an even chance of having had both a circumcised and unaltered male partner. However, women do not procure their sexual partners randomly. Most sexual partners are found within a fairly close social network [22]. Likewise, circumcision does not occur randomly; within some of these networks, circumcision rates can approach 100%. For a woman to have a sexual partner with an anatomically complete penis involves having partners outside her immediate social network, which is uncommon. For these reasons, a median number of partners of 10 is not unexpected.

While this study shows clearly that women prefer the surgically unaltered penis, it does have shortcomings. The respondents were not selected randomly and several were recruited using a newsletter of an anti-circumcision organization. However, when the responses from respondents gathered from the mailing list of the anti-circumcision organization were compared with those of the other respondents, there were no differences. This selection bias may be compensated to the degree that each respondent acted as her own control, using her subjective criteria on both types of penises. The findings cannot be completely attributed to selection bias.

In asking women to evaluate their experience based on all of their lifetime sexual partners, there may be an element of recall bias, but the circumcision status of the most current sexual partner did not significantly alter the findings. Because the surveys were not completed 'face-to-face', not all questions were completed by all respondents. There were also several questions that were misunderstood by the respondents, but these were only a very small proportion of the respondents. Women who preferred vaginal orgasms had a strong preference for unaltered partners. Women who preferred circumcised partners were half as likely to prefer vaginal orgasms, but there were too few women preferring circumcised partners to make any valid statistical claims. This would suggest that the foreskin makes the most positive impact during vaginal intercourse.

Table 2 Ratings of experiences with circumcised men compared with experiences with normal men (uncircumcised). All difference were significant at $P < 0.001$

Item	Mean (SD) rating Circumcised	Intact	Z value
Number of partners	10.36 (11.21)	3.61 (5.81)	6.16
Vaginal fluid secretions *	-0.23 (0.79)	0.60 (0.58)	-9.47
Vaginal discomfort **	2.01 (0.87)	0.85 (0.83)	10.93
Likelihood of vaginal orgasm (%) see next line	34.7 (35.2)	60.6 (36.2)	6.16
Refigured in book, SEX..., women unable to orgasm with either type were eliminated from analysis.			
Orgasm frequency rating **	1.68 (1.13)	2.39 (1.02)	-5.39
Multiple orgasm frequency rating **	0.96 (1.11)	1.59 (1.27)	-4.32
Duration of coitus (minutes)	10.72 (9.55)	14.85 (10.46)	-3.36
Number of responses to:			
irritable ¶ [article misprinted not irritable]	5.99 (4.73)	1.31 (2.54)	10.04
distanced ¶¶ [article misprinted not distanced]	5.10 (3.75)	0.84 (1.11)	10.81
Positive postcoital feelings §	1.95 (2.88)	5.01 (2.88)	-9.05
Overall rating (range -10 to +10)	1.81 (6.17)	8.03 (3.17)	10.33

* The responses were scored as 'increased'= 1, 'stayed about the same'= 0, 'lessened'= -1.

** The responses were scored as 'mostly yes'= 3, 'mostly no'= 2, 'rarely' = 1, 'never'= 0.

¶ Positive responses from 14 possibilities. (See Table 3, Set 1)

¶¶ Positive responses from 13 possibilities. (See Table 3, Set 2)

§ Positive responses from 8 possibilities. (See Table 3, Set 3)

Table 3 Comparison of the responses for circumcised partners with normal partners

Item	Odds ratio (95% CI)
Set 1:	
irritability	9.39 (4.65-18.95)
unappreciated	9.06 (4.67-17.57)
sexually violated	5.57 (2.80-11.10)
aggravated	7.51 (3.55-16.30)
out of sync	13.12 (6.17-27.90)
partner cared little about me	10.05 (5.33-18.94)
other than my vagina partner wouldn't know I was there	10.10 (4.57-22.30)
'bitchy'	4.16 (1.96-8.82)
'guilty'	4.52 (2.20-9.29)
having separate experiences	8.67 (4.76-15.80)
thrusting out of sync	7.31 (3.98-13.44)
'I was a masturbating object'	4.16 (2.36-7.33)
incomplete as a woman	7.07 (3.03-16.51)
glad it's over	10.53 (5.65-19.62)
Set 2:	
distanced	10.22 (4.62-22.58)
my mind wanders	7.21 (3.92-13.26)
he's working awfully hard	34.19 (13.15-88.89)
he's concentrating on his needs	13.01 (5.90-28.68)
he's working hard for an orgasm	7.68 (3.88-15.21)
disinterested	23.10 (8.07-66.13)
my vagina doesn't like this	7.68 (3.88-15.21)
his pumping might hurt me	17.62 (7.27-42.72)
we're having separate experiences	4.08 (2.07-8.05)
wide awake 'on alert'	2.87 (1.28-6.46)
frustrated	10.15 (3.86-26.76)
discomfort	11.41 (4.95-26.31)
discontent	8.45 (3.81-18.75)
Set 3:	
relaxed	0.19 (0.11-0.32)
peace	0.22 (0.13-0.38)
human warmth and closeness	0.19 (0.11-0.32)
mutual satisfaction	0.18 (0.11-0.31)
complete as a woman	0.25 (0.15-0.42)
afterglow	0.24 (0.12-0.34)
'gee that was great'	0.25 (0.15-0.42)
'what a lover'	0.10 (0.05-0.19)

Another weakness of the survey is its preoccupation with vaginal intercourse. Several respondents commented that the foreskin also makes a difference in foreplay and fellatio. Although this was not directly measured, some respondents commented that unaltered men appeared to enjoy coitus more than their circumcised counterparts. The lower rates of fellatio, masturbation and anal sex among unaltered men [5] suggests that unaltered men may find coitus more satisfying [20].

Clearly, the anatomically complete penis offers a more rewarding experience for the female partner during coitus. While this study has some obvious methodological flaws, all the differences cannot be attributed to them. It is important that these findings be confirmed by a prospective survey of a randomly selected population of women with experience with both types of men. It would be useful to examine the role of the foreskin in other sexual activities. Because these findings are of interest, the negative effect of circumcision on the sexual enjoyment of the female partner needs to be part of any discussions providing 'informed consent' before circumcision.

References

1. Taylor JR, Lockwood AP, Taylor AJ. The prepuce: specialized mucosa of the penis and its loss to circumcision. *Br J Urol* 1996; **77**: 291-5
2. Hodges F. A short history of the institutionalization of involuntary sexual mutilation in the United States. In: Denniston GC, Milos MF, eds. *Sexual Mutilations: a Human Tragedy*. New York: Plenum Press, 1997: 17-40
3. Money J, Davison J. Adult penile circumcision: erotosexual and cosmetic sequelae. *J Sex Res* 1983; **19**: 289-92
4. Valentine RJ. Adult circumcision: a personal report. *Med Aspects Human Sex* 1974; **8**: 31-55
5. Laumann EO, Masi CM, Zuckerman EW. Circumcision in the United States: prevalence, prophylactic effects, and sexual practice. *JAMA* 1997; **277**: 10527
6. Lumia AR, Sachs BD, Meisel RL. Sexual reflexes in male rats: restoration by ejaculation following suppression by penile sheath removal. *Physiol Behav* 1979; **23**: 273-7
7. Caroom D, Bronson FH. Responsiveness of female mice to preputial attractant: effects of sexual experience and ovarian hormones. *Physiol Behav* 1971; **7**: 659-62

8. Orsulak PJ, Gawienowski AM. Olfactory preferences for the rat preputial gland. *Biol Reprod* 1972; **6**: 219-23
9. Hucklebridge FH, Nowell NW, Wouters A. A relation between social experience and preputial gland function in the albino mouse. *J Endoc* 1972; **55**: 449-50
10. Ninomiya K, Kimura T. Male odors that influence the preference of female mice: roles of urinary and preputial factors. *Physiol Behav* 1988; **44**: 791-5
11. Ninomiya K, Brown RE. Removal of the preputial glands alters the individual odors of male MHCcongenic mice and the preferences of females for these odors. *Physiol Behav* 1995; **58**:191-4
12. Chipman RK, Albrecht ED. The relationship of the male preputial gland to the acceleration of oestrus in the laboratory mouse. *J Reprod Fert* 1974; **38**: 91-6
13. Halata Z, Munger BL. The neuroanatomical basis for the protopathic sensibility of the human glans penis. *Brain Res* 1986; **371**: 205-30
14. Masters W, Johnson V. *Human Sexual Response.* Boston, MA: Little Brown & Co 1966
15. Williamson ML, Williamson PS. Women's preferences for penile circumcision in sexual partners.] Sex *Educ Therapy* 1988; **14**: 81-2
16. Epps GMR, Morgan D, Dolenzal Zelzer D. Personal attitudes toward circumcision. October 1997 http://www.gepps.com/survey/results/patc.htm.
17. Moses Maimonides. (1135-1204). *The Guide for the Perplexed.* New York: Dover Publications 1956: 378
18. Cold CJ, Taylor JR. The prepuce. *BJU Int* 1999; **83** (Suppl. 1); 34-44
19. Cold CJ, Tarara RP. Penile and clitoral prepuce mucocutaneous receptors in *Macaca mulatta. Vet Pathol* 1997; **34**: 506
20. Van Howe RS, Cold CJ. Advantages and disadvantages of neonatal circumcision. *JAMA* 1997; **278**: 203
21. Hughes GK. Circumcision--another look. *Ohio Med* 1990; **86**: 92
22. Laumann E0, Gagnon JH, Michael RT, Michaels S. *The Social Organization of Sexuality. Sexual Practices in the United States.* Chicago, IL: The University of Chicago Press 1994

Appendix 1

Questions asked in the survey to assess the level of intimacy.

Set 1
During or after most intercourse, have you noticed yourself having any of the feelings listed below?
irritability
unappreciated
sexually violated
emotionally aggravated
a general 'out of sync' feeling
he cared very little about my sexual satisfaction
except for my vagina, he didn't seem to know I was there
bitchy, argumentative
we had two separate experiences (no feeling of sexual unison)
our thrusting rhythms were 'out of sync'
felt like I was being used as a masturbating object
incomplete as a woman
I'm glad it's over
NONE of the above

Set 2
During intercourse with most (circumcised/natural) men, do any of these thoughts generally cross your mind?
he seems to be distanced from what I'm feeling
my mind wanders to other things
he seems to be working too hard at it
he seems to concentrate on his sexual needs more than mine
he seems to have to work too hard at achieving his orgasm
I seem to be becoming disinterested
my vagina doesn't seem to be enjoying this
sometimes when he really gets pumping, I'm afraid its going to start hurting me
we seem to be engaging in two separate experiences
I feel wide awake, 'on alert'
frustration

discomfort
a general feeling of discontentment
NONE of the above

Set 3

How would you describe your general feelings after having sex with most (circumcised/natural) men?

a feeling of relaxation
a feeling of being at peace with myself and my surroundings
a sense of human warmth and closeness to my partner
a sense of completeness and wholeness as a woman
a wonderful positive-feeling afterglow
'gee, that was really great'
'what a lover!!'
NONE of the above

Appendix F

SURVEY QUESTIONNAIRE

COPYRIGHT © 2000 Kristen O'Hara. All Rights Reserved.

Women were given a brief introduction to the survey and were presented with line drawings of the two types of penises, both flaccid and erect, including the erection process of the natural penis.

AGE____

1. How many TOTAL men have you had sexual intercourse with?

    Please Circle 1 2 3 4 5 6 7 8 9 10+

    Note: It might be helpful for you to write down, on a separate piece of paper, the names (or in the case of a one-night stand where you might not remember the name, the place/circumstance) for each relationship as a reference aid for answering this questionnaire.

2. How many CIRCUMCISED men have you had sexual intercourse with? If you are absolutely unsure as to the circumcised or natural status of a particular partner, please eliminate him from this question and succeeding questions. Indicate only those you are reasonably certain about.

    Please Circle   1 2 3 4 5 6 7 8 9 10+

3. How many of the CIRCUMCISED men in question 2 were:
    one-night stands___   under 2 months___   2 months to 1 year___
    longer than 1 year___ (but less than 5 yrs)   longer than 5 years___

4. Of your CIRCUMCISED intercourse experiences, how many men USUALLY (50-100% of the time) had their orgasm within 2-3 minutes after insertion?
    number of men ____

5. How many NATURAL (i.e., uncircumcised) men have you had sexual intercourse with?   Please Circle   1 2 3 4 5 6 7 8 9 10+

6. How many of the NATURAL men in the above question were:
    one-night stands___   under 2 months___   2 months to 1 year___
    longer than 1 year___ (but less than 5 yrs)   longer than 5 years___

7. Of your NATURAL intercourse experiences, how many men USUALLY (50-100% of the time) had their orgasm within 2-3 minutes after insertion?
    number of men ____

8. EXCLUDING your CIRCUMCISED intercourse experiences that only lasted 2-3 minutes, how long would you say your average CIRCUMCISED intercourse lasts (intercourse time only, NOT foreplay, etc.). This should be an overall estimated average.

9. EXCLUDING your NATURAL intercourse experiences that only lasted 2-3 minutes, how long would you say your average NATURAL intercourse lasts (intercourse time only, NOT foreplay, etc.). This should be an overall estimated average.

Questions 10-21 pertain to vaginal orgasm so I would like to be sure you understand how it is being defined.

A VAGINAL ORGASM is an orgasm that occurs during intercourse, brought about by your partner's penis and its accompanying pelvic movements and body contact, along with your own pelvic movements, with no simultaneous stimulation of the clitoris by hand. What happens during FOREPLAY is NOT OF CONCERN. But once serious intercourse thrusting begins, a vaginal orgasm is one which you feel was brought about by genital/pelvic movements and body contact/pressure.

10. In your experiences with CIRCUMCISED men, have you been able to achieve VAGINAL orgasm through intercourse movements alone (with no simultaneous stimulation of the clitoris by the hands)? (Check one)

   mostly yes____   mostly no____   rarely____   never____

11. With how many CIRCUMCISED men have you been able to achieve a VAGINAL orgasm?   number of men ____

12. In your experiences with CIRCUMCISED men with whom you had a vaginal orgasm, approximately what percent of the time would you say you were able to achieve vaginal orgasm?
(Very important to give an overall estimated percentage) ____ %

13. If you are capable of achieving vaginal orgasm during your CIRCUMCISED intercourse experiences, have you generally been able to achieve MULTIPLE vaginal orgasms? (Check one)

   mostly yes____   mostly no____   rarely____   never____

14. Switching to NATURAL, in your experiences with NATURAL men, have you been able to achieve VAGINAL orgasm through intercourse movements alone (with no simultaneous stimulation of the clitoris by the hands)? (Check one)   mostly yes____   mostly no____   rarely____   never____

15. With how many NATURAL men have you been able to achieve a VAGINAL orgasm?   number of men ____

16. In your experiences with NATURAL men with whom you had a vaginal orgasm, approximately what percentage of the time would you say you were able to achieve vaginal orgasm?
(Very important to give an overall estimated percentage) ____ %

Survey Questionnaire

17. If you are capable of achieving vaginal orgasm during your NATURAL intercourse experiences, have you generally been able to achieve MULTIPLE vaginal orgasms? (Check one)
    mostly yes____   mostly no____   rarely____   never____

18. With which type of partner did you first experience *vaginal orgasm*?
    circumcised_____   natural_____

19. Before you had your first vaginal orgasm, how many CIRCUMCISED men did you <u>previously</u> have intercourse with?
    0 1 2 3 4 5 6 7 8 9 10+

20. Before you had your first vaginal orgasm, how many NATURAL men did you <u>previously</u> have intercourse with?
    0 1 2 3 4 5 6 7 8 9 10+

21. If you have been vaginally orgasmic with both circumcised and natural men, with which type of partner can you achieve it more easily?
    circumcised_____   natural_____   Comments:

22. Are you aware that your natural intercourse experiences are somehow different from your circumcised intercourse experiences? YES NO Comments:

23. During those intercourses with CIRCUMCISED men which lasted 5 minutes or longer, as intercourse progressed, did the amount of vaginal lubrication
    (circle one)   lessen   stay about the same   increase

24. During those intercourses with NATURAL men which lasted 5 minutes or longer, as intercourse progressed, did the amount of vaginal lubrication
    (circle one)   lessen   stay about the same   increase

25. Of the following three types of orgasms, which do you prefer to receive from your partner, taking into consideration which gives you the greatest overall satisfaction (including build-up to orgasm). Please rank them:
    1 (favorite)   2 (second)   3 (third)
    ___ vaginal orgasm   ___ orally-induced orgasm
    ___ hand-induced orgasm (no vibrator or mechanical device)

26. Regarding CIRCUMCISED intercourse, have you experienced vaginal discomfort during sex (or after having sex)? Please circle one.
    often   occasionally   rarely   never   Comments?

27. Regarding NATURAL intercourse, have you experienced vaginal discomfort during sex (or after having sex)? Please circle one.
    often   occasionally   rarely   never   Comments?

28. Do you tend to agree or disagree with the following:

In general, intercourse with the CIRCUMCISED man is more rough—they tend to pound or bang away and the penis feels discomfortingly harder during intercourse thrusting.

In contrast, the NATURAL man has gentler and more sensually tender sexual movements, and the penis does *not* feel discomfortingly hard during intercourse thrusting.

Please circle AGREE if you tend to agree with this entire statement, or underline those parts you tend to agree with. Comments:

If you disagree with this entire statement, circle DISAGREE, and explain in what way your experiences differ. Comments:

Author's Note: **The above question was changed (in the last third of the surveys) to 29a and 29b below:**

29a. This question will ask you to GENERALIZE about your CIRCUMCISED intercourse experiences. Granted, there can be individual differences in how men perform sexually and exceptions can exist, nevertheless, please try to answer the question as it applies to your circumcised experiences in general. In the statements below, first read the statement on the left, then read the statement on the right. Check one or the other (or neither), but not both.

Which of the following characteristics tend to describe your CIRCUMCISED intercourse experiences, in general.

___ thrusting actions are rougher and tougher than natural   ___ thrusting actions are gentler and more tender than natural

___ penis feels almost too hard, or even discomfortingly hard   ___ penis feels comfortable and sensuous

___ penis sometimes feels like it's poking the vagina   ___ penis feels deliciously wonderful in me

___ partner seems to bang or pound away at my genitals   ___ body contact with my genitals is gentle and tender

___ my vagina feels tensed-up and/or tightened   ___ my vagina feels soft, relaxed

___ penis seems to discomfort my vagina more than I think it should   ___ our sex organs seem to melt into one another

Comments?

29b. This question will ask you to GENERALIZE about your NATURAL intercourse experiences. Granted, there can be individual differences in how men perform sexually and exceptions can exist; nevertheless, please try to answer the question as it applies to your natural experiences in general. In the statements below, first read the statement on the left, then read the statement on the right. Check one or the other (or neither), but not both.

Which of the following characteristics tend to describe your NATURAL intercourse experiences, in general.

___ thrusting actions are rougher and tougher than circumcised   ___ thrusting actions are gentler and more tender than circ'd
___ penis feels almost too hard, or even discomfortingly hard   ___ penis feels comfortable and sensuous
___ penis sometimes feels like it's poking the vagina   ___ penis feels deliciously wonderful in me
___ partner seems to bang or pound away at my genitals   ___ body contact with my genitals is gentle and tender
___ my vagina feels tensed-up and/or tightened   ___ my vagina feels soft, relaxed
___ penis seems to discomfort my vagina more than I think it should   ___ our sex organs seem to melt into one another

Comments?

30a. Do you tend to agree or disagree with the following: The NATURAL man's pubic area stays in closer contact with the woman's clitoral area during intercourse because he generally uses shorter strokes in his thrusting movements. He seems to gently "grind" or "jiggle" more, resulting in a pleasant pressuring of the woman's clitoral area which gives her greater pleasure.

Please circle AGREE if you tend to agree with this entire statement, or underline those parts you tend to agree with. Comments:

If you disagree with this entire statement, circle DISAGREE and then explain in what way your experiences differ. Comments:

30b. On the other hand, the CIRCUMCISED man's pubic area makes less contact with the woman's clitoral area during intercourse because he seems to use longer strokes in his thrusting movements. These longer thrusts result in less physical contact between his pubic mound and the woman's clitoral area.

Please circle AGREE if you tend to agree with this entire statement, or underline those parts you tend to agree with. Comments:

If you disagree with the statement, circle DISAGREE & explain why.

31. During which type of sex — CIRCUMCISED or NATURAL — do YOU feel more relaxed, comfortable, and at ease?
    circumcised____   natural____   Comments?

32. For YOU, regardless of your vaginal-orgasmic capabilities, which type of intercourse simply feels better during the overall experience?
    circumcised____   natural____   Comments?

33. Of your CIRCUMCISED experiences where the time of ACTUAL intercourse lasted for 8-10 minutes or more, as intercourse progressed,

Did you OFTEN start wishing to just get it over with?   YES   NO
—OR—
Did you OFTEN really get into it and want it to continue?   YES   NO
Which reaction was more PREDOMINANT—wanting to get it over with? or really getting into it? Please underline those words which apply. Comments?

34. Of your NATURAL experiences where the time of ACTUAL intercourse lasted for 8-10 minutes or more, as intercourse progressed,

Did you OFTEN start wishing to just get it over with?   YES   NO
—OR—
Did you OFTEN really get into it and want it to continue?   YES   NO
Which reaction was more PREDOMINANT—wanting to get it over with? or really getting into it? Please underline those words which apply. Comments?

35. During or after many CIRCUMCISED intercourses, have you noticed yourself having any of the feelings below? If so, indicate with (S)ometimes or (O)ften

    irritability____   unappreciated____   sexually violated____
    emotionally aggravated____   general out of sync feeling____
    he cared very little about my sexual satisfaction____
    except for my vagina, he didn't seem to know I was there____
    bitchy, argumentative____   guilty____
    we had two separate experiences (no feeling of sexual unison)____
    our thrusting rhythms were out of sync____
    felt like I was being used as a masturbating object____
    incomplete as a woman____   I'm glad it's over____
    none of the above____   Comments?

36. During or after many NATURAL intercourses, have you noticed yourself having any of the feelings below? If so, indicate with (S)ometimes or (O)ften

    irritability____   unappreciated____   sexually violated____
    emotionally aggravated____   general out of sync feeling____
    he cared very little about my sexual satisfaction____
    except for my vagina, he didn't seem to know I was there____
    bitchy, argumentative____   guilty____
    we had two separate experiences (no feeling of sexual unison)____
    our thrusting rhythms were out of sync____
    felt like I was being used as a masturbating object____
    incomplete as a woman____   I'm glad it's over____
    none of the above____   Comments?

37. During intercourse with most CIRCUMCISED men, do any of these thoughts often cross your mind? Please check all those that apply.

    __ he seems to be distanced from what I'm feeling
    __ my mind wanders to other things
    __ he seems to work too hard at it (like he's on an exercise machine)
    __ he seems to concentrate on his sexual needs more than mine
    __ he seems to have to work too hard at achieving his orgasm
    __ I seem to be becoming disinterested
    __ my vagina doesn't seem to be enjoying this

___ sometimes when he really gets pumping, I'm afraid it's going to start hurting me
___ we seem to be engaging in two separate experiences
___ I feel "on alert"   ___ frustration
___ discomfort   ___ a general feeling of discontentment
___ none of the above   Comments?

38. During intercourse with most NATURAL men, do any of these thoughts often cross your mind? Please check all those that apply.
___ he seems to be distanced from what I'm feeling
___ my mind wanders to other things
___ he seems to work too hard at it (like he's on an exercise machine)
___ he seems to concentrate on his sexual needs more than mine
___ he seems to have to work too hard at achieving his orgasm
___ I seem to be becoming disinterested
___ my vagina doesn't seem to be enjoying this
___ sometimes when he really gets pumping, I'm afraid it's going to start hurting me
___ we seem to be engaging in two separate experiences
___ I feel "on alert"   ___ frustration
___ discomfort   ___ a general feeling of discontentment
___ none of the above   Comments?

39. How would you describe your GENERAL feelings after having sex with most CIRCUMCISED men? Please check all those that apply.
___ a feeling of relaxation
___ a feeling of being at peace with myself and my partner
___ a sense of human warmth and closeness to my partner
___ a sense of a mutually satisfying experience
___ a sense of completeness and wholeness as a woman
___ a wonderful positive-feeling afterglow
___ gee, that was really great
___ what a lover!!
___ none of the above   Comments?

40. How would you describe your GENERAL feelings after having sex with most NATURAL men? Please check all those that apply.
___ a feeling of relaxation
___ a feeling of being at peace with myself and my partner
___ a sense of human warmth and closeness to my partner
___ a sense of a mutually satisfying experience
___ a sense of completeness and wholeness as a woman
___ a wonderful positive-feeling afterglow
___ gee, that was really great
___ what a lover!!
___ none of the above   Comments?

41. This question will ask you to assess your overall impression of sexual intercourse with CIRCUMCISED men, rating it as either a positive or negative experience. You may only indicate ONE number in your response.

If your OVERALL impression of intercourse with most CIRCUMCISED men was a NEGATIVE experience, circle a negative number (-).

If your OVERALL impression of intercourse with most CIRCUMCISED men was a POSITIVE experience, circle a positive number (+).

(circle one number only)

-10 -9 -8 -7 -6 -5 -4 -3 -2 -1 +1 +2 +3 +4 +5 +6 +7 +8 +9 +10

lowest   <<<< NEGATIVE   POSITIVE >>>>   highest
rating   rating

42. This question will ask you to assess your overall impression of sexual intercourse with NATURAL men, rating it as either a positive or negative experience. You may only indicate ONE number in your response.

If your OVERALL impression of intercourse with most NATURAL men was a NEGATIVE experience, circle a negative number (-).

If your OVERALL impression of intercourse with most NATURAL men was a POSITIVE experience, circle a positive number (+).

(circle one number only)

-10 -9 -8 -7 -6 -5 -4 -3 -2 -1 +1 +2 +3 +4 +5 +6 +7 +8 +9 +10

lowest   <<<< NEGATIVE   POSITIVE >>>>   highest
rating   rating

43. You have been shipwrecked and washed ashore onto a deserted paradise island in the Pacific. Your rescue ship won't be by to pick you up for five years. On this island is only one other person — a man — a very attractive man, who is interesting to be with and is very likeable. Because you are in paradise, you will probably be having sex fairly often. When you get around to your first lovemaking encounter and you are slowly undoing his belt and pants, would you be wishing that he is

Please circle: Circumcised   Natural   Comments?

44. How long ago was your last CIRCUMCISED intercourse experience? Comment?

45. How long ago was your last NATURAL intercourse experience? Comment?

46. Which type of man are you presently in a relationship with?
Circumcised___   Natural___

47. Do you have any final comments?

Author's Note: The newer, current version of the survey has been slightly revised to improve wording on a few questions. Also, a few questions have been added and a few deleted.

COPYRIGHT © 2000 Kristen O'Hara. All Rights Reserved.

Glossary

Anesthesia. Insensibility induced by drugs before surgery and other painful procedures. Circumcision, although surgery, is performed without general anesthesia, due to the risks involved. Recently, but only recently, some doctors have begun using analgesia to *relieve* the pain during circumcision

Circumcised Intercourse. The term coined to refer to sexual intercourse wherein the penis has been surgically altered by circumcision.

Circumcision. The amputation of all or part of the foreskin (prepuce) of the male or female. Anti-circumcision activists (intactivists) prefer to use the term "male genital mutilation (MGM)" instead of circumcision.

Clitoral Mound (Female). The term coined to refer to the entire area surrounding the clitoris (the outer vulvar lips, the pubic mound and the clitoris itself), which are sexually excited through body contact and pressuring by the male pubic mound during intercourse. Although the female pubic mound and vulvar lips are erogenous in themselves, importantly, they serve to transmit cushioned pressure to the female clitoris during intercourse. In effect, this entire area works as a unit to build up sexual excitement during intercourse, combined with penile stimulation of the vagina.

Clitoris (Male). The organ within the penis responsible for erection; homologous to the female clitoris. Medically identified as the corpora cavernosa. The tip of the male clitoris (Lowndes crown) is located *interiorly* underneath the glans. From there, the overall clitoris continues down the entire length of the penis into the pelvic region, where it branches into two distinct tracts. The entire male clitoris abounds with pressure-sensitive nerves.

Clitoridectomy. Removal of the female glans clitoris (i.e., the tip or Lowndes crown of the clitoris).

Coital Orgasm. See **Vaginal Orgasm.**

Corona. The prominent, elevated, circular border of the glans penis. The outermost rim of the glans.

Coronal ridge. The area of the penis where the shaft meets the penile head, extending outward from the shaft to the corona. The projection between the corona and the penile shaft.

DDD. See **Desire Deficiency Disorder.**

Denial. A defense mechanism involving refusal to acknowledge certain aspects of reality.

Desire Deficiency Disorder. A lack of sexual desire for one's partner.

FGM. See **Female Genital Mutilation.**

Female Genital Mutilation (FGM). Excision of any part of the female genitalia. Sometimes referred to as female circumcision.

Flaccid Penis. The non-erect penis.

Foreskin. The prepuce. The retractable fold of skin that covers the glans of the natural (uncircumcised) penis. The skin covering of the female clitoris. On the female, sometimes called the hood.

Frenulum (Frenum). The hinge of highly erogenous tissue on the underside of the glans that attaches the foreskin inner lining to the penis. During intercourse, it serves to restrain the penis from thrusting forcefully. In the United States, *frenulum* is the preferred term.

Frictionize. To rub and cause friction, which can cause irritation and chafing; common in circumcised intercourse.

Glans Penis (Glans). (Derived from the Latin word for "acorn" due to physical resemblance.) The head of the penis. Normally, the glans is covered by the foreskin and is an internal organ.

Intact. Untouched, especially by anything that harms or diminishes. The natural, uncircumcised penis. The adjective "intact" is currently being used to describe a male who has his foreskin. Also referred to colloquially as "uncut."

Intactivist. Someone who actively works to enlighten others on the importance of intact genitalia.

Keratinization. The process whereby the skin cells of the circumcised penis form layers of callused, unfeeling tissue to cover those parts of the penis that would normally be protected by the foreskin. The circumcised glans becomes keratinized due to lack of moisture and constant friction from clothing.

Lanofore. Author's suggested term to describe the lubricating fluid produced by the foreskin (and glans).

Lowndes Crown. Josephine Lowndes Sevely's name for tip of the male clitoris; also, her name for the female glans clitoris.

Male Clitoris. See **Clitoris (Male)**.

Male Genital Mutilation (MGM). The term currently being used by many intactivists instead of circumcision, since it more accurately describes its consequences.

MGM. See **Male Genital Mutilation**.

Mohel (Mohelet). A Jewish ritual circumciser, usually a rabbi, who has special training and certification to do this operation. In former times mohelim (pl.) learned from each other. In modern times, mohelim usually train in hospitals and use the same clamps and devices that are used by the medical profession. (Orthodox Jews, however, prohibit the use of clamps, as they believe that not enough blood is shed with these devices.)

Mutilate. To damage, injure, or otherwise make imperfect, especially by removing an essential part or parts.

Natural. As provided by nature.

Natural penis. A penis with a foreskin; the penis that nature equips a male with at birth.

Natural Intercourse. The term coined to refer to sexual intercourse wherein the penis is either intact as nature provided, or restored, surgically or non-surgically.

Neonatal. Of or pertaining to babies during the first four weeks of life.

Paraphimosis. A condition in which the infant's normally tight foreskin, when forcefully retracted beyond the glans, constricts and becomes stuck. The tourniqueted glans then swells and the foreskin cannot be easily replaced.

Phimosis. A condition, in adulthood, in which the foreskin is either adhered to the glans penis or tightly constricted over the glans and cannot be retracted; a rare condition. Phimosis in adulthood is correctable *without* circumcision, even without surgery of any kind. Be aware that prior to adulthood, foreskin retractability may develop gradually, in stages, for some males, who may not achieve full retractabilty until the late teens. This slow, though normal, development should not be mistakenly diagnosed as phimosis.

Phimosis (Acquired). Phimosis caused by forcefully retracting a child's foreskin before it has naturally separated from the glans. Forced retraction causes tissue tears, which may, in the process of healing, fuse the glans to the foreskin, resulting in acquired phimosis.

Premature Ejaculation. As defined in this book, the male ejaculates within 2-3 minutes after insertion of the penis into the vagina.

Prepuce. The medical term for the foreskin.

Primary Pleasure Zone. As discussed herein, the area of the penis where a man experiences most of his pleasure *during intercourse*. For the natural penis, this area is the upper area of the penis; for the circumcised penis, it is the middle and base area of the penis.

Reconstruction, of the Foreskin. More recently reserved to refer to surgical re-creation of the foreskin.

Restoration, of the Foreskin. Refers to any form of foreskin re-creation. More recently, re-creation by non-surgical means (i.e., stretching techniques).

Ridged Band. A tightly pleated (or ridged) zone of erogenous tissue at the tip of the foreskin inner lining, rich in touch-sensitive (i.e., fine-touch) nerves. When the natural penis is flaccid, the muscle tissue associated with the ridged band works to narrow the foreskin opening, enabling the glans and the foreskin's inner lining to remain moist. Formerly referred to as the frenar band.

Smegma. The visible substance that collects beneath the foreskin of the penis and around the female clitoris and labia, postulated in this book as largely a waste residue of dairy products that exude through the skin.

Softly-stiff Natural Penis. The term coined to describe the resilient, giveable characteristic of the erect natural penis, especially the glans. The shaft, also, is resilient to the touch—firm, but somewhat giveable.

Sulcus. See **Coronal Ridge**.

UTI. Urinary tract infection.

Vagina. The female genital canal.

Vaginal Orgasm. Defined in this book as an orgasm that occurs while the penis is in the vagina, brought about by the partners' genital and pelvic movements and body pressure, with no simultaneous stimulation of the clitoris by hand. (Note: Wording above differs slightly from survey's wording. I refined the defintion for the book, but for accuracy, I reported the original survey definition in the survey chapter.)

Vaginismus. An involuntary constriction of the muscles of the vagina, making penis entry and intercourse exceedingly difficult or impossible.

Venereal Disease. Disease transmitted by sexual contact.

Vulva. The visible, external parts of the female genitalia.

Resources

STAY INFORMED ON NEWS AND INFORMATION

Email registry: To be notified of important upcoming events and info about the anti-circumcision topic, send an email to *majordomo@cirp.org*. Indicate "subscribe Intact-N" in the body of your message.

ACTIVIST INFORMATION

To subscribe to Against Circ, an internet discussion and support group, visit *http://groups.yahoo.com/group/againstcirc* and follow the directions.

NOHARMM Market Place
Posters, buttons, T-shirts, bumper stickers, genital integrity ribbons, pens, postcards, and more.
www.noharmm.org/market.htm

FORESKIN RESTORATION

TugAhoy™
New invention for restoring the foreskin. Tapeless. Easy-on. Easy off. Excellent results in a reasonable time. Restored foreskin photos at this site are a must see.
www.tugahoy.com

RECAP-EZ
Tapeless restoration device that comes highly recommended.
Http://communities.msn.com/RECAP or email the inventor at *recap_ez@hotmail.com* for details.

Restore Yourself! A Handy Taping Kit for Circumcised Men
If tightly circumcised, you may need this starter kit to gain enough skin for the above-mentioned inventions to work.
NOCIRC of Michigan, POB 333, Birmingham, MI 48012
www.RestoreYourself.com

R2K (ForeSkin Natural Restorer 2000)
Applies tension to existing penile skin, producing new skin that will grow into a functioning foreskin. Requires use of tape. The amount of tension is adjustable by user.
http://www.4restore.com

Largest Foreskin Restoration Support Group on the Internet
http://restoringmen.net (Click on Restoration Club to join.)

Foreskin Restoration Internet Discussion Group
This is an internet discussion and support group for men interested in or already restoring. To subscribe, send an email to: *restore-list-request@eskimo.com.* Indicate "subscribe" in the subject line.

National Organization of Restoring Men (NORM) Southern California
Informative site. Dynamite presentation.
www.norm-socal.org

National Organization of Restoring Men (NORM)
www.norm.org
For an initial information packet, send $5.00 to cover printing and postage. For information on joining the support network or to learn the location of regional NORM groups, send request with a SASE to
R. Wayne Griffiths
3205 Northwood Dr., #209, Concord, CA 94520-4506
Tel: (510) 827-4077   Fax: (510) 827-4119

Information on surgical restoration as it develops.
www.foreskinrestoration.org

The Joy of Uncircumcising! (A restoration manual and more)
by Jim Bigelow, Ph.D.
Any man interested in restoring should read this book. Originally published in 1992, presently being prepared for Internet publishing. For details send a self-addressed stamped envelope to Jim Bigelow, PO Box 52138, Pacific Grove, CA 93950

BOOKS

To order additional copies of *Sex As Nature Intended It*
(Activists may order 5 copies at $14 each, shipping included, or 10 copies at $12 each, shipping included, by contacting Turning Point Publ. below.)

For individual copies, order from your favorite bookstore or send $19.95 + $3.50 S/H to: Turning Point Publications, PO Box 486, Hudson, MA 01749. Or visit

www.SexAsNatureIntendedIt.com

You Call This Love? The Real Reason Women Don't Like Sex
by Lisa Bisque. Published 2001. Order from your favorite bookseller.

Doctors Re-examine Circumcision
By Thomas J. Ritter, M.D. and George C. Denniston, M.D. publ'd 2002.
Order from your favorite bookstore or from Lisa Stefan, POB 103,
Mountville, PA 17554, $15 shipping included.

Circumcision: The Hidden Trauma
by Ronald Goldman, Ph.D., published 1997, $18.95 + $3 S/H
Available from Vanguard Publications
PO Box 8055, Boston, MA 02114, or order from your favorite bookstore.

Questioning Circumcision: A Jewish Perspective
by Ronald Goldman, Ph.D., published 1998, $11.95 + $3 S/H
Available from Vanguard Publications
PO Box 8055, Boston, MA 02114, or order from your favorite bookstore.

Circumcision Exposed: Rethinking a Medical and Cultural Tradition
by Billy Ray Boyd, published 1999, $14.95 + $4 S/H
The Crossing Press, POB 1048, Freedom, CA 95018, or order from your
favorite bookstore.

Circumcision: A History of the World's Most Controversial Surgery
by David L. Gollaher, published 2000, now available in paperback.
Order from your favorite bookstore; may be in stock.

Circumcision: A Book for Victims and Activists
by Sean B. Keen, published 1999, $13.50 + $ 3 S/H
Supernova Press, POB 14422, Albuquerque, NM 89191-4422

The Joy of Uncircumcising! (A restoration manual and more)
by Jim Bigelow, Ph.D. Originally published in 1992, presently being
prepared for Internet publishing. For details send self-addressed stamped
envelope to Jim Bigelow, PO Box 52138, Pacific Grove, CA 93950

VIDEOS

Whose Body, Whose Rights?
56 min. VHS $34.95 plus $5 postage in U.S. (CA residents add $3 sales tx)
Tim Sally, 3801 Market St., #2, San Francisco, CA 94131
More information at *www.noharmm.org/wbwr.htm*

Circumcision? Intact Facts.
18-minute VHS edited for childbirth educators from the 56-minute video
"Whose Body Whose Rights?" $44.95.
Injoy Productions, 3970 Broadway, Suite B4, Boulder, CO 80304

Resources

ORGANIZATIONS FROM JEWISH PERSPECTIVE

Circumcision Resource Center (CRC), Ronald Goldman, Ph.D.
Send $5 for information packet.
P.O. Box 232, Boston, MA 02133, Tel/Fax: (617) 523-0088
Information and resources.
www.circumcision.org/question.htm

WEBSITES

Doctors Opposing Circumcision
www.DoctorsOpposingCircumcision.org

Nurses for the Rights of the Child
www.cirp.org/nrc

Mothers Against Circumcision
www.mothersagainstcirc.org

Attorneys for the Rights of the Child
www.arclaw.org/

Official Website of this Book
www.SexAsNatureIntendedIt.com

Circumcision Information and Resource Pages
www.cirp.org

National Organization of Circumcision Information Resource Centers (NOCIRC)
www.nocirc.org

Circumcision Resource Center
General information and Jewish perspective
www.circumcision.org

National Organization of Restoring Men—Southern California
www.norm-socal.org

National Organization of Restoring Men (NORM)
www.norm.org

National Organization to Halt the Abuse & Routine Mutilation of Males
NOHARMM
www.noharmm.org

Circumcision Information Resource Centre
www.infocirc.org/top.htm

Dr. Dean Edell's crusade against circumcision
Log on and search for *circumcision*
http://cgi.myprimetime.com

Children's Integrity Network
www.childrensintegrity.net

Human Body, Human Pyschology, and Human Rights Education
www.wicked-envy.com

Canadian based website educating against circumcision
www.intact.ca

Stop Infant Circumcision
www.sicsociety.org

MUSIC (Musicians United to Stop Involuntary Circumcision)
www.musiciansunited.org

Men's Health Info: Circumcision = Genital Mutilation = Child Abuse
http://members.easyspace.com/magic999/pubservice.html

Circumstitions
www.circumstitions.com

In Memory of the Sexually Mutilated Child
www.sexuallymutilatedchild.org

Foreskin photos and more
www.foreskin.org

Circumcision: The Step to Becoming a REAL Man
josh.bakehorn.net/circ.html

Muslims Opposed to Circumcision
www.moslem.org/khatne.htm

Notes

Chapter 1 The Secret Enters the Spotlight

1. Zilbergeld, Bernie, Ph.D., MALE SEXUALITY: A GUIDE TO SEXUAL FULFILLMENT, Boston, Little, Brown & Co., 1978, p. 3-4.

2. Ibid., p. 6.

3. Ritter, Thomas J., M.D., SAY NO TO CIRCUMCISION! 40 COMPELLING REASONS, 2nd ed., Aptos, CA, Hourglass Book Publishing, 1996, p. 18-1 (each chapter of book numbered separately).

4. Taylor, J.R., Lockwood, A.P., Taylor, A.J., "The prepuce: specialized mucosa of the penis and its loss to circumcision," BRITISH JOURNAL OF UROLOGY, vol. 77, no. 2, 1996, p. 292.

5. According to the Health Care Investment Analysts, which maintains the health care industry's largest database, as reported in NOCIRC (see Resources) Annual Report, Spring 2000, vol. 14, page 1.

6. Wallerstein, Edward, CIRCUMCISION: AN AMERICAN HEALTH FALLACY, New York, Springer Publishing Co., 1980, pp. 89-99.

7. Ibid.

8. Ibid., pp. 32-33.

Chapter 2 Something is Missing

1. Jacoby, Susan, "Why sex matters so much," COSMOPOLITAN, July, 1996, pp. 146-149.

2. Kalter, Joanmarie, "Couples therapy: It could be just what you need." COSMOPOLITAN, August, 1993, pp. 82-86.

3. Berkeley, Bud and Joe Tiffenbach, FORESKIN: ITS PAST, ITS PRESENT, &....ITS FUTURE, private publication, 1983, pp. 54-56.

4. Walsh, Anthony, Ph.D., THE SCIENCE OF LOVE, Buffalo, NY, Prometheus Books, 1991, pp. 179-229.

5. Taylor, J.R., Lockwood, A.P., Taylor, A.J., "The prepuce: specialized mucosa of the penis and its loss to circumcision," BRITISH JOURNAL OF UROLOGY, vol. 77, no. 2, 1996, pp. 291-295.

6. Ritter, Thomas J., M.D., SAY NO TO CIRCUMCISION! 40 COMPELLING REASONS, 2nd ed., Aptos, CA, Hourglass Book Publishing, 1996, p. 11-1 thru 11-2 (each chapter of book is numbered separately).

7. Letters on file at NOCIRC, UNCIRC, and NOHARMM.

8. United Nations, 1993 Demographic Yearbook, (New York: Author, 1995), pp. 557-559, as cited by Ronald Goldman, Ph.D., CIRCUMCISION: THE HIDDEN TRAUMA, Boston, Vanguard Publications, 1997, p. 146.

Chapter 3 Making Love Last: The Tie That Binds

1. Laumann, Edward O., et al., "Sexual dysfunction in the United States," JAMA, Feb. 10, 1999, vol. 281, no. 6, p. 538.

2. Cameron, P. and Fleming, P., "Self-reported degree of pleasure associated with sexual activity across the adult life-span," St. Mary's College of Maryland mimeographed research report, 1975, as cited by Anthony Walsh, Ph.D., THE SCIENCE OF LOVE, Buffalo, NY, Prometheus Books, 1991, p. 219.

3. Hite, Shere, THE HITE REPORT: A NATIONWIDE STUDY OF FEMALE SEXUALITY, New York, Dell Publishing, 1976, p. 229.

4. Hayden, Naura, HOW TO SATISFY A WOMAN EVERY TIME...AND HAVE HER BEG FOR MORE!, New York, Bibli O'Phile Publishing Co., 1982, p. 15-16.

5. Bakos, Susan Crain, "Just when you thought you knew all there is to know about orgasm," COSMOPOLITAN, August, 1996.

Chapter 4 A Sexual Comparison of the Natural and Circumcised Penis

1. Ritter, Thomas J., M.D., SAY NO TO CIRCUMCISION! 40 COMPELLING REASONS, 2nd ed., Aptos, CA, Hourglass Book Publishing, 1996, p. 11-4 (each chapter of book is numbered separately).

2. Foley, John M., M.D., "The unkindest cut of all," FACT magazine, vol. 3, no. 4, July-Aug., 1966, p. 3-9, as cited by Rosemary Romberg in CIRCUMCISION: THE PAINFUL DILEMMA, South Hadley, MA, Bergin & Garvey Publishers, Inc., 1985, p. 171. "Normally the surface of the glans is composed of a smooth, glistening membrane only a few cells in thickness. The surface cells are alive, and naked nerve-endings are distributed among these cells. After circumcision, when the glans is exposed to soiled diapers and rough clothing, this membrane becomes ten times thicker, and the free nerve-endings disappear. The surface becomes covered with an adherent layer of dead cells, rough, dry, and insensitive."

3. Cold, C.J., and Taylor, J.R., "The prepuce," BJU INTERNATIONAL, vol. 83, Supplement 1, 1999, p. 41.

4. Taylor, J.R., Lockwood, AP, Taylor, A.J. "The prepuce: specialized mucosa of the penis and its loss to circumcision," BRITISH JOURNAL OF UROLOGY, vol. 77, no. 2, 1996, pp. 291-295. "The prepuce is much more complex than the 'simple fold of skin' described in textbooks. Its inner, mucosal surface contains a tightly pleated zone, near the tip, rich in nerve endings, particularly large mucocutaneous endorgans that are also described in the glans....the prepuce is specialized junctional tissue with a special sensory function."

5. Winkelman, R.K., "Erogenous zones: their nerve supply and its significance," Mayo Clinic, 1959, as cited by Bud Berkeley in FORESKIN: A CLOSER LOOK, Boston, Alyson Publications, Inc., 1993, p. 91.

6. Ritter, Thomas J., M.D., SAY NO TO CIRCUMCISION! 40 COMPELLING REASONS, 2nd ed., p. 18-1 (each chapter is numbered separately).

7. Taylor, J.R., Lockwood, AP, Taylor, A.J. "The prepuce: specialized mucosa of the penis and its loss to circumcision," BRITISH JOURNAL OF UROLOGY, vol. 77, no. 2, 1996, p. 292.

8. Ritter, Thomas J., M.D., SAY NO TO CIRCUMCISION!, p. 18-1 (each chapter of book is numbered separately).

9. Ibid.

Chapter 5 The Gliding Mechanism of the Natural Penis vs. the Friction Action of the Circumcised Penis

1. Hagar, Scher, "Doing it! Sex do's & don'ts," GLAMOUR, January, 1999, p. 161.

Chapter 6 A Further Sexual Comparison of the Natural and Circumcised Penis

1. Lamb, Lawrence E., M.D., DEAR DOCTOR: IT'S ABOUT SEX.... New York, Dell Publishing, 1973, pp. 184-186.

2. Masters, William H. and Johnson, Virginia E., HUMAN SEXUAL RESPONSE, New York, Bantam Books, 1966, p. 78 (figure 6-7).

3. Berkeley, Bud and Joe Tiffenbach, FORESKIN: ITS PAST, ITS PRESENT, &....ITS FUTURE, private publication, 1983, pp. 54-56.

4. Sevely, Josephine Lowndes, EVE'S SECRETS: A NEW THEORY OF FEMALE SEXUALITY, New York, Random House, 1987, p. 21, also pp. 46-47 female's urethra/prostate bulge, and its pleasuring pp. 112-113.

5. Ibid., p. 101.

6. Berkeley, Bud, FORESKIN: A CLOSER LOOK, Boston, Alyson Publications, Inc., 1993, p. 188.

7. Carper, Jean, "Foods that make you smarter and happier," LADIES HOME JOURNAL, July, 1993, p. 73.

8. Sevely, Josephine Lowndes, EVE'S SECRETS: A NEW THEORY OF FEMALE SEXUALITY, p. 145.

9. Ibid., p. 146.

Chapter 8 A: The Normal Thrusting Rhythm of the Natural Penis vs. the Abnormal Thrusting Rhythm of the Circumcised Penis

1. Swift, Rachel, HOW TO HAVE AN ORGASM...AS OFTEN AS YOU WANT, New York, Carroll & Graf Publishers, Inc., 1993, condensed in LADIES HOME JOURNAL, July, 1993, p. 79.

2. Kronhausen, Phyllis and Eberhard, THE SEXUALLY RESPONSIVE WOMAN, New York, Ballantine Books, 1964, pp. 65-66.

Chapter 8 B: Male Clitoris: Its Discovery, Pleasurement, and How It Affects the Thrusting Rhythm

1. Sevely, Josephine Lowndes, EVE'S SECRETS: A NEW THEORY OF FEMALE SEXUALITY, New York, Random House, 1987, p. 17.

2. Ibid.

3. Ibid., p. 17, 19.

4. Ibid., p. 17, 18, 21.

5. Ibid., p. 21.

6. Ibid., p. 22. *Author's note:* Since Sevely identifies the female and male clitorises as homologues, then the **next 2 references**, which confirm the presence of pressure-sensitive nerves (Pacinian corpuscles) in the female clitoris, apply in all probability to the male clitoris as well. Also, see my brief discussion of Pacinian corpuscles in Chapter 10.

Masters, William H. and Johnson, Virginia E., HUMAN SEXUAL

RESPONSE, New York, Bantam Books, 1966, p. 61: "...pacinian corpuscles located within the individual [female] clitoral glans and shaft. Since *the assigned role of pacinian corpuscles is* that of proprioceptive *response to deep pressure* (receptor role), the great variety in female automanipulative techniques ranging from demand for severe to insistence upon the lightest touch may be explained." [Emphasis added]

Cold, C.J., and Taylor, J.R., "The prepuce," BJU INTERNATIONAL, vol. 83, Supplement 1, 1999, p. 38: "In females, the glans clitoris...has a much denser concentration of Vater-Pacinian corpuscles than either the glans penis or the male prepuce."

7. Krause, W., HANDBUCH DER MENSCHLICHEN ANATOMIE, Hannover, Germany: Hahn, 1841, also Krause, W., "Die anatomie des kaninchens." in TOPOGRAPHISCHER UND OPERATIVE RUCH-SICHT, Leipzig, Gemanany: Engelman, 1868, as cited by Masters and Johnson, HUMAN SEXUAL RESPONSE, p. 46: "Pacinian corpuscles [pressure-sensitive nerves] are distributed irregularly throughout the autonomic system nerve fibers both in the glans [head of the female clitoris] and the corpora [shaft of the female clitoris] but usually have *greatest concentration in the glans [head of the female clitoris]*." (Emphasis added)

8. Sevely, Josephine Lowndes, EVE'S SECRETS: A NEW THEORY OF FEMALE SEXUALITY, p. 139.

9. Ibid., p. 141.

10. Masters, William H. and Johnson, Virginia E., HUMAN SEXUAL RESPONSE, p. 63.

11. AWAKENINGS: A Preliminary Poll of Circumcised Men—Revealing the Long-Term Harm and Healing the Wounds of Infant Circumcision. A publication of NOHARMM (see Resources for website). Later published as Hammond, T., "A preliminary poll of men circumcised in infancy or childhood." BJU INTERNATIONAL, vol. 83, suppl. 1, 1999, pp. 85-92.

12. Taylor, J.R., Lockwood, AP, Taylor, A.J. "The prepuce: specialized mucosa of the penis and its loss to circumcision," BRITISH JOURNAL OF UROLOGY, vol. 77, no. 2, 1996, p. 291.

13. Ibid.

14. Swift, Rachel, HOW TO HAVE AN ORGASM...AS OFTEN AS YOU WANT, New York, Carroll & Graf Publishers, Inc., 1993, condensed in LADIES HOME JOURNAL, July, 1993, p. 79.

Chapter 9 Why Does the Circumcised Man Thrust Hard or Bang and Pound Away?

1. Hayden, Naura, HOW TO SATISFY A WOMAN EVERY TIME...AND HAVE HER BEG FOR MORE!, New York, Bibli O'Phile Publishing Co., 1982, pp. 36-37.

2. Hayden, Naura, ISLE OF VIEW: SAY IT OUT LOUD, New York, Arbor Publishing Company, 1980, p. 43.

3. Hayden, Naura, HOW TO SATISFY A WOMAN EVERY TIME...AND HAVE HER BEG FOR MORE!, p. 19.

4. Ibid., p. 20.

5. Ibid., p. 55.

6. Berkeley, Bud, FORESKIN: A CLOSER LOOK, Boston, Alyson Publications, Inc., 1993, pp. 195-196.

7. Swift, Rachel, HOW TO HAVE AN ORGASM...AS OFTEN AS YOU WANT, New York, Carroll & Graf Publishers, Inc., 1993, p. 248.

Chapter 10 It's Over In a Flash! But What If It Lasts? And Desire Deficiency: Hers, His

1. Pearson, Durk and Shaw, Sandy, LIFE EXTENSION: A PRACTICAL SCIENTIFIC APPROACH, New York, Warner Books Company, 1982, p. 204.

2. Pfeiffer, Carl C., Ph.D., M.D., et al., MENTAL AND ELEMENTAL NUTRIENTS, New Canaan, CT, Keats Publishing, Inc., 1975, pp. 469-471.

3. Ibid., p. 470.

4. Ibid., pp. 469-470.

5. Stonehouse, Bernard, M.D., THE WAY YOUR BODY WORKS, Bonanza Books, New York, 1974, p. 20.

6. Winkelman, R.K., "Erogenous zones: their nerve supply and its significance," *Proc Mayo Clinic,* 1959, vol. 34, pp. 38-47, as cited by Bud Berkeley in FORESKIN: A CLOSER LOOK, Boston, Alyson Publications, Inc., 1993, p. 91.

7. Tortora, Gerard J., PRINCIPLES OF ANATOMY AND PHYSIOLOGY, 6th edition, Biological Sciences Textbooks, Inc, Div. of Harper & Row, Publishers, Inc, New York, 1990, p. 428.

8. Taylor, John, M.D., Lockwood, A.P., Taylor, A.J., "The prepuce, specialized mucosa of the penis, and its loss to circumcision," BRITISH JOURNAL OF UROLOGY, vol. 77, no. 2, February, 1996, p. 294.

9. Ibid., p. 293

10. Tortora, Gerard J., PRINCIPLES OF ANATOMY AND PHYSIOLOGY, 6th edition, p. 428.

11. DORLAND'S ILLUSTRATED MEDICAL DICTIONARY, 27th edition, W.B. Saunders Company, London, 1985, p. 1277.

12. Letter to the Editor, MOTHERING, July, 1994.

13. Knopf, Jennifer, M.D., Seiler, Michael, M.D., with Meltsner, Susan, INHIBITED SEXUAL DESIRE, New York, Warner Books, 1991, p. 7.

14. Ibid., pp. 7-8.

Chapter 11 My Personal Story

1. Laura Markowitz, "How women learn to make love," GLAMOUR, July, 1993, pp. 146-149.

Chapter 12 Joining the Foreskin Restoration Revolution & the Personal Stories of Two Men Who Restored

1. From a correspondence on file at NOHARMM. (See Resources.)

2. THE INTACT NETWORK (Newsletter), Spring, 1999, Private Publication edited by Ken Derifield, p. 1.

3. Ibid., pp. 2-3.

4. Bigelow, Jim, Ph.D., THE JOY OF UNCIRCUMCISING!, 2nd ed., Aptos, CA, Hourglass Book Publishing, 1995, p. 51.

5. Personal correspondence on file at UNCIRC headquarters as cited by Jim Bigelow, Ph.D., in THE JOY OF UNCIRCUMCISING!, 2nd ed., p. 51.

6. Paul Tardiff, circumcised at 30, NOCIRC CONFERENCE VIDEO, by Marilyn Milos, RN, & Sheila Curran, RN. (See NOCIRC in Resources.)

7. R. T. from Denver, CO [quoted] by Thomas J. Ritter, MD, in SAY NO TO CIRCUMCISION! 40 COMPELLING REASONS, 2nd ed., Aptos, CA, Hourglass Book Publishing, 1996, p. 12-4 (each chapter numbered separately).

8. Letter on file at NOCIRC. (See Resources.)

9. Comments received in response to AWAKENINGS: A Preliminary Poll of Circumcised Men Revealing the Harm and Healing the Wounds of Infant Circumcision, NOHARMM (see Resources for website). Later published as Hammond, T., "A preliminary poll of men circumcised in infancy or childhood." BJU INTERNATIONAL, vol. 83, suppl. 1, 1999, 85-92.

10. Greer, Donald M., Jr. and Mohl, Paul C., M.D., "Foreskin reconstruction: a preliminary report," SEXUAL MEDICINE TODAY, April, 1982, pp. 17, 21. (Note: Physicians interested in updated refinements to Greer's procedure should contact Turning Point Publications--see copyright page.)

Greer, Donald M., Jr., et al., "A technique for foreskin reconstruction and some preliminary results," THE JOURNAL OF SEX RESEARCH, vol. 18, no. 4, November, 1982, pp. 324-330.

11. Winkelman, R.K., "Erogenous zones: their nerve supply and its significance," *Proc Mayo Clinic,* 1959, vol. 34, pp. 38-47.

Chapter 14 How Americans Came to be Routinely Circumcised

1. Snowman, Leonard V., "Circumcision," ENCYCLOPEDIA JUDAICA, Jerusalem, Israel: Macmillan Co., 1971, vol. 5, p. 568, as cited by Edward Wallerstein in CIRCUMCISION: AN AMERICAN HEALTH FALLACY, New York, Springer Publishing Company, 1980, p. 7.

2. Berkeley, Bud, FORESKIN: A CLOSER LOOK, Boston, Alyson Publications, Inc., 1993, p. 53.

3. Berkeley, Bud and Joe Tiffenbach, FORESKIN: ITS PAST, ITS PRESENT, &....ITS FUTURE?, private publication, 1984, p. 29.

4. Berkeley, Bud, FORESKIN: A CLOSER LOOK, p. 66.

5. Ibid., p. 51.

6. Ibid., p. 52-53.

7. Edwardes, Allen , THE JEWEL IN THE LOTUS: A HISTORY SURVEY OF THE SEXUAL CULTURE OF THE EAST, New York, The Julian Press, 1959, p. 95, as cited by Bud Berkeley in FORESKIN: A CLOSER LOOK, p. 67.

8. Berkeley, Bud, FORESKIN: A CLOSER LOOK, p. 72.

9. Spitz, Rene A., M.D., "Authority and masturbation: some remarks on a bibliographical investigation," cited by Irwin M. Marcus, M.D. & John J. Francis, M.D., in MASTURBATION: FROM INFANCY TO SENESCENCE, New York, International Universities Press, Inc., 1975, p. 386.

Notes

10. Bullough, Vern L., SEXUAL VARIANCE IN SOCIETY AND HISTORY, New York, Wiley, 1976, p. 542, as cited by Edward Wallerstein in CIRCUMCISION: AN AMERICAN HEALTH FALLACY, New York, Springer Publishing Company, 1980, p. 32.

11. Rush, Benjamin, MEDICAL INQUIRIES AND OBSERVATIONS UPON THE DISEASES OF THE MIND, Philadelphia, Kimber and Richards, 1812, p. 347, as cited by Edward Wallerstein in CIRCUMCISION: AN AMERICAN HEALTH FALLACY, New York, Springer Publishing Company, 1980, p. 32.

12. Graham, Sylvester, A LECTURE TO YOUNG MEN ON CHASTITY, INTENDED ALSO FOR THE SERIOUS CONSIDERATION OF PARENTS AND GUARDIANS, 10th Edition, Boston, C.H. Pierce, 1848, as cited by Edward Wallerstein in CIRCUMCISION: AN AMERICAN HEALTH FALLACY, New York, Springer Publishing Company, 1980, p. 33.

13. Duffy, John, "Masturbation and clitoridectomy," JOURNAL OF THE AMERICAN MEDICAL ASSOCIATION, vol. 186, no. 3, Oct., 19, 1963, p. 246, as cited by Edward Wallerstein in CIRCUMCISION: AN AMERICAN HEALTH FALLACY, New York, Springer Publishing Company, 1980, p. 36.

14. Bullough, Vern L., SEXUAL VARIANCE IN SOCIETY AND HISTORY, p. 545, as cited by Edward Wallerstein in CIRCUMCISION: AN AMERICAN HEALTH FALLACY, New York, Springer Publishing Company, 1980, pp. 33-34.

15. Ibid., p. 545, as cited by Edward Wallerstein in CIRCUMCISION: AN AMERICAN HEALTH FALLACY, New York, Springer Publishing Company, 1980, p. 34.

16. Remondino, P.C., M.D., HISTORY OF CIRCUMCISION, New York, The F.A. Davis Co., Publishers, 1900, pp. 254-255, as cited by Jim Bigelow, Ph.D. in THE JOY OF UNCIRCUMCISING!, 2nd edition, Aptos, CA, Hourglass Book Publishing, 1995, p. 71.

17. Melendy, Mary R., M.D., THE IDEAL WOMAN—FOR MAIDENS, WIVES AND MOTHERS, 1903, as cited by Jim Bigelow, Ph.D. in THE JOY OF UNCIRCUMCISING!, 2nd edition, Aptos, CA, Hourglass Book Publishing, 1995, p. 69.

18. Wallerstein, Edward, CIRCUMCISION: AN AMERICAN HEALTH FALLACY, New York, Springer Publishing Company, 1980, p. 217.

19. NOCIRC, P.O. Box 2512, San Anselmo, CA 94979 (see Resources).

20. NOCIRC Annual Report, vol. 14, Spring 2000. Figures come from HCIA (Health Care Investment Analysts) which maintains the healthcare industry's largest database.

Chapter 15 35 Reasons Why You Should Not Circumcise Your Son

1. Bigelow, Jim, Ph.D., THE JOY OF UNCIRCUMCISING!, 2nd ed., Aptos, CA, Hourglass Book Publishing, 1995, p. 19.

2. Wallerstein, Edward, CIRCUMCISION: AN AMERICAN HEALTH FALLACY, New York, Springer Publishing Company, 1980, p. 218.

3. Ibid.

4. Peron, James E., "Ten very good reasons why your baby boy should not be circumcised," Richland, PA, Childbirth Education Foundation, 1981, p. 1.

5. Bigelow, Jim, Ph.D., THE JOY OF UNCIRCUMCISING!, 2nd ed., pp. 26, 21, and 27.

6. American Academy of Pediatrics, NEWBORNS: CARE OF THE UNCIRCUMCISED PENIS, January, 1994, Publications Division, 141 Northwest Point Blvd., P.O. Box 927, Elk Grove Village, IL 60009.

7. Goldman, Ronald, Ph.D., CIRCUMCISION: THE HIDDEN TRAUMA, Boston, Vanguard Publications, 1997, pp. 82-123.

8. Berkeley, Bud, FORESKIN: A CLOSER LOOK, Boston, Alyson Publications, Inc., 1993, p. 110.

9. Ibid., p. 92.

Chapter 17 Common Myths that Popularized Circumcision

1. Bigelow, Jim, Ph.D., THE JOY OF UNCIRCUMCISING!, 2nd ed., Aptos, CA, Hourglass Book Publishing, 1995, p. 72.

2. Diamond, Harvey and Marilyn, FIT FOR LIFE, New York, Warner Books, 1985, pp. 81-86.

3. Imamura, E., "Phimosis of infants and young children in Japan," ACTA PAEDIATR JPN, 1997, vol. 39, pp. 403-5, as cited by Cold, C.J., and Taylor, J.R., "The prepuce," BJU INTERNATIONAL, vol. 83, Supplement 1, 1999, p. 40.

4. Pomeranz, Virginia E., M.D. & Schulta, Dodi, THE MOTHERS' MEDICAL ENCYCLOPEDIA, New York, Signet Books, 1972, p. 99.

5. Wilkes, Edward T., M.D., "Should your son be circumcised?," PARENTS' MAGAZINE, vol. 34, no. 2, February, 1959, p. 50.

6. Rutherford, Frederick W., M.D., YOU AND YOUR BABY, New York, Signet Books, 1971, p. 100.

7. Schlosberg, Charles, M.D., "Thirty years of ritual circumcision," CLINICAL PEDIATRICS, vol 10, no. 4, April, 1971, p. 205.

8. Isenberg, Seymour & Elting, L.M., CONSUMER'S GUIDE TO SUCCESSFUL SURGERY, cited by Edward Wallerstein in CIRCUMCISION: AN AMERICAN HEALTH FALLACY, New York, Springer Publishing Company, 1980, p. 136.

9. Goldman, Ronald, Ph.D., CIRCUMCISION: THE HIDDEN TRAUMA, Boston, Vanguard Publications, 1997, pp. 19-24.

10. Stang, Howard J., M.D., et al., "Local anesthesia for neonatal circumcision," JOURNAL OF THE AMERICAN MEDICAL ASSOCIATION, vol. 259, no. 10, March 11, 1988, p. 1510.

11. Marchbanks, Howard, M.D., Interview with Rosemary Romberg, cited by Rosemary Romberg in CIRCUMCISION: THE PAINFUL DILEMMA, South Hadley, MA, Bergin & Garvey Publishers, Inc., 1985, p. 134.

12. Wallerstein, Edward, CIRCUMCISION: AN AMERICAN HEALTH FALLACY, New York, Springer Publishing Company, 1980, p. 127.

13. NOCIRC Newsletter, fall, 1991. (See Resources.)

14. Parkash, Satya, "Phimosis and its plastic correction," JOURNAL OF THE INDIAN MEDICAL ASSOCIATION, vol. 58, no. 10, May 16, 1972, pp. 389-390.

Ohjimi, Toshihide, M.D. & Ohjimi, Hiroyuki, M.D., "Special surgical techniques for relief of phimosis," THE JOURNAL OF DERMATOLOGIC SURGERY AND ONCOLOGY, vol. 7, no. 4, April 1981, pp. 326-330.

Emmett, Anthony J.J., "Z-plasty reconstruction for preputial stenosis- a surgical alternative to circumcision," AUSTRALIAN PAEDIATRIC JOURNAL, vol.. 18, 1982, pp. 219-220.

Hoffman, S., et al., "A new operation for phimosis: prepuce saving technique with multiple y-v-plasties," BRITISH JOURNAL OF UROLOGY, vol.. 56, 1984, pp. 319-321.

Wåhlin, Nils, "'Triple incision plasty'. A convenient procedure for preputial relief," SCANDINAVIAN JOURNAL OF UROLOGY AND NEPHROLOGY, vol. 26, no. 2, 1992, pp. 107-110.

Cuckow, Peter M., et al., "Preputial plasty: A good alternative to circumcision," JOURNAL OF PEDIATRIC SURGERY, vol.. 29, no. 4, April 1994, pp. 561-563.

15. Ying H, Xiu-hua Z (Changzheng Hosp. Shanghai), "Balloon dilation treatment of phimosis in boys: report of 512 Cases," CHINESE MEDICAL JOURNAL, 104, 1991, pp. 491-493, as cited in PEDIATRICS, 19th edition, 1991, edited by Abraham M. Rudolph, et al., pp. 298-300.

16. Beaugé, Michel, M.D., "Conservative treatment of primary phimosis in adolescents (Traitement médical du phimosis congénital de l'adolescent)," Thesis for the University Diploma of Andrology, Director of Studies Professor G. Arvis, Faculty of Medicine, Saint-Antoine University, Paris Vl, University Year 1990-1991. Fourteen pages of French text and 9 pages with 17 color photographs of phimosed penises before, during and after gentle stretching with speculums, plus 10-page English translation by J. P. Warren (contact NOCIRC—see Resources).

17. Wallerstein, Edward, CIRCUMCISION: AN AMERICAN HEALTH FALLACY, p. 128.

18. Bigelow, Jim, Ph.D., THE JOY OF UNCIRCUMCISING!, 2nd ed., p. 33.

19. Personal conversation with Carolyn Kolbaba at American Academy of Pediatrics, May 21, 1992.

20. American Academy of Pediatrics, NEWBORNS: CARE OF THE UNCIRCUMCISED PENIS, January, 1994 Publications Division, 141 Northwest Point Blvd., P.O. Box 927, Elk Grove Village, IL 60009.

21. Bigelow, Jim, Ph.D., THE JOY OF UNCIRCUMCISING!, 2nd ed., p. 44.

22. Peron, James E., "Ten very good reasons why your baby boy should not be circumcised," Richland, PA, Publication of Childbirth Education Foundation, 1981, p. 2.

23. Denton, John, M.D., et al., "Circumcision complication," CLINICAL PEDIATRICS (Phila.), vol. 17, no. 3, March, 1978, p. 285-286, as cited by Edward Wallerstein in CIRCUMCISION: AN AMERICAN HEALTH FALLACY, p. 149.

24. Ibid.

25. Snyder, James L., M.D., FACS, Presentation to the California Med. Assc. Scientific and Educational Activities Committee, 118th Annual Session and Western Scientific Assembly, Anaheim, CA, March 4, 1989.

26. Money, John, Ph.D., & Tucker, Patricia, SEXUAL SIGNATURES, Boston, MA, Little, Brown and Company, 1975, pp. 91-98.

27. Seabrook, Charles, "Lawyers: $22.8 million to be paid over botched circumcision," The ATLANTA CONSTITUTION, March 12, 1991, pp. A1 and A6.

28. Romberg, Rosemary, CIRCUMCISION: THE PAINFUL DILEMMA, South Hadley, MA, Bergin & Garvey Publishers, Inc., 1985, p. 161.

29. Peron, James E., "Ten very good reasons why your baby boy should not be circumcised," p. 2.

30. Streitfeld, Hank, M.D., "Should circumcision be routine?," PARENTS' PRESS, March 5, 1991, p. 5.

Chapter 18   Medical Myths Perpetuate Circumcision in America

1. Bigelow, Jim, Ph.D., THE JOY OF UNCIRCUMCISING!, 2nd edition, Aptos, CA, Hourglass Book Publishing, 1995, p. 29.

2. McMillen, S.I., M.D. NONE OF THESE DISEASES, Westwood, NJ, Fleming H. Revell Co., 1963, p. 20.

3. Silber, Sherman J., M.D., THE MALE, New York, Charles Scribner's Sons, 1981, p. 118.

4. Lewis, Alfred Allen, et al., THE MALE: HIS BODY, HIS SEX, Garden City, NY, Anchor Press/Doubleday, 1978, p. 106.

5. McMillen, S.I., M.D., NONE OF THESE DISEASES, p. 19.

6. Silber, Sherman J., M.D., THE MALE, pp. 115-116.

7. Bigelow, Jim, Ph.D., THE JOY OF UNCIRCUMCISING!, 2nd edition, p. 39.

8. McMillen, S.I., M.D., NONE OF THESE DISEASES, 2nd ed., Old Tappan, NJ, Fleming H. Revell Co., 1984, p. 91.

9. Wallerstein, Edward, CIRCUMCISION: AN AMERICAN HEALTH FALLACY, New York, Springer Publishing Company, 1980, p. 95.

10. Ibid., p. 99.

11. Denniston, George C., M.D., MPH, "First, do no harm," First International Symposium on Circumcision, Anaheim, CA, March 1-3, 1989.

12. Wallerstein, Edward, CIRCUMCISION: AN AMERICAN HEALTH FALLACY, p. 106.

13. http://www3.cancer.org/cancerinfo/load_cont.asp?st=pr&ct=35

14. Eiger, Marvin S., M.D., "The case for circumcision," TODAY'S HEALTH, vol. 50, no. 4, April, 1972, p. 15.

15. Apt, Adolf, "Circumcision and prostatic cancer," ACTA MEDICA SCANDINAVICA, vol. 178, fasc. 4, 1965, pp. 493-504.

16. Preston, E. Noel, Captain, M.C., USAF, "Whither the foreskin?," JOURNAL OF THE AMERICAN MEDICAL ASSOCIATION, vol. 214, no. 11, September 14, 1970, p. 1857.

17. Wallerstein, Edward, CIRCUMCISION: AN AMERICAN HEALTH FALLACY, p. 104.

18. Grossman, Elliot, M.D. & Posner, Norman Ames, M.D., "Surgical circumcision of neonates: a history of its development," OBSTETRICS AND GYNECOLOGY, vol. 55, no. 2, August, 1981, p. 245.

19. Vermooten, Vincent, M.D., cited by Jane E. Brody in "A restudy urged on circumcision," NEW YORK TIMES, September 20, 1970, p. 19.

20. Eiger, Marvin S., M.D., "The case for circumcision," TODAY'S HEALTH., p. 15.

21. Ravich, Abraham, M.D., PREVENTING V.D. AND CANCER BY CIRCUMCISION, New York, Philosophical Library, 1973.

22. Reuben, David, M.D., HOW TO GET MORE OUT OF SEX, New York, Bantam Books, 1975, p. 6.

23. Fink, Aaron J., M.D., "In defense of circumcision," cited by Edward Wallerstein in "Circumcision: Information, Misinformation, Disinformation," Private Publication, p. 4, as cited by Jim Bigelow, Ph.D., in THE JOY OF UNCIRCUMCISING!, 2nd edition, Aptos, CA, p. 36.

24. Bigelow, Jim, Ph.D., THE JOY OF UNCIRCUMCISING!, 2nd edition, p. 37.

25. Ibid.

26. Ibid.

27. Wallerstein, Edward, CIRCUMCISION: AN AMERICAN HEALTH FALLACY, p. 87.

28. Center of Disease Control, Recorded Message, May 3, 1993. Telephone 888-232-3228 or visit websites www.ashastd.org or www.cdc.gov. The telephone number is a general number with a series of prompts to direct you, or call 800-227-8922 between 8 a.m.-11 p.m. to speak with a live operator, also 404-332-4555.

29. Ibid.

30. Ibid.

31. Personal telephone conversation at Center for Disease Control, Sexually Communicated Diseases statistics, Melinda Lochner, May 20, 1992.

32. Swadey, John, M.D., Personal correspondence cited by Marilyn Milos, R.N., in NOCIRC Newsletter, vol. 2 , no. 1, Winter 1987, pp. 1 and 3.

33. AWAKENINGS: A Preliminary Poll of Circumcised Men Revealing the Harm and Healing the Wounds of Infant Circumcision. A publication of NOHARMM (see Resources for website). Later published as Hammond, T., "A preliminary poll of men circumcised in infancy or childhood." BJU INTERNATIONAL, vol. 83, suppl. 1, 1999, 85-92.

34. Silberner, Joanne & Carey, Joseph, "Circumcision," U.S. NEWS & WORLD REPORT , May 30, 1988, p. 68.

35. Wiswell, Thomas E., Major, MC., USA & Roscelli, John D., LTC, MC, USA, "Corroborative evidence for the decreased incidence of urinary tract infections in circumcised male infants," PEDIATRICS, vol. 78, no. 1, July, 1986, pp. 96-99.

36. Altschul, Martin S., M.D., "Cultural bias and the urinary tract infection (UTI) circumcision controversy," First International Symposium on Circumcision, Anaheim, CA, March 1-3, 1989.

37. Ibid.

38. Marino, Leonard J., M.D., Letter to the Editor, CONTEMPORARY PEDIATRICS, November, 1989.

39. Altschul, Martin S., M.D., Letter to the Editor, PEDIATRICS, vol. 80, no. 5, November, 1987, p. 763.

40. Winberg, Jan, et al., "The prepuce: a mistake of nature?," THE LANCET, March 18, 1989, p. 598.

41. Romberg, Rosemary, personal correspondence cited by Billy Ray Boyd in CIRCUMCISION: WHAT IT DOES, San Francisco, CA, Taterhill Press, 1990, p. 17.

42. Pearce, Joseph, "The magical child," Third Intl. Symposium on Circumcision, University of Maryland, College Park, MD, May 18-22, 1994.

43. American Academy of Pediatrics Work Group on Breastfeeding, "Breastfeeding and the use of human milk (RE9729)," PEDIATRICS, 1997, vol. 100, no. 6, pp. 1035-1039. http://www.aap.org/policy/re9729.html

44. Canadian Paediatric Society, Fetus and Newborn Committee, "Neonatal circumcision revisited," CANADIAN MEDICAL ASSOCIATION JOURNAL, 1996, vol. 154, no. 6, pp. 769-780.

45. Denniston, George C., M.D., MPH, "First, do no harm," First International Symposium on Circumcision, Anaheim, CA, March 1-3, 1989.

46. American Academy of Pediatrics Task Force, "Circumcision policy statement (RE9850)," PEDIATRICS, vol. 103, no. 3, March, 1999, pp. 686-693. http://www.aap.org/policy/re9850.html.

47. Highlights and selected comments about the AAP "Circumcision Policy Statement," as reported in the 1999 NOCIRC Annual Report, vol. 13, p.1.

Chapter 19 Will the Jewish People Disavow Circumcision?

1. Donin, Rabbi Hayim Halevy, TO BE A JEW, New York, Basic Books, Inc., Publishers, 1972, p. 58, as cited by Rosemary Romberg in CIRCUMCISION: THE PAINFUL DILEMMA, South Hadley, MA, Bergin & Garvey Publishers, Inc., 1985, p. 58.

2. Wallerstein, Edward, CIRCUMCISION: AN AMERICAN HEALTH FALLACY, New York, Springer Publishing Company, 1980, pp. 154-163.

3. Ibid., p. 163.

4. Ibid., pp. 154-163.

5. Wallerstein, Edward, "The case of the marble foreskin," FORUM, September, 1983, pp. 53-55.

6. Rapoport, Judith, L., M.D., THE BOY WHO COULDN'T STOP WASHING: The Experience and Treatment of Obsessive-Compulsive Disorder, New York, E. P. Dutton, 1989, p. 240. This section of her book describes how spiritual leaders try to deal with religious scrupulosity, an illness wherein zealots compulsively make vows to God which they cannot keep.

7. Ibid., p. 241

8. Ibid., p. 242.

9. Ibid.

10. Ibid.

11. Ibid.

12. Ibid., p. 243

13. Goldman, Ronald, Ph.D., CIRCUMCISION: THE HIDDEN TRAUMA, Boston, Vanguard Publications, 1997, pp. 220-221.

Index

A

AAP. *See* American Academy of Pediatrics
AIDS and circumcision 331–333, 337, 354
Altschul, Martin 334, 417
American Academy of Pediatrics
    analgesia recommended to reduce circumcision pain 312
    breastfeeding prevents urinary tract infection 335
    care and cleaning of the intact penis 306, 318, 412
    circumcision is "amputation of the foreskin" 63
    policy statement on circumcision 13, 327, 329
        full text of statement and discussion, websites 338
        summary of 1999 policy statement 337–338
    retracting a child's foreskin, advice on 306, 335
    their policy endorsed by ACOG (see below) 292–293
American College of Obstetricians & Gynecologists 292
Apt, Adolf 328, 416

B

Bauman, Eli 324
Beaugé, Michael 414
Berkeley, Bud 300, 403, 405, 406, 408, 410, 412
BIG BANG explained by Naura Hayden 157–158
Bigelow, Jim 215, 325, 330, 409, 411, 412, 414, 415, 416
BJU (British Journal of Urology) *Intl.* reprint 371–384. *See* surveys: *Sex As Nature Intended It*
Bobbitt, John and Lorena 32–33
Boyd, Billy Ray 417
breastfeeding to prevent UTI 335
Bullough, Vern 411

C

Canadian Medical Association Journal 417
Cameron and Fleming study ranking sex 46, 404
Carper, Jean 406
Center for Disease Control 331, 416

circumcised penis. *See also* circumcision (male) listings
  abnormal thrusting rhythm during intercourse 123, 221–223
  anatomical drawing of 5
  arousal. *See* muscle contractions: circumcised & natural induce differently
  bang-away thrusting, reasons for. *See also* circumcised penis: rough, hard thrusting
    excites pressure-sensitive nerves 160–162
    summary of reasons and effects 169
  cleaner than natural? 305–307, 337
  Desire Deficiency Disorder, a cause of 184–188
  devastation to upper penis 147–149, 208–209
  discomforts the male during intercourse 95–96
    friction irritation and chafing 74, 95, 220–221
  elongated stroke characteristic of 8, 121, 152–153
  masturbation and oral sex 220
  premature ejaculation 177, 363–364. *See also* reasons for, below
    exposed frenulum theory 180
    histamine theory 174–177
    over-reliance on pressure-sensitive nerves 177–180
  primary pleasure zone 121, 151, 161–162
  rough, hard thrusting. *See also* circumcised penis: bang-away thrusting, reasons for
  sexually detrimental to female partner 8
    bang-away, pound-away thrusting 158–159
    friction irritation 77
    "jams" the vagina with a hard-pressing action 153–155
    lessens her frequency desire. *See also* Desire Deficiency Disorder
    male takes too long to reach orgasm 183–184
    man tightens his abdominal muscles 154–155, 162, 169
    out-of-sync abnormal thrusting rhythm 153, 221–223
    painful or discomforting intercourse 161–162, 254, 276–277
    penis feels too hard 161
    rough, hard thrusting 7, 66, 67–68, 147, 154, 245–246
    scrapes the tissue of vaginal walls 90–91, 232
    she just wants it over with 181, 243
    vagina not relaxed, abnormally tenses up 93, 261
    vaginal lubrication, effect on 75–79, 94, 253
  sexually detrimental to male partner. *See* circumcision (male): sexually detrimental to male
  skin loss
    erection too tight 62
circumcised-sex syndrome 99–100

circumcision (male). *See also* circumcised penis
   A.M.A. Code of Ethics, violates principles of 353
   AIDS, circumcision does not protect U.S. men 331–333, 337, 354
      tight circumcision may spread HIV 332–333
   American medical origins of
      anti-masturbation mania 284–287
      Brit Royal College of Surgeons masturbation paper 284
      reasons for widespread acceptance 287–288
   America's rate of 15, 288–289
   Australian rate presently at 10 percent 305
   British mercantilism results in spread of 282–285
      company agents and Brit. soldiers forcibly circ'd 283
      Crusades and King Richard 282–283
      England ultimately abandons it "overnight" 290
   Canadian rate presently at 20 percent 305
   controversy 13, 53, 324, 336–337
   doctors too quick to recommend in U.S. 314
   erection too tight 333
   genital mutilation, considered as 211
   harm caused by 10, 211, 324, 332
      men's voices 161–162, 204–208, 208–209, 210–211, 294–295
   human rights violation 312–313
   Jewish religious ritual 281
      Abrahamic covenant 325, 339, 340, 341
      changes through history 341, 343
      David's foreskin by Michelangelo, importance of 341–342
      end it, a call to 339–340, 341, 343, 347
      Jewish Reform Movement opposed to 339
      not for health reasons 340–341
      Talmudic Laws as a means to disavow circumcision 344–346
      venereal disease, Jews compared to others 330
   medical benefits?
      AAP Task Force reviews 40 years of literature 337
   men circumcised in adulthood 209–210
   Moslem (Muslim) cultural tradition 282
      British empire adopts from Moslems 283
      Koran makes no reference to 282
      uncircumcised penis an affront to Allah 282–283
   myths
      cancers alleged to be linked with natural penis 298, 325, 338
      circumcision does no harm? 319–322, 338
      cleanliness 305–307, 337
      foreskin is superfluous, unnecessary? 323
      foreskin should retract at birth? 316
      infant pain 299, 310–312, 338

circumcision (male) *continued*
    parents' right to amputate healthy tissue? 312, 354
    sooner or later circumcision is needed? 313–314
    urinary-tract infection (UTI) preventative? 333, 337
    venereal disease more likely with intact penis? 329
  origins of 281, 339
  practiced where, by whom 12, 281
  psychological repercussions of 32–34, 96
    brain's pleasure centers suffer deprivation 30–40, 97–98
    female bitchiness: caused by the man or the penis? 126–129
    sex is incomplete and unfulfilling 185–186
  reasons not to
    brothers don't need to match 292
    cancer of the penis risk is insignificant 298, 338
    cervical cancer link invalid 298
    childbirth educators are increasingly against 293
    doesn't need to be done later in life 297–298
    father and son don't have to match 291
    foreskin gives penis a fuller look 299
    foreskin needed for comfortable erection 297
    foreskin protects the glans from abrasive clothing 299
    foreskin's mobile skin more fun for sexual play 297
    human right to retain one's genitals 292, 294, 338, 354
    insurance companies are refusing to pay for 299
    internal organ is made an external organ 294
    locker room look is changing to natural 292
    masturbation practice unaffected by circumcision 297
    medical authorities deem it unwarranted surgery 292–293
    natural penis sexually superior 294
    nature knows best 52–53, 292
    pain is traumatic for the newborn 299
    premature ejaculation, may be a cause of 294
    Princess Di opts for intact and breaks tradition 293
    psychological scars left on circumcised men 294–295
    regret and grievous guilt over wrong decision 295
    restoration expense and hassle avoided later 300
    serious medical complications and risk 299
    son may never forgive you 295
    thrill of an unsheathing erection denied 300
    unmutilated natural penis will become "the look" 295–296
    urinary-tract infection (UTI) rare & disputed 298, 333–338, 337
    venereal disease not prevented by circumcision 298
    world norm is natural 292
  reasons practiced in America 13, 14, 16
  relationship discord 21–22, 35–37, 93, 98, 165, 186, 196

Index 423

circumcision (male) *continued*
  risk and possible complications 299, 319–322
    circumcision does no harm? 338
    sex-change case, TV show topic 321
  sexual effects on female partner 29, 57, 62–63, 66, 67, 77–78, 90–91, 92–93, 93–94, 119, 121–122, 152–153, 154–156, 157–159, 163–165, 168–169, 169, 239–267
  sexual importance: an overview 7
  sexually detrimental to male 57, 62–63, 68
    clitoral tip not massaged 138–140
    desensitized glans 56–57
    devastates functioning of upper penis 147–149, 208–209, 294
    devastation to upper penis 147–149, 208–209
    female partner is not pleased 171–172
    friction irritation and chafing 74–76, 95–96, 220–222
    lack of gliding mechanism 69–79
    must work harder to achieve orgasm 96–97, 232
    overly tight erection. *See* circumcision (male): skin loss
    scraping of coronal ridge 95–96
    shaft tissue abnormally compressed 62–64
    takes too long to reach orgasm 183–184, 294, 365
    too long to orgasm - a solution 365
    too much continuous stimulation to upper penis 95
  sexually transmitted diseases, not protective of 329–336
  skin loss
    amount of 12, 63–64
    erection too tight 62–63, 220–221, 319
  world's per cent of men 4, 12
Circumcision: An American Health Fallacy. See Wallerstein, Edward
Circumcision: The Hidden Trauma 347
Circumcision: The Painful Dilemma 311, 321
Clinical Pediatrics 413, 414
clitoris, male. *See* male clitoris
Cold, C.J. 405, 407, 412
coronal ridge, "the hook" 25–26, 82–91, 98
  allows foreskin to bunch-up 83
  compacted coronal ridge scrapes vaginal walls 90–91
  giveable natural glans allows it to flex 83
  male is discomforted 95–96
  picture of 25
  term's origin described 82
corpora cavernosa. *See* male clitoris
Cosmopolitan 21, 403
Cuckow, Peter M. 414

D

dairy products as a cause of smegma. *See* smegma
DDD. *See* Desire Deficiency Disorder
Denniston, George C. 327, 335, 415, 418
  Afterword 353–355
Denton, John 320, 414
Derifield, Ken 409
Desire Deficiency Disorder 93, 184–188
Diamond, Harvey and Marilyn 412. *See Fit For Life*
diddling. *See* jiggling
divorce
  America's rate vs. W. Europe 37
  circumcision contributes to? 49, 99
Doctors Opposing Circumcision (D.O.C.) 337, 353
Donin, Rabbi Hayim Halevy 418
Duffy, John 411

E

Edwardes, Allen 283, 410
Eiger, Marvin S. 328, 329, 415, 416
Elting, L. M. 310
endorphins. *See* nerves: endorphins can numb pain
Eve's Secrets. See male clitoris

F

female genital mutilation (FGM) 17
Fink, Aaron J. 330, 416
Fit For Life, dairy products discussion 307–308
Foley, John M. 404
foreskin (male)
  benefits to female partner 7, 8–10, 55, 58–59
    bunching/unbunching sexually exciting 85–86, 88–89
    clitoral mound is rhythmically pleasured 118–119, 132, 138, 359
    cushions coronal ridge hook 28, 83
    gentler intercourse 160, 165–166, 167–168, 169, 233
    gliding mechanism of natural penis 69–74
    lubrication retained 72
    relationship happiness 166
    softly-stiff natural penis more pleasurable 60–62, 89, 269
    vagina relaxes 261
  benefits to male
    assists in bringing on orgasm 141–143
    bunching and unbunching excites penis 86–87, 87–88

Index 425

comfortable erection 59–62
cushions coronal ridge 27–28, 83–85
general 59–60
gliding mechanism 71–72
masturbation and oral sex 231
maximizes clitoral tip stimulation 137–140
nerves of glans protected 54–56
skin abundance 59–60
Table of Sexual Benefits 234
thrill of erection and "the stretch" 224–225, 300
care of intact penis 318
masturbation and oral sex 73–74, 220
purpose of: general discussion 3–4, 7, 10–11
retractability is gradual process 316–318
touch-sensitive nerves 178, 179–180
foreskin restoration 3, 172
benefits of being restored 58–59, 79, 96, 140, 185, 211–212, 232–233. *See* forekin (male): benefits to male
penis enlargement 212
temperature-sensitive nerves reawaken 225
what sex is like after you're restored 58–59, 224
compensating for loss of foreskin nerves,. *See* nipple twiddling
facing up to the truth: you want foreskin back 223, 234
methods of 212–217
Dr. Donald Greer's surgical technique 215–217, 218
recommended book: *The Joy of Uncircumcising!* 215
non-surgical restoration
photos of restored foreskin website 234
tapeless inventions 213
NORM (National Organization of Restoring Men) 215
personal accounts
non-surgical restoration, one man's story 230–233
surgically restored, Jeff's story 217–225
testimonials 89, 203–204
relationship happiness benefited by 50–51
sexual benefits, Table of 234
surgical restoration
caveat 216
vitamins & nutrients beneficial 214–215
women's issue 6, 8, 17, 17–18, 58–59, 182, 233
author's sex life and marriage affected by 199–200
Foreskin Restoration Revolution 6, 11, 30, 188
Foreskin: A Closer Look 300
frenar band. *See* ridged band of foreskin
front-door tipping, the ultimate sexual ecstasy 230

G

genital cleaning methods
   soap recommended: Dove original 306
   vegetable oil 306–307
Glamour 405, 409
   Sharon surprised she didn't like sex 192
glans
   circumcised
      abnormally hard 56–57, 90
      corona may flares out more than natural 90
      dried-out, keratinized 232
      sensitivity decreased 161, 209, 232
   natural is more pliable 82–83
   natural is softer, yet erection is firm 23–24, 55, 231
Glasser, William 404
gliding mechanism of natural penis 69–74
   arm/hand simulation of natural intercourse 73
   finger simulation of circumcised intercourse 74
   finger simulation of natural intercourse 70
Goldman, Ronald 347, 404, 412, 413, 418
Graham, Sylvester 285, 411
Greer, Donald 410. *See also* foreskin restoration: methods of
Grossman, Elliot 329, 416

H

Hagar, Scher 405
Hayden, Naura 404, 408. *See also* BIG BANG explained. *See* surveys: women faking orgasm
histamine as a cause of premature ejaculation 174–177
   natural and circumcised penis different 175
Hite Report 46
Hoffman, S. 413

I

Ideal Women—For Maidens, Wives And Mothers, The 286
Imamura, E. 412
Isenberg, Seymour 310, 413

J

Jeff's personal story 217–225
Jewish religious circumcision. *See* circumcision: Jewish religious ritual
jiggling (or diddling) 118–119, 359
Joy of Uncircumcising!, The 215

K

Kellogg, John 285
Klein, Fred 324
Knopf, Jennifer 184, 409
Koran. See circumcision: Moslem (Muslim) cultural tradition
Krause, W. 407
Kronhausen, Drs. Phyllis & Eberhard 406. *See* transference effect

L

Ladies Home Journal 406
Lamb, Lawrence E., Dr. 405
    advice column discusses foreskin 81–82
Lancet, The 417
lanofore 55, 307, 309
Laumann, Edward O., report 46, 404
leg muscle analogy to penis 163
Lewis, Alfred Allen 324, 415
love bond, the
    circumcision erodes love bond 99–100, 186–188, 196
    natural penis promotes love bond 170–172, 200
Lowndes crown. *See* male clitoris: location of
lubrication, vaginal. *See* vaginal fluids

M

male clitoris
    compared to female clitoris 133–134, 137
        Lowndes Crown Theory excerpts from *Eve's Secrets* 367–370
    corpora cavernosa, same as 134
    erection, process of 134–137
    location of 134
        excerpts from *Eve's Secrets* 368
        tip (Lowndes crown) 134
    massaged by glans 137–138
    pressure-responsive nerves 137
Marchbanks, Howard 311, 413
Marcus, Irwin M. 410
Marino, Leonard 335, 417
Masters, William and Johnson, Virginia 82, 139, 405, 406, 407
Mayo Clinic study 228, 405, 408, 410. *See* nerves: touch-sensitive nerves of the foreskin
McMillen, S. I. 323, 325, 326, 415
Meissner's corpuscles. *See* nerves: touch-sensitive nerves of the foreskin
Melendy, Mary R. 286, 411

Men's Health 46, 404
Mental and Elemental Nutrients 175, 214
Money, John 321, 414
mosquito-bite sex 24–25, 96
Mothering 409
muscle contractions
  circumcised and natural penis induce differently 143, 146–147, 162–163
    natural induced by actions in upper penis 143–146
  orgasm brought about by 143, 144–145
  Trousseau's phenomenon 179

N

natural penis
  anatomical drawing of 5
  compatible thrusting rhythm and 122–123
  nature, as provided by 5, 13, 48, 53, 54
  premature ejaculation and 175–176
  primary pleasure zone of 120–121, 129–130, 145
  retraction of foreskin for infant, child, adult 306
  secondary pleasure zone at base of penis 131
  sexual benefits of. *See* foreskin (male): benefits to male
  sexual benefits to female. *See* foreskin (male): benefits to female partner
  sexual benefits to male. *See* forekin (male): benefits to male
  shorter thrusting stroke, why 132
  upper penis is primary pleasure zone 133
  world popularity of 12
nerves
  endorphins can numb pain 91, 91–92
  pressure-sensitive 87–88, 137, 178–179
    Pacinian corpuscles 178
    Trousseau's phenomenon 179
    two penis types pleasured differently upper penis 150–151
  rest/recharge concept 87, 123–124, 148–149
    circumcised nerves denied rest/recharge 151
    circumcised nerves overstimulated 150
    foreskin action rests pressure-sensitive nerves 150–151
    foreskin cloaking rests touch-sensitive nerves 149
  touch-sensitive nerves, different kinds of 177–178, 179–180
nipple twiddling of male
  enhances pleasure 228–229
  helps man to maintain erection 358
  helps man to orgasm 365
NOCIRC 398, 409, 411, 412, 413
nutrients to enhance skin elasticity 210

O

orgasm
    faking 2, 46, 48–49
    men who have difficulty, a solution 365
    secrets to achieving vaginal orgasm 359–360
    side-by-side position for intercourse 360
    sneeze, similar to 144–145
    vaginal orgasm
        defined 47
        success rates of 247–250

P

Pacinian corpuscles 178
paraphimosis 315, 317
Pearce, Joseph 417
Pearson, Durk, and Sandy Shaw 408
Pediatrics 414, 417, 418
penis. *See* circumcised penis, natural penis
penis enlargement 212
penis head. *See* glans
Peron, James E. 412, 414, 415
Pfeiffer, Carl 175, 214, 407, 408
phimosis
    acquired phimosis 317
        case example 321–322
    cause of, suggestion for finding 316
    circumcision in adulthood 209–210
    correcting without circumcision 314–316
        balloon catheter stretching, China method 315
        minimal surgical techniques 315
        steroidal, non-steroidal topical ointments 315
        stretching with graduated speculums 315
    rare condition 315
Pomeranz, Virginia 412
Posner, N. A. 329
premature ejaculation 174
    circumcised more prone to 177, 178–179
    solution using the "tap me" technique 363–364
Preston, E. Noel 328, 416
Princeton Bio Center 175
psychological repercussions. *See* circumcision (male): psychological repercussions of
Psychology Today survey 2
pubic hair, purpose of during intercourse 131

R

Rapoport, Judith 418
Ravich, Abraham 330, 416
restoration. *See* foreskin restoration
Reuben, David 330, 416
rhythm of the thrusting penis
    controlled by the penis, not the man 124, 128
    distorted rhythm of circumcised penis 119, 155–156, 157–159, 168
    importance to woman's orgasm 117–118, 156
        circumcised long stroke lessens pubic contact 152–153
        circumcised penis is out of sync with her needs 153
        side-by-side position, best control in 359
    natural penis more consistently regular 118–119, 145–146
ridged band of foreskin
    compensating for loss of nerves 227–229
    functions of 141–143, 151
    location of 141
Ritter, Thomas J. 64, 403, 404, 405, 409
Romberg, Rosemary 321, 404, 413, 415, 417, 418
rooming in promotes newborn's immunity 335
Rush, Benjamin 284, 411
Rutherford, Frederick W. 310, 413

S

Schlosberg, Charles 310, 413
Seabrook, Charles 415
Sevely, Josephine Lowndes 406, 407. *See also* male clitoris
sexual techniques
    front-door tipping, the ultimate sexual ecstasy 230
    man takes too long to orgasm - a solution 365
    nipple twiddling of male 228–229
    side-by-side intercourse position 357–361
    "Tap Me" secret to prolonging intercourse 363–364
sexually transmitted diseases (STDs) 331
Sharon's story in *Glamour* magazine. *See Glamour* magazine
side-by-side position for intercourse 357–360
    used in front-door tipping 230
Silber, Sherman J 324, 325, 415
sinusoids 136
smegma
    dairy waste product of the body 307–309

Is it a problem? 307–309
   solution 309
   lanofore, distinguished from. *See* lanofore
smegmalith 309
Snowman, Leonard 410
Snyder, James L. 320, 321, 414
Spitz, Rene A. 410
Stang, Howard J. 311, 413
STDs. *See* sexually transmitted diseases (STDs)
Stonehouse, Bernard 408
Strand, John 223. *See also* dedication page
stre-t-c-h, the ultimate male experience 215, 300
Streitfeld, Hank 415
survey questionnaire, complete transcript of 385
surveys
   importance of sex rated by women and men 46
   Iowa survey, women preferred circumcised
      conclusions misleading, reasons for 265–267
   Psychology Today 2
   Sex As Nature Intended It 47
      age of participants 258
      duration of intercourse 252–253
      general info 239, 240
      get into it or get it over question 181–183
      natural overwhelmingly preferred 242–243
      negative thoughts correlated with intercourse 254–257
      not a random sampling of women, why 263–265
      overview of findings 240–241
      penis types perform differently 244–246
      positive thoughts correlated with intercourse 257
      questionnaire, full transcript of 385
      questions on your mind 258–265
      small number of participants, why 262
      special terms used in 101
      vaginal discomfort comparison 254
      vaginal lubrication comparison 253
      vaginal-orgasmic success compared 247–252
      women who preferred circumcised, why 258–260
      women's comments about circumcised 274–278
      women's comments regarding natural 269–273
      women's personal stories 101–115
   women faking orgasm 46–47
Swadey, John 332, 417
Swift, Rachel 406, 408

T

Table of Sexual Benefits for restored foreskin 234
"Tap Me" secret to prolonging intercourse 363–364
Taylor, John R. 403, 405, 407, 409, 412. *See* ridged band
tipping. *See* front-door tipping
Tortora, Gerard J. 408, 409
touch-sensitive nerves. *See* nerves: touch-sensitive nerves, different kinds of
transference effect 35, 126
Trousseau's phenomenon. *See* muscle contractions: Trousseau's phenomenon
Tucker, Patricia 321, 414

U

uncircumcised penis. *See* natural penis
Uncut Society of America 300
urinary-tract infections (UTI) and circumcision 333–338, 337
UTI. *See* urinary-tract infections (UTI) and circumcision

V

vaginal dryness. *See* vaginal fluids
vaginal fluids 76, 78–79
vaginal orgasm
   controversiality of the term 48
   definition of 47
   rate of success due to penis type 47, 48, 241, 247–252
vaginal wall ribbings 83, 85
vaginismus 78
   author's personal story 197–199
vegetable oil. *See* genital cleaning methods
Vermooten, Vincent 329, 416
vitamin B6. *See* nutrients to enhance skin elasticity
vitamin C. *See* nutrients to enhance skin elasticity

W

Wåhlin, Nils 413
Wallerstein, Edward
   313, 319, 326, 327, 329, 331, 340, 342, 403, 411, 412, 413, 414, 415, 416, 418
Walsh, Anthony 403
waterbed improves sexual intercourse 360–361
   Land and Sky Quality Sleep mattress 361
Wilkes, Edward T. 310, 413
Winberg, Jan 417

Winkelman, R. K. 405, 408, 410
Wiswell, Thomas E. 333, 335, 336, 417
Woody Allen 188
 Bananas 19, 37–38

Y

Ying H, Xiu-hua 414

Z

Zilbergeld, Bernie 2, 403
zinc. *See* nutrients to enhance skin elasticity